ANGINA PECTORIS: ETIOLOGY, PATHOGENESIS AND TREATMENT

T0401116

ANGINA PECTORIS: ETIOLOGY, PATHOGENESIS AND TREATMENT

ALICE P. GALLO

AND

MARGARET L. JONES

EDITORS

Nova Biomedical Books

New York

Library of Congress Cataloging-in-Publication Data

Angina pectoris : etiology, pathogenesis, and treatment / Alice P. Gallos and Margaret L. Jones (editors).   p. ; cm.
Includes bibliographical references and index.
ISBN 978-1-60456-674-1 (hardcover)
1. Angina pectoris. 2. Angina pectoris--Treatment. 3. Coronary heart disease. I. Gallos, Alice P. II. Jones, Margaret L.
[DNLM: 1. Angina Pectoris--etiology. 2. Angina Pectoris--therapy. 3. Atherosclerosis. 4. Coronary Artery Disease.
WG 298 A58825 2008] RC685.A6A54   2008
616.1'22--dc22   2008014837

Published by Nova Science Publishers, Inc. ✦ New York

Contents

Preface

This new book provides up-to-date research on angina pectoris which and is a chest pain due to ischemia (a lack of blood and hence oxygen supply) of the heart muscle, generally due to obstruction or spasm of the coronary arteries (the heart's blood vessels). Coronary artery disease, the main cause of angina, is due to atherosclerosis of the cardiac arteries. It is common to equate severity of angina with risk of fatal cardiac events. There is a weak relationship between severity of pain and degree of oxygen deprivation in the heart muscle (i.e. there can be severe pain with little or no risk of a heart attack, and a heart attack can occur without pain).

Expert Commentary - *Introduction*: Low-molecular-weight heparins are an attractive option for patients with acute coronary syndromes without ST-segment elevation [ACS-NSTE]. Their pharmacokinetic and pharmacodynamic characteristics provide efficacy and safety in treatment of ACS-NSTE, reducing the ischemic events. The anti-Xa activity is used as a marker to assess anticoagulation and it has shown to be correlated with the administrated dose as well as the clinical outcomes.

Objectives: The authors evaluated the relationship between the level of anti-Xa activity and the onset of clinical end-points of enoxaparin in treatment of ACS-NSTE.

Methods: A total of 30 patients with ACS-NSTE were treated with Enoxaparin 1mg/kg s.c twice daily. The anti-Xa activity was measured six hours after the initial dose, and then every 6 h. The end-points were recurrent angina [RA], myocardial infarction [MI], heart failure [HF], the onset of cerebrovascular insult [ICV], performing of coronary artery by-pass graft [CABG], need of percutaneous coronary intervention [PCI] and death at day 180. Pearson Product Moment Correlation was used for relationship between anti-Xa activity and outcomes.

A p value < .05 was considered to indicate significance.

Results: Six hours after the initial dose of enoxaparin, 19 patients [63.3%] were into the target level of anti-Xa activity [0.6-1.0 IE/L]. Eight patients [26%] were below 0.5 IE/L and 3 patients [10%] were above 1.01 IE/L. Further dynamic of anti-Xa activity was calculated and mean concentration of anti-Xa activity was 0.7 IE/L. The authors did not note statistically significant differences between the number of platelets at the time of admission and 6 h after the enoxaparin application [Z=0,00, p=1,00].

For 180 day follow-up, the incidence of end-points RA, MI, HF, ICV, CABG, PCI, death and minor bleeding were 36.6%, 3.0%, 13.3%, 3.3%, 13.3%, 3.3%, 90% and 16.7%. Pearson Product Moment Correlation showed positive correlation between the level of anti-Xa activity and the day of onset of RA [r=0.21], MI [r=0.21], HF [r=0.98], CABG [r=0.63] and the minor bleeding [r=0.81]. The authors did not find correlation between the level of anti-Xa activity and the day of PCI [r=0.07].

Conclusion: Anti-Xa activity is an independent predictor of adverse cardiac events in patients with acute coronary syndromes without ST-segment elevation, treated with enoxaparin.

Chapter I - Chest pain is one of the most common complaints of patients who are seen in an emergency room and ambulatory practice. The major early objective in the diagnosis of such patients is to separate noncardiac from cardiac pain.

The primary care provider plays a critical role in the management and the long-term care of patients who have coronary heart disease (CHD). Such care is focused on reducing symptoms and long-term complications. This reviews the details of management of chronic stable angina, and unstable angina.

Chronic stable angina pectoris includes predictable and reproducible left anterior chest discomfort after physical activity, emotional stress, or both; symptoms are typically worse in cold weather or after meals and are relieved by rest or sublingual nitroglycerin. The presence of one or more obstructions in major coronary arteries is likely; the severity of stenosis is usually greater than 70 percent.

Unstable angina is commonly classified by use of simple clinical descriptors, such as the presence or absence of ischemic chest discomfort at rest, as well as ECG changes and biochemical markers of myocardial injury during and after ischemic episodes. Although these clinical descriptors are helpful in estimating prognosis and are used widely in determining the intensity of treatment, they provide little information regarding the cause of the syndrome.

Chapter II - In patients with stable angina, endothelial function has been found to be impaired and closely related from the early steps of atheromatosis. In this article the authors will review the association of stable angina pectoris and endothelial dysfunction, focusing on classical and novel risk factors that predispose to endothelial dysfunction, while suggesting potential therapeutic approaches of improving vascular endothelium status. Classical risk factors include hypercholesterolemia-dyslipidemia, diabetes mellitus, hypertension, cigarette smoking, while novel risk factors refer to inflammation-infection, hyperhomocysteinemia and genetics. Classical therapeutic approaches such as statin treatment and angiotensin converting enzyme inhibitors (ACE-I) treatment are nowadays accompanied by novel therapies including insulin sensitizers and antioxidant vitamins and others still under investigation such as folic acid supplementation.

Chapter III – Background: The concurrence of acute coronary syndromes with hypersensitivity reactions as well as anaphylactic or anaphylactoid insults is increasingly in clinical practice and there are several reports associating mast cell activation with acute cardiovascular events.

Definition: Kounis syndrome is the coincidental occurrence of acute coronary syndromes with hypersensitivity reactions involving activation of interrelated and interacting inflammatory cells and including allergic or hypersensitivity and anaphylactic or anaphylactoid insults. It is caused by inflammatory mediators such as histamine, neutral proteases, arachidonic acid products, platelet activating factor and a variety of cytokines and chemokines released during the hypersensitivity insult. All these inflammatory cells participate in a vicious inflammatory cycle and via multidirectional signals mast cells can enhance T cell activation, T cells can mediate mast cell proliferation and activation, inducible macrophage protein-1α can activate mast cells, mast cells can activate macrophages, and T cells can regulate macrophage activity. Clinical and experimental findings show that there is a common pathway between allergic and non allergic coronary events, because the same mediators from the same cells are present in both hypersensitivity episodes and acute coronary syndromes.

Variants: Type I variant: includes patients with normal coronary arteries without predisposing factors for coronary artery disease in whom the acute release of inflammatory mediators can induce either coronary artery spasm without increase of cardiac enzymes and troponins or coronary artery spasm progressing to acute myocardial infarction with raised cardiac enzymes and troponins.

Type II variant: includes patients with culprit but quiescent pre-existing atheromatous disease in whom the acute release of inflammatory mediators can induce either coronary artery spasm with normal cardiac enzymes and troponins or plaque erosion or rupture manifesting as acute myocardial infarction.

Cardiac Actions of Main Mediators: Tryptase and chymase actions: Activate the zymogen forms of metalloproteinases such as interstitial collagenase, gelatinase, and stromelysin and can promote plaque disruption or rupture.

Furthermore, chymase converts angiotensin I to angiotensin II and angiotensin II receptors are found in the medial muscle cells of human coronary arteries. Thus, angiotensin II generated by chymase could act synergistically with histamine and aggravate the local spasm of the infarcted coronary artery.

Leukotrienes are powerful arterial vasoconstrictors and their biosynthesis is enhanced in the acute phase of unstable angina. Thromboxane is a potent mediator of platelet aggregation with vasoconstricting properties. Platelet activating factor: In myocardial ischemia acts as proadhesive signalling molecule or via activation of leucocytes and platelets to release other mediators. In experimental anaphylaxis reproduces the electrical and mechanical effects observed in allergic reactions such as ST changes and arrhythmias acting either through the release of leukotrienes or as a direct vasoconstrictor.

Histamine can induce: coronary vasoconstriction, intimal thickening, inflammatory cell modulation, platelet activation, proinflammatory cytokine production, p-selectine upregulation, sensitization of nerve ending in coronary plaques, tissue factor expression.

Clinical and Therapeutic Implications: Today, concern has been raised that intracoronary stents could be associated with in stent thrombosis, paradoxical coronary vasoconstriction and hypersensitivity reactions. Components of currently used DES have been reported to induce either separately or synergistically hypersensitivity reactions and in some occasions hypersensitivity cardiac events. Stent-activated intracoronary mast cells could release histamine, arachidonic acid metabolites, proteolytic enzymes such as tryptase and chymase, as well as a variety of cytokines -chemokines and platelet activating factor leading to local inflammation and thrombosis. These events may be more common than suspected because it is hard to document them, unless they become systemic, in which case they manifest as the Kounis syndrome. Recognition of this problem may lead to better vigilance, as well as new stent with mast cell blocking molecules that may also be disease modifying.

So far, attempts have been made to counteract the actions of the inflammatory mediators by using mediator antagonists, inhibitors of mediator biosynthesis and mediator receptor blockers. However, in the medical armamentarium there are drugs and natural molecules that are capable to stabilize and protect mast cell surface which could prevent also acute thrombotic events , at least in some instances. This has already been achieved experimentally.

Chapter IV - Atherosclerosis is a chronic inflammatory disease that affects medium and large-sized arteries. It begins after birth and the progression depends on several factors – traditional triad: hypertension, hyperlipidemia and diabetes mellitus, then age, sex, smoking and sedentary life-style. At the beginning atherosclerosis is asymptomatic and the authors cannot estimate appropriately its frequency, but its complications – coronary artery diseases, cerebrovascular diseases, peripheral arterial diseases, which occur late, are responsible for more than half of the yearly mortality in the world. Unfortunately, sudden cardiac death may be the first clinical manifestation.

The incipient event is endothelial dysfunction, as a result of injury, caused by high level of cholesterol [especially low-density-lipoprotein LDL], hyperglycemia, hypertension, smoking, infectious agents, and toxins. Endothelial cells overexpress adhesion molecules – vascular cell adhesion molecule–1 [VCAM-1] and increases recruitment of inflammatory cells– monocytes [Mo], T-cells and subsequent release of monocyte chemo–attractant protein–1 [MCP-1] that results in additional leucocytes recruitment. Injured endothelium allows migration of inflammatory cells that release cytokines and lipids into the intima. That leads to cytokine-mediated progression of atherosclerosis and oxidation of LDL. Macrophages [MP] take up oxi-LDL and form foam-cell. They have metabolic activity and produce cytokines, proliferation of smooth muscle cells and formulate athero-fibrose plaque. Atherosclerotic plaque is composed of superficial layer – fibrose cap and lipid core, that consists of foam cells, extracellular lipid and necrotic cellular debris. It progresses as a result of accumulation of lipid and proliferation of smooth muscle cells and results in luminal narrowing of the arteries which leads to compromised blood and oxygen supply to the tissues. The gradually growing atherosclerotic plaques have thick fibrose cap and are stable. They cause symptoms of stable angina. Rapidly growing plaques cause unstable coronary artery disease. These plaques are mainly composed of lipids and have tiny fibrose cap that is prone to fissuring or rupture. Intraplaque hemorrhage from microvessels in plaque initiate platelet adhesion and activation of coagulation cascade that leads to platelet thrombus formation, i.e. promote thrombogenesis.

Knowledge of the pathogenesis of the atherothrombosis modifies the diagnostic and therapeutic approach.

Conclusion: Our attention should be focused on the management of three points:

1. Endothelial dysfunction [correction of modified risk factors: hypertension, hyperlipidemia, diabetes mellitus, life-style-smoking, physical activity and food],
2. Atherosclerosis [modification of the inflammatory cascade, i.e. elimination of inflammatory pathways and inhibition of oxidation of LDL],

3. Thrombogenesis [inhibition of platelet adhesion, activation and aggregation].

Chapter V - *Background/Aims:* Despite the reported benefits of cardiac rehabilitation, attendance at these programs is particularly poor among coronary artery disease patients following surgery. Very little is known about the role that psychosocial factors may play in patients' decision to attend a cardiac rehabilitation program post surgery. In a prospective study, the authors aimed to determine if psychosocial factors are independent predictors of cardiac rehabilitation attendance.

Methods: A consecutive sample of private hospital cardiac patients (n=146) with angina who had undergone surgical intervention including either angioplasty (*n*=61) or coronary artery bypass surgery (*n*=25) were invited to participate (response rate 58.9%; n=86). Patients were classified according to confirmed rehabilitation records into attendees (*n*=56) and non-attendees (*n*=30). Patients completed a self report valid questionnaire on anxiety, depression, social support, coping, illness perceptions, neuroticism, optimism and quality of life (QOL).

Results: Patients who decided to attend rehabilitation were significantly different compared with non-attenders with regards to having greater trait anxiety (P=0.01) and use of self blame as a coping mechanism (P=0.05). Attenders were more likely to label their condition as unpredictable (*P*< .01), perceived greater subsequent effects from their illness (*P* = .01), reported difficulty emotionally dealing with the circumstances (*P* = .04), and had less understanding of their illness (*P* = .02). In terms of QOL, attenders reported significantly greater emotional interference (*P* = .04), and subsequently greater impairment to their mental health (*P* = .04), compared with non-attenders. None of these factors however were independently associated with attendance. Depression, social support, coping, optimism and neuroticism did not significantly differentiate between the two groups.

Conclusions: Psychosocial factors including trait anxiety, a maladaptive coping style, impaired illness perceptions and poorer quality of life may play a role in patient's decision to attend a cardiac rehabilitation program following surgery, although other factors are likely to be more important.

Chapter VI - Rho-kinase has been identified as one of the effectors of the small GTP-binding protein Rho. In a series of experimental and clinical studies, it has been demonstrated that Rho-kinase is substantially involved in the pathogenesis of coronary spasm. Intracoronary administration of fasudil or its metabolite, hydroxyfasudil, both of which are Rho-kinase inhibitors, markedly inhibited coronary spasm in animal models. Importantly, the inhibition of Rho-kinase with fasudil/hydroxyfasudil was associated with the suppression of enhanced myosin light chain (MLC) phosphorylations at the spastic coronary segments in those models. The activity and the expression of Rho-kinase were enhanced at the inflammatory/arteriosclerotic coronary lesions, thereby suppressing myosin phosphatase through phosphorylation of its myosin-binding subunit with a resultant increase in MLC phosphorylations and coronary spasm. In patients with vasospastic angina, intracoronary fasudil markedly inhibited acetylcholine-induced coronary spasm and related myocardial ischemia, demonstrating that Rho-kinase pathway is substantially involved in the pathogenesis of coronary spasm in humans as well. Fasudil was also effective in treating patients with microvascular angina, indicating an involvement of Rho-kinase-mediated hyperreactivity of coronary microvessels. Intracoronary administration of fasudil was effective in reducing tachypacing-induced myocardial ischemia even in patients with stable effort angina without changing heart rate or blood pressure, suggesting that inappropriate coronary microvascular vasoconstriction is involved in the pathogenesis of effort angina. Intracoronary fasudil also was effective for the treatment of intractable coronary spasm resistant to maximal vasodilator therapy with calcium channel blockers and nitrates after coronary artery bypass surgery. These lines of evidence indicate that Rho-kinase is an important therapeutic target for the treatment of the spasm.

Chapter VII - Identification of the specific cause for pain or distress in the chest in clinical practice is ordinarily more difficult than the specific treatment for it becomes after proper recognition. At least 100 different disorders have been identified that produce pain or discomfort in the chest. The diagnosis is certain to be overlooked if that disorder is not considered. Such oversight has been responsible for most of the treatment failures that have come to my attention is consultation practice.

With broad perspective and recognition that pain felt to be within the chest may actually originate in the wall of the chest or from disorders in the head, neck, or abdomen, diagnosis may ordinarily be fairly simply established when the significant details from the clinical history taking, from physical examination, and from laboratory investigation are adequately evaluated. Sometimes, special investigations, ordinarily available in university and diagnostic centers become essential although details of readily available diagnostic facilities ordinarily are more important safeguards for correct diagnosis than are the reports from specialized facilities.

Chapter VIII - *Aims*: The aim of this study was to determine how the location and symptoms of angina pectoris differed among those presenting with acute chest pain.

Methods: The sample consisted of individuals who presented to Nepean Hospital Emergency Department with acute chest pain. At initial presentation, patients who elected to undergo further diagnostic tests were assessed according to a standard protocol. All patients were asked to fill out the Chest Pain Questionnaire (CPQ). A cluster analysis was undertaken to determine any pattern in the angina pectoris location and symptoms described by patients.

Results: This study recruited 212 subjects with acute chest pain (aged 21-90, mean 57, SD: 14). The prevalence of angina pectoris was 39% (n=75). Cluster analysis identified three distinct angina pectoris locations: 1) mid-left chest; 2) central chest and left arm; and 3) central and upper left chest.

Conclusions: Angina pectoris is a heterogenous condition. There is significant overlap of chest pain symptoms and locations among angina pectoris, thus making differentiation from other 'causes' difficult.

Chapter IX - During the past decades, ischemic cardiopathy has been extensively studied. Nonetheless it has been an important advance in its diagnostics and its treatment; this illness is a currently public health challenge in developed countries. Moreover, in emerging economies, ischemic cardiopathy has also started to follow the same trend as in developed countries. Epidemiological studies on ischemic cardiopathy have shown important genetic and ambient risk factors. In particular, it is well recognized that atherosclerosis, a suffering of large arteries, is the primary cause of ischemic cardiopathy. Atherosclerosis is characterized by an immunologic mechanism; where adaptive and innate immune response are involved. One of the most common triggering events for this response is an accumulation of minimally oxidized LDL molecules. This event involves mainly the endothelial cells; which produce pro-inflammatory molecules. Other cells involved here and in progressive thrombosis are T and B cells. Lately, infection by cytomegalovirus and elevated homocysteine, have been also recognized as another triggering events for immune response activation. As a consequence, nowadays the atherosclerosis has been clearly recognized as a chronic inflammation that could promote severe clinical consequences due to atherosclerotic plaque and thrombosis. This is in high contrast with the previously understanding; where atherosclerosis and atherome were considered just as probable degenerative sufferings related with age. A thrombus can cause an abrupt diminishing of blood flow through the affected blood vessels as well as a complete blood flow interruption. As a result, the oxygen cell distribution is affected and an ischemic clinical condition is promoted. The ischemic cardiopathy diagnostic and prognostic can be done by several biomarkers. Some of them can also point out the future occurrence of ischemic cardiopathy. Although some pharmacological treatments have been focused on the acute ischemic cardiopathy, the importance of pharmacological treatments where the immunological modulation of inflammatory process plays an essential role has been recently increased. The recognition of immunologic mechanisms involved in ischemic cardiopathy is undoubtedly necessary. Drugs acting at this level enhance the possibilities for a good prognostic of ischemic cardiopathy.

Chapter X - Coronary heart disease is the single most common cause of illness and death in the developed world.

Coronary atherosclerosis is by far the most frequent cause of ischemic heart disease, and plaque disruption with superimposed thrombosis is the main cause of the acute coronary syndromes of unstable angina, myocardial infarction, and sudden death. Atherosclerosis is the result of a complex interaction between blood elements, disturbed flow, and vessel wall abnormality, involving several pathological processes: inflammation, with increased endothelial permeability, endothelial activation, and monocyte recruitment; growth, with smooth muscle cell proliferation, migration, and matrix synthesis; degeneration, with lipid accumulation; necrosis, possibly related to the cytotoxic effect of oxidized lipid; calcification/ossification, which may represent an active rather than a dystrophic process; and thrombosis, with platelet recruitment and fibrin formation.

Approximately one third of patients with CAD do not have traditional risk factors. New evidence shows that systemic markers of inflammation are a strong predictor of cardiovascular events, adding independently to traditional risk factors. Inflammation systemically or locally within atherosclerotic plaque is believed to play a major role in the initiation and progression of CAD and the precipitation of acute coronary events. Cardiovascular events may most commonly arise from sites of "nonsignificant" stenosis, suggesting that plaque instability rather than the degree of stenosis is the key risk factor. This plaque instability is believed related to inflammation within the plaque, with activated macrophages releasing inflammatory mediators, activating matrix metalloproteinases, and breaking down the protective fibrous cap. The source of this inflammation may include noninfectious triggers (e.g., oxidized low-density lipoprotein [LDL], oxidation products of smoking, endothelial injury, genetics, etc.) or from a number of proposed infectious triggers.

Now it is known that local and systemic inflammatory processes play an important role in the genesis and development of atheroclerotic lesions and in the pathophysiology of acute coronary syndromes. This hypothesis is supported by findings of elevated parameters of the inflammatory reaction in the blood of atherosclerotic patients and of histopathological characteristic of unstable plaque (thin fibrous cap, large necrotic core, less smooth muscle cells and abundant foamy cells and lymphocytes). Besides several studies have demonstrated that inflammation has an determining role in the rupture of the coronaric plaque, and have been carried out to identify the etiopatogenetic moment of the inflammation itself, trying to correlate coronaric atherosclerosis and its development with some infectious agents.

Potentially, acute or chronic infections could initiate and promote CAD in the absence of traditional risk factors. More likely, infections act to augment CAD risk in the presence of other risk factors. A number of mechanisms have been proposed which could link infection to atherosclerosis.

Understanding the pathogenesis of atherosclerosis and the role of inflammation, first requires knowledge of mentions of the structure and biology of the normal artery and its indigenous cell types.

Chapter XI - Nitrates, apart from beta-blockers and calcium antagonists, are the mainstays of antianginal drug therapy in patients with stable angina pectoris. All patients with angina should receive a prescription for sublingual nitroglycerin (NTG) and instructions on its use. The pharmacological and physiological benefits of nitrates in coronary artery disease, and also some potentially harmful mechanisms are discussed in the paper. Organic nitrates are considered as valuable symptomatic agents, improving the quality of life of patients with angina pectoris. Although, these nitrates are effective anti-anginal drugs during initial treatment, their therapeutic value is compromised by the rapid development of tolerance during sustained therapy. Thus, their major disadvantage is connected with the occurrence of tolerance, which means that their clinical efficacy is decreased during long-term use. A widely accepted method of preventing tolerance is intermittent administration. Sublingual tablets or sprays are suitable for the immediate relief of effort or rest angina and can be used prophylactically before exercise. In patients with stable angina treated with high doses of oral nitrates in long-term therapy, sublingual NTG maintains its full anti-ischemic effect both after initial oral ingestion and after intermittent long-term oral administration (eg once daily). However, sublingual NTG attenuates this effect during continuous treatment (eg administration every 6h), when tolerance to oral nitrates occurs, and this is called cross-tolerance between sublingual and long-lasting nitrates. The relationship between nitrate tolerance and cross-tolerance is a positive phenomenon. Thus, when high doses of nitrates in sustained-release medications are chosen, they should be given once daily. This method of treatment should be used not only to maintain antianginal efficacy of nitrate in the prophylaxis of angina pectoris, but also to effectively relieve angina after sublingual NTG ingestion during chest pain. Long-acting nitrates are considered third-line therapy because a nitrate-free interval is required to avoid the development of tolerance. Therefore, nitrates should be considered for patients who cannot tolerate or fail to respond adequately to beta-blockers and calcium antagonists. All long-acting nitrates seem to be equally effective, but the duration of antianginal effects of pentaerythritol tetranitrate (PETN) in lower doses are not known. A relatively recent development is the suggestion that organic nitrates vary considerably in their potential to induce the development of tolerance. In particular, it has been suggested that PETN may induce minimal release of a superoxide anion, and hence may result in minimal tolerance. During long-lasting nitrate therapy (except PETN), one can observe the development of reactive oxygen species (ROS) inside the muscular cell of a vessel wall, and these bind with nitric oxide (NO). This leads to decreased NO activity, thus, nitrate tolerance. PETN has no tendency to form ROS, and therefore nitrate tolerance is absent. One would expect that prolonged exposure to PETN does not lead to diminution of responses to other organic nitrates such as sublingual NTG. Thus, during long-term PETN therapy, there is probably no tolerance or cross-tolerance, as during treatment with other organic nitrates.

Chapter XII - Tako-tsubo cardiomyopathy (TC) is a recently described acute cardiac syndrome that mimics acute myocardial infarction and is characterized by ischemic chest symptoms, an elevated ST segment on electrocardiogram, increase levels of cardiac disease markers and transient left apical and middle ventricular walls disfunction (apical "ballooning"). In contrast to the acute coronary arterial syndromes (ACS), patients with TC have no angiographically detectable or nonobstructive coronary arterial disease.

This syndrome can be triggered by profound psychological stress and is also known as "stress cardiomyopathy" or "broken-heart syndrome".

The TC was initially recognized in the Japanese population (first described in 1991) but has recently been reported in the USA and Europe. The term "tako-tsubo" was proposed by Dote et al and means "fishing pot for trapping octopus," and the left ventricle disfunction, in this syndrome, resembles that shape. The true prevalence of the apical ballooning syndrome remains uncertain. In the last few years, the number of published reports of patients presenting with this syndrome is constantly increasing. Only six series assessed the prevalence of this syndrome among consecutive patients presenting with suspected ACS.

In: Angina Pectoris: Etiology, Pathogenesis and Treatment
Editors: A. P. Gallo, M. L. Jones

Expert Commentary

Anti-Xa Activity and the Onset of Clinical End-Points of Enoxaparin in Treatment of Acute Coronary Syndromes

Slavica Mitrovska[1] and Silvana Jovanova[2]
[1]Military Hospital, Department of Cardiology, Skopje, Macedonia
[2]Institute for Heart Disease, Clinical Center, Skopje, Macedonia

Abstract

Introduction: Low-molecular-weight heparins are an attractive option for patients with acute coronary syndromes without ST-segment elevation [ACS-NSTE]. Their pharmacokinetic and pharmacodynamic characteristics provide efficacy and safety in treatment of ACS-NSTE, reducing the ischemic events. The anti-Xa activity is used as a marker to assess anticoagulation and it has shown to be correlated with the administrated dose as well as the clinical outcomes.

Objectives: We evaluated the relationship between the level of anti-Xa activity and the onset of clinical end-points of enoxaparin in treatment of ACS-NSTE.

Methods: A total of 30 patients with ACS-NSTE were treated with Enoxaparin 1mg/kg s.c twice daily. The anti-Xa activity was measured six hours after the initial dose, and then every 6 h. The end-points were recurrent angina [RA], myocardial infarction [MI], heart failure [HF], the onset of cerebrovascular insult [ICV), performing of coronary artery by-pass graft [CABG], need of percutaneous coronary intervention [PCI] and death at day 180. Pearson Product Moment Correlation was used for relationship between anti-Xa activity and outcomes.

A p value < .05 was considered to indicate significance.

Results: Six hours after the initial dose of enoxaparin, 19 patients [63.3%] were into the target level of anti-Xa activity [0.6-1.0 IE/L]. Eight patients [26%) were below 0.5

---

* Address for correspondence: Mitrovska Slavica M.D. Mr.Sci.Med, ul.Sole Stojcev br.1-2-8 1000 Skopje, Macedonia, tel: 0038971634494, e-mail: mitrovska2000@yahoo.com.

IE/L and 3 patients [10%] were above 1.01 IE/L. Further dynamic of anti-Xa activity was calculated and mean concentration of anti-Xa activity was 0.7 IE/L. We did not note statistically significant differences between the number of platelets at the time of admission and 6 h after the enoxaparin application [Z=0,00, p=1,00].

For 180 day follow-up, the incidence of end-points RA, MI, HF, ICV, CABG, PCI, death and minor bleeding were 36.6%, 3.0%, 13.3%, 3.3%, 13.3%, 3.3%, 90% and 16.7%. Pearson Product Moment Correlation showed positive correlation between the level of anti-Xa activity and the day of onset of RA [r=0.21], MI [r=0.21], HF [r=0.98], CABG [r=0.63] and the minor bleeding [r=0.81]. We did not find correlation between the level of anti-Xa activity and the day of PCI [r=0.07].

Conclusion: Anti-Xa activity is an independent predictor of adverse cardiac events in patients with acute coronary syndromes without ST-segment elevation, treated with enoxaparin.

Keywords: *Anti-Xa Activity, Acute Coronary Syndrome Without ST Segment Elevation, Low-Molecular-Weight Heparin.*

Introduction

Antithrombotic therapy has a prominent role in the treatment of acute coronary syndromes. Low-molecular-weight heparins [LMWH], are the potential new class in the treatment of non-ST-segment elevation acute coronary syndromes [ACS-NSTE] [1]. They are isolated from standard heparin by chemical or enzymatic depolymerization and have better pharmacokinetic and pharmacodynamic characteristics over unfractionated heparin. Enoxaparin has a low molecular weight of 4500 D, high anti-Xa activity [>100 IE/mg], low anti-IIa activity [28 IE/mg], bioavailability of 96% and longer plasma half-life of 4-6 h. Stable anticoagulant response, less platelet activation, resistance to inactivation by platelet factor 4, lower rate of thrombocytopenia, provide no need of laboratory monitoring [2]. These properties provide good therapeutic response and significant diminution in frequency of the adverse clinical outcomes-recurrent angina [RA], myocardial infarction [MI], heart failure [HF], the onset of cerebrovascular insult [ICV], performing of coronary artery by-pass graft [CABG], need of percutaneous coronary intervention [PCI] and death [3]. It is difficult to measure LMWH concentrations directly, and anti-Xa activity is used as biological effect markers which has been shown to be correlated with the administrated dose as well as the clinical effect [4].

Objectives: We evaluated the relationship between the level of anti-Xa activity and the onset of clinical end-points of enoxaparin in treatment of ACS-NSTE.

Methods: The study was prospective, randomised, open-labeled two-centered study. A total of 30 patients with ACS-NSTE were randomised to receive LMWH-Enoxaparin [Clexane®, Aventis Pharma] 1mg/kg twice daily, s.c application.

The anti-Xa activity has been used as a marker to assess anticoagulation. It was measured 6 hours after the initial dose of subcutaneous administration of enoxaparin, and then every 6 h. The blood specimens were collected in siliconized Vacutainer tubes [Belliver Industrial Estate, Plymouth, UK] with 3.3% acidum citricum. The analyses were performed with

Humaclot analyzer, Berichrom Heparin, at the Institute for Transfusiology, Medical faculty, Skopje, Macedonia.

Further dynamic of anti-Xa activity was calculated and mean concentartion of anti-Xa activity was 0.7 IE/L. Also, we counted the platelet at the time of admission and 6 h. after the initial dose of enoxaparin. We evaluated the relationship between the level of anti-Xa activity and the day of onset of RA, MI, HF, ICV, CABG, death and PCI at 180 day. Also we followed the incidence of hemorrhagic complications.

Statistical analysis: The statistical analyses were performed by using the commercial statistical package, Statistica for Windows, Version 6.0. The Kruskal-Wallis ANOVA analyse was used for nonparametric variables, Wilcoxon Matched Pairs Test for two dependent samples, and Pearson Product Moment Correlation was used for relationship between anti-Xa activity and outcomes. A p value $< .05$ was considered to indicate significance.

Results: Six hours after the initial dose of enoxaparin, 19 patients [63,3%] were into the target level of anti-Xa activity of 0.6-1.0 IE/L. Below the target level [0,5 IE/L] were 8 patients [26%] and 3 patients [10%] achieved a level higher than 1.01 IE/L (Figure1). Further dynamic of anti-Xa activity was calculated and mean concentration of anti-Xa activity was 0.7 IE/L. The number of platelets was counted at the time of admission and 6 h after the initial dose of enoxaparin. We did not find statistically significant differences between the number of platelets at the time of admission and 6 h after the enoxaparin application [Z=0.00, p=1.00] (Figure 2).

For 180 day follow-up, the incidence of end-points were 11 patients with RA [36.6%], 9 patients with MI [30%], 4 patients with HF [13.3%], 1 patient with ICV [3.3%], 4 patients with CABG [13,3%], 27 patients with PCI [90%], 1 patient died [3.3%], and 5 patients with minor bleeding [16.7%] (Table1).

Pearson Product Moment Correlation showed positive correlation between the level of anti-Xa activity and the day of onset of recurrent angina [r=0.21), myocardial infarction [r=0.21], heart failure [r=0.98], performing of coronary artery by-pass graft [r=0.63] and minor bleeding [r=0.81].

Table 1. Adverse cardiac outcomes at day 180

Adverse cardiac outcomes	patients
Recurrent angina	11 (36.6%)
Myocardial infarction	9 (30%)
Heart failure	4 (13.3%)
Insultus cerebrovascularis	1 (3.3%)
CABG	4 (13.3%)
PCI	27 (90%)
Death	1 (3.3%)
Minor bleeding	5 (16.7%)

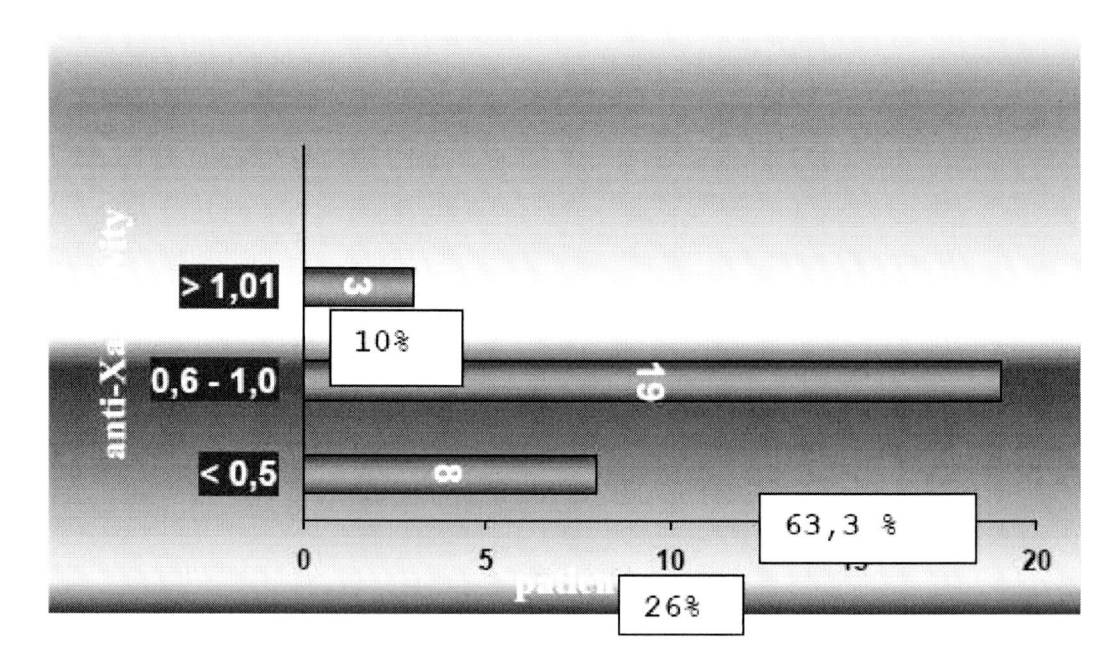

Figure 1. Anti-Xa activity 6 h after the first s.c application of enoxaparin.

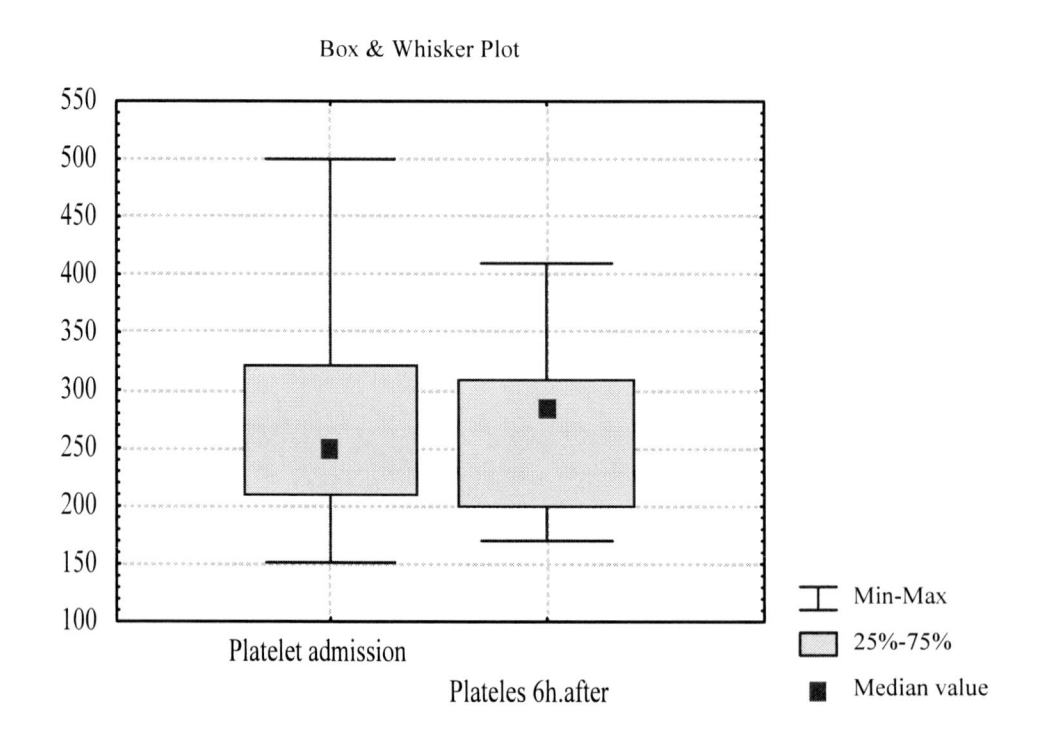

Figure 2. The difference between the number of platelets at the time of admission and 6h after the application of Enoxaparin.

This means the earlier onset of RA, MI, HF, CABG and bleeding correlated with lower anti-Xa activity. We did not find correlation between the level of anti-Xa activity and the day of PCI [r=0.07] (Figure 3, Figure 4, Figure 5, Figure 6, Figure 7, Figure 8).

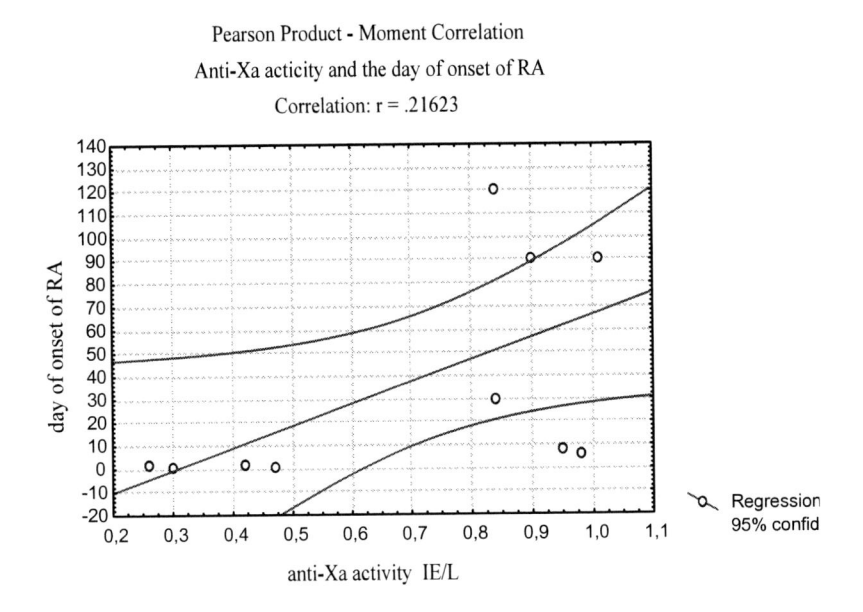

Figure 3. Pearson Product Moment Correlation between the level of anti-Xa activity and the day of onset of recurrent angina .

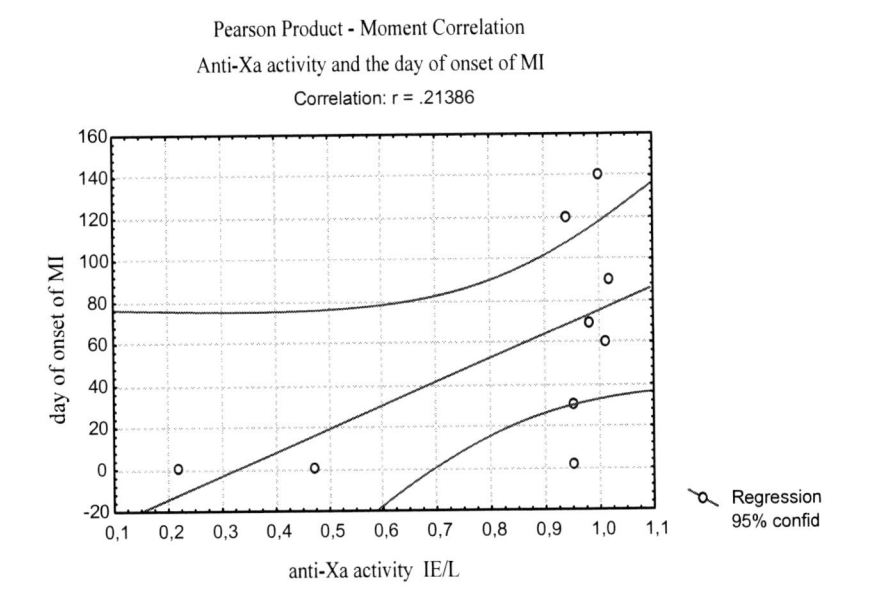

Figure 4. Pearson Product Moment Correlation between the level of anti-Xa activity and the day of onset of myocardial infarction.

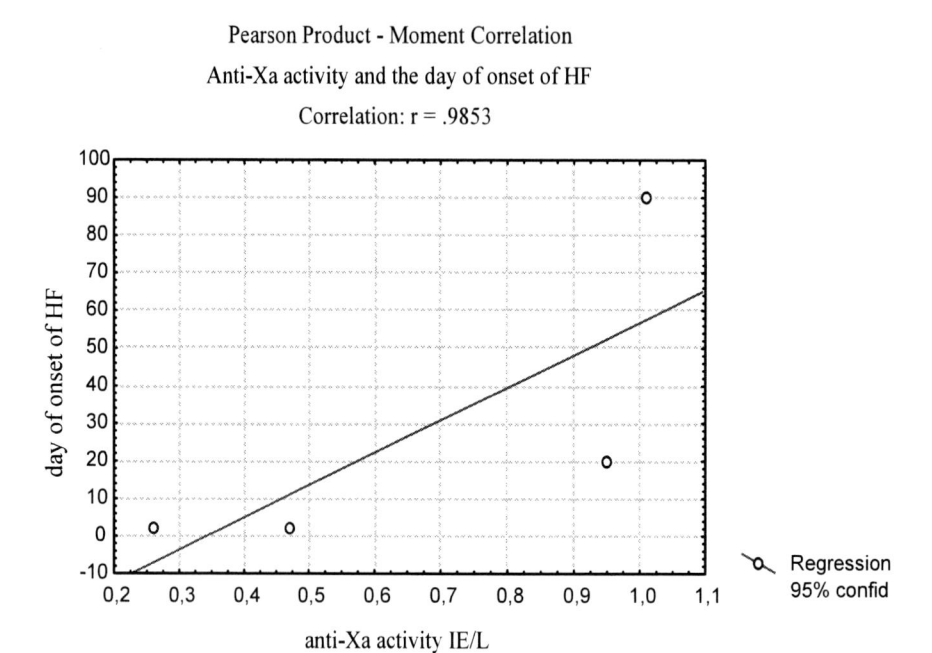

Figure 5. Pearson Product Moment Correlation between the level of anti-Xa activity and the day of onset of heart failure.

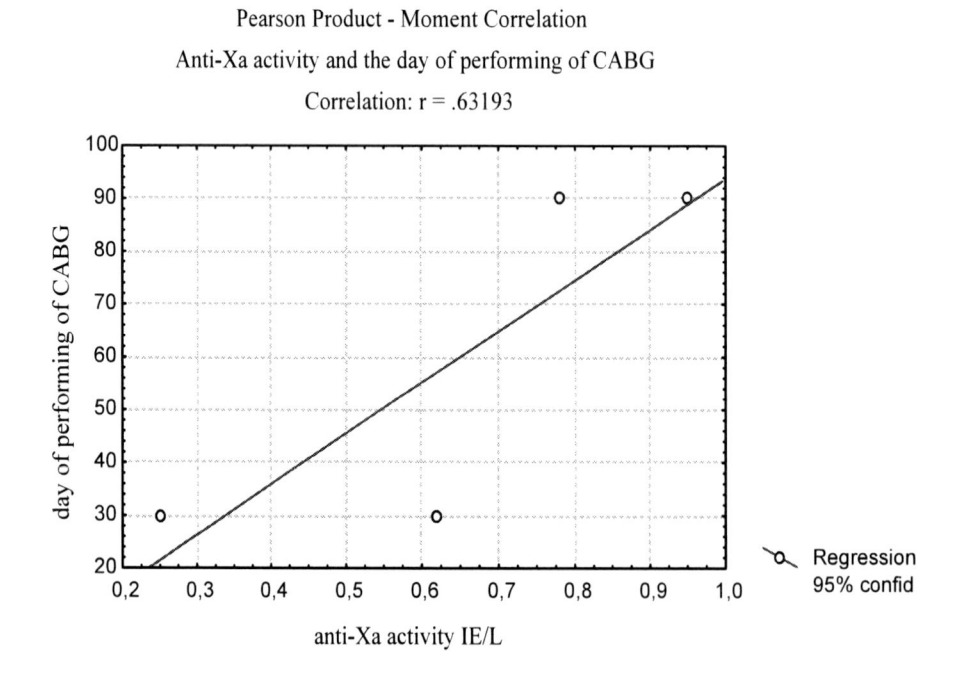

Figure 6. Pearson Product Moment Correlation between the level of anti-Xa activity and the day of performing of CABG.

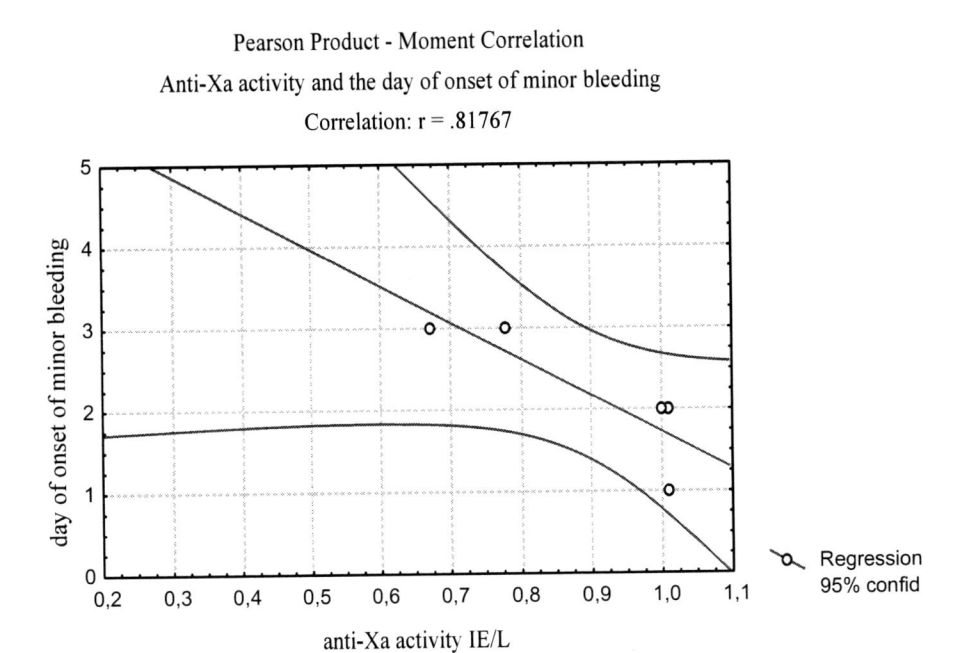

Figure 7. Pearson Product Moment Correlation between the level of anti-Xa activity and the day of onset of minor bleeding.

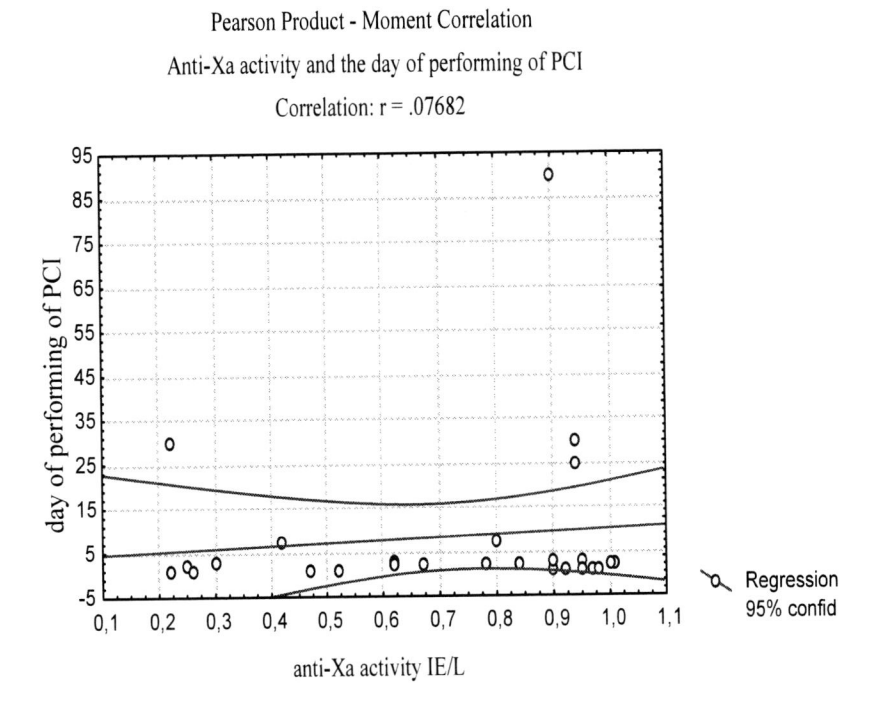

Figure 8. Pearson Product Moment Correlation between the level of anti-Xa activity and the day of PCI.

Discussion: In recent years a number of new agents have been used and have contributed to the better treatment of patients with acute coronary syndromes without ST-segment elevation. Combination of antiplatelet and antithrombin therapy is a potential new strategy that promises favorable results. Of the available antithrombins, low-molecular-weight heparins, mainly Enoxaparin, possess several advantages over unfractionated heparin. It has pharmacokinetic and pharmacodynamic characteristics making it an attractive option for use and resulting in favorable clinical outcomes [5].

To achieve optimal anticoagulation Food and Drug Administration recommends the dose regimen for Enoxaparin of 1mg/kg/12 h. s.c application. Four applications of this dose provide adequate anticoagulation and good clinical outcomes.

PEPCI study makes a comparison between the predictable and the actual level of anti-Xa activity. The actual level is approximately 10% of the predictable level [0.6-1.8 IE/ml] and it is achieved in 96% of patients [6].

In our study, 63.3% achieved the target level of anti-Xa activity of 0.6-1.0 IE/L. Below the target level [0.5 IE/L] were 8 patients [26%] and 3 patients [10%] achieved a level higher than 1.01 IE/L. These data served as an indicator of good anticoagulation, achieved with recommended dose regimen for Enoxaparin of 1mg/kg/12 h. s.c application.

The fact that there is no statistically significant differences between the number of platelets at the time of admission and 6 h after the enoxaparin application, indicate no platelet activation, lower rate of thrombocytopenia and safe use of enoxaparin.

Concerning the onset of adverse ischemic events, a positive correlation was noted between the level of anti-Xa activity and the day of onset of recurrent angina [r=0.21], myocardial infarction [r=0.21], heart failure [r=0.98], performing of coronary artery by-pass graft [r=0.63] and minor bleeding [r=0.81]. This means the earlier onset of RA, MI, HF, CABG and bleeding correlated with lower anti-Xa activity. We did not find correlation between the level of anti-Xa activity and the day of PCI [r=0.07]. The PCI were performed independent of the level of anti-Xa activity. In these cases, the level of heparinization was no indicator of real need of PCI. When interpreting these results, some other points must be taken into consideration. Thus, we explain this inverse relationship with the influence of the subjective factor i.e. the type of cardiologists-clinicians or interventionalists and their tendency to use interventional strategies.

Conclusion

Anti-Xa activity is an independent predictor of adverse cardiac events in patients with acute coronary syndromes without ST-segment elevation, treated with enoxaparin.

References

[1]   Bertrand ME, Simoons ML, Fox KA et al: Management of acute coronary syndromes: acute coronary syndromes without persistent ST segment elevation. Recommendation of the Task Force of the European Society of Cardiology. *Eur. Heart J.* 2000; 83:361-6

[2]   Frydman A. Low-molecular-weight heparins: an overview of their pharmaco-dynamics, pharmacokinetics and metabolism in humans. *Haemostasis.* 1996;26 Suppl 2:24-38.

[3]   Kereiakes DJ, Tcheng J, Fry ETA: Pharmacoinvasive Management of Acute Coronary Syndrome in the Setting of Percutaneous Coronary interventions: Evidence-Based, Site nad Spectrum-of-Care Strategies for Optimizing Patient Outcomes in NSTE-ACS. *J. Invasive Cardiol.* 2003; 15(9): 536-553

[4]   Gosselin R. Variability of Plasma Anti-Xa Activities with Different Lots of Enoxaparin. *The Annals of Pharmacotherapy* 2004; Vol.38(4): 563-568.

[5]   Mark DB, Cowper PA, Berkowitz SD, et al. Economic assessment of low-molecular-weight heparin (enoxaparin) versus unfractionated heparin in acute coronary syndrome patients: results from the ESSENCE randomized trial: Efficacy and Safety of Subcutaneous Enoxaparin in Non-Q wave Coronary Events [unstable angina or non-Q-wave myocardial infarction]. *Circulation,* 1998;97:1702-7

[6]   Martin JL, Fry ETA, Serano A, et al. Pharmacokinetic study of enoxaparin in patients undergoing coronary intervention after treatment with subcutaneous enoxaparin in acute coronary syndromes: the PEPCI study (abstract). *Eur. Heart J.* 2001; 22:14

In: Angina Pectoris: Etiology, Pathogenesis and Treatment
ISBN: 978-1-60456-674-1

Editors: A. P. Gallo, M. L. Jones
© 2008 Nova Science Publishers, Inc.

Chapter I

Angina Pectoris: Etiology, Pathogenesis, Clinical Feature and Treatment

Nidal A. Asaad and Jassim M. Al-Suwaidi*

Department of Cardiology and Cardiovascular Surgery, Hamad General Hospital and
Weill Cornell Medical College, Doha, Qatar

Introduction

Chest pain is one of the most common complaints of patients who are seen in an emergency room and ambulatory practice. The major early objective in the diagnosis of such patients is to separate noncardiac from cardiac pain.

The primary care provider plays a critical role in the management and the long-term care of patients who have coronary heart disease (CHD). Such care is focused on reducing symptoms and long-term complications. This reviews the details of management of chronic stable angina, and unstable angina.

Chronic stable angina pectoris includes predictable and reproducible left anterior chest discomfort after physical activity, emotional stress, or both; symptoms are typically worse in cold weather or after meals and are relieved by rest or sublingual nitroglycerin. The presence of one or more obstructions in major coronary arteries is likely; the severity of stenosis is usually greater than 70 percent.

Unstable angina is commonly classified by use of simple clinical descriptors, such as the presence or absence of ischemic chest discomfort at rest, as well as ECG changes and biochemical markers of myocardial injury during and after ischemic episodes.[1] Although these clinical descriptors are helpful in estimating prognosis and are used widely in

---

* Correspondence: Nidal A. Asaad MBBS, FRCPC, From the department of cardiology and cardiovascular surgery, Hamad General Hospital,P.O.BOX 3050, Doha, Qatar, Fax:+9744392454, e-mail:nasaad@uottawa.ca.

determining the intensity of treatment, they provide little information regarding the cause of the syndrome.

Etiology

Chronic stable angina increases in myocardial oxygen demand and may result from tachycardia, fever, thyrotoxicosis, endogenous and exogenous hyperadrenergic states, and elevations of left ventricular afterload—systemic hypertension and various forms of aortic stenosis.

In unstable angina, it appears to be possible to distinguish 5 different causes. These are summarized in the (Table 1).

Nonocclusive Thrombus on Preexisting Plaques

Unstable angina results from an imbalance between myocardial oxygen supply and demand. Probably the most common cause is reduced myocardial perfusion resulting from a nonocclusive thrombus on a fissured or eroded atherosclerotic plaque that often had caused only mild to moderate obstruction previously.[2] Nonocclusive thrombi in patients with unstable angina have been demonstrated by coronary angioscopy and arteriography.[3] They occur most commonly on complex, irregular lesions.[4] Plaques that have undergone disruption often have a core that is rich in cholesteryl esters and tissue factor. They have a thin fibrous cap; disruption is caused by shear forces acting on the shoulder of the plaque. In patients with unstable angina, products of aggregating platelets are released into the coronary circulation,[5] and there appears to be continued thrombus formation, often for months, after the index event.[6] Nonocclusive coronary thrombi often become organized and incorporated into the growing plaque.

Treatment with antithrombotic agents (unfractionated heparin[7] and low-molecular-weight heparin[8]) and antiplatelet agents (aspirin,[7] ticlopidine,[9] and glycoprotein IIb/IIIa inhibitors[10]) is beneficial in this form of angina. Perhaps tissue factor inhibitors will prove useful as well.

Dynamic Obstruction

A second form of unstable angina is caused by dynamic obstruction, ie, coronary vasoconstriction.

Four subgroups are recognized. (1) The first is Prinzmetal's variant angina, with intense focal spasm of a segment of an epicardial coronary artery not involved by coronary atherosclerosis. (2) In the second, also called Prinzmetal's angina, the spasm occurs adjacent to a nonobstructive atheromatous plaque. Both of these forms of vasospastic angina appear to be due to hypercontractility of vascular smooth muscle and endothelial dysfunction occurring

Table 1. Causes of Unstable Angina

1. Nonocclusive thrombus on preexisting plaque.
2. Dynamic obstruction (coronary spasm or vasoconstriction)
3. Progressive mechanical obstruction.
4. Inflammation and/or infection.
5. Secondary unstable angina.

in the region of spasm. They are characterized by ST-segment elevation accompanying rest pain and can often be provoked by stimuli such as ergonovine, acetylcholine, or hyperventilation. Rarely, vasospastic angina is caused by allergic reactions, with mediatorssuch as histamine or leukotrienes acting on coronary vascular smooth muscle. (3) The third subgroup results from nonfocal constriction of major coronary arteries containing atherosclerotic plaques.11 Such coronary vasoconstriction may be caused by adrenergic stimuli, cold immersion, or cocaine. Most commonly, coronary vasoconstriction may also occur when shear stress and/or humoral stimuli such as thrombin and substances released from platelets, including serotonin and thromboxane A2, act on dysfunctional coronary endothelium, with reduced production of relaxing factors and increased release of endothelin, causing contraction of coronary vascular smooth muscle. (4) The fourth is microcirculatory angina. In this condition, the ischemia is secondary to constriction of the small intramural coronary resistance vessels,[11,12] which in some instances is also caused by endothelial dysfunction. The epicardial coronary arteries appear normal on coronary arteriography, but the clearance of contrast material from the myocardium may be prolonged.[13] Dynamic obstruction often responds to coronary vasodilators: nitrates and calcium antagonists.

Progressive Mechanical Obstruction

The third form of unstable angina results from severe, organic luminal narrowing; perhaps its "purest" form is the restenosis after percutaneous transluminal coronary angioplasty and other forms of catheter-based revascularization. However, serial angiographic studies in many patients without previous intracoronary procedures have shown progressive luminal narrowing of the culprit vessel in the period just preceding the onset of unstable angina.[14] In such cases, progressive coronary obstruction causes the severe imbalance between myocardial oxygen supply and demand that is responsible for this form of unstable angina. Treatment of this cause of unstable angina consists of transcatheter or surgical revascularization. The benefit of mechanical revascularization is directly proportional to the contribution of the organic obstruction to the ischemia.

Inflammation and/or Infection

There is increasing evidence that arterial inflammation plays a role in atherogenesis and is responsible for thrombogenesis in some patients with unstable angina and other acute coronary syndromes. There may be an increase of circulating activated lymphocytes, as well as of neutrophil and monocyte adhesion molecules.[15] Macrophages and T lymphocytes are present at the shoulder of atherosclerotic plaques.[16] These cells may increase the expression of metalloproteinases and other enzymes that cause thinning of the fibrous cap, thereby predisposing to plaque rupture. Mononuclear cells exhibit enhanced secretion of cytokines, such as tumor necrosis factor (TNF)-a and g-interferon. Elevations of acute-phase reactants, such as C-reactive protein and serum amyloid A, portend a poor prognosis in patients with unstable angina.[17,18] Taken together, these observations suggest that inflammation may precipitate unstable angina.[19]

There is serological evidence that infection with organisms such as *Chlamydia pneumoniae*, virulent strains of *Helicobacter pylori*,[20] herpes simplex virus, and cytomegalovirus are common in patients with chronic atherosclerosis and acute coronary syndromes[15];*C pneumoniae* has been repeatedly identified in atherosclerotic plaques. It has been postulated that these organisms induce the production of cytokines, such as TNF-a and several interleukins, which may unfavorably alter local lipid metabolism, destabilize coronary plaques, stimulate platelet activation, and enhance thrombus formation.

The ability to recognize an inflammatory or infectious origin of unstable angina is still primitive, but the inflammatory markers C-reactive protein and serum amyloid A, as well as antibodies to *C pneumoniae*, are becoming more widely available. These might form the basis for the management of patients with unstable angina in whom inflammation and/or infection plays an important role. It has been suggested that the increased leukocyte adhesiveness observed in some patients with unstable angina identifies those who will benefit from treatment with anti-inflammatory agents.[21] Two small studies suggest that macrolide antibiotics reduce the incidence of recurrent events in patients with unstable angina[22] and acute myocardial infarction.[23] Anti-inflammatory drugs, including the new COX II inhibitors; antibiotics that are effective against *C pneumoniae* and *H pylori*; and drugs that are effective against the other putative infectious organisms may prove useful in patients with unstable angina in whom an infectious and/or inflammatory component plays an important pathogenetic role.

Secondary Unstable Angina

This form of unstable angina is precipitated by conditions that are extrinsic to the coronary vascular bed. It can be caused by conditions that increase myocardial oxygen demand and those that impair oxygen supply, occurring against the background of coronary stenosis and chronic stable angina. Increases in myocardial oxygen demand may result from tachycardia, fever, thyrotoxicosis, endogenous and exogenous hyperadrenergic states, and elevations of left ventricular afterload—systemic hypertension and various forms of aortic stenosis. Unstable angina secondary to impaired oxygen delivery can result from anemia, hypoxemia, and hyperviscosity states. Hypotension can reduce coronary perfusion pressure and impair myocardial perfusion distal to an atherosclerotic obstruction, thereby causing severe ischemia. In most cases, the cause of secondary unstable angina can be recognized and corrected. β-Adrenergic receptor blockers are often effective in reducing excess myocardial oxygen demands.

Pathogenesis

The endothelium plays an integral role in the defense against atherosclerosis and in modulating vascular tone and preventing thrombosis in blood vessels. These endothelial functions are affected by the presence of CAD risk factors, even before atherosclerosis is evident. In the earliest stages, circulating monocytes adhere to the endothelial cells (through adhesion molecules) and migrate into the intima of the blood vessel, where they ingest oxidatively modified low-density lipoprotein (LDL) and are trapped as foam cells. Collections of foam cells, known as fatty streaks, have been found in early childhood. Foam cells die, leading to the development of a lipid core, and smooth muscle cells are signaled to migrate from the media, destroying the internal elastic lamina of the vessel in the process. Calcification of the plaque occurs early and can be visualized with techniques such as CT and MRI. The arterial wall begins to thicken and remodel. Based on intravascular ultrasonographic studies, the encroachment of plaque into the lumen of a coronary artery is a late process and reflects advanced disease (the arterial cross-sectional area is reduced by 40% before a lesion is visible as luminal narrowing at catheterization). The progression of atherosclerosis is accelerated by three processes: endothelial dysfunction, inflammation, and thrombosis. The advanced atherosclerotic lesion has a core of lipid and necrotic tissue surrounded by a fibrous cap. This cap contains collagen, and its characteristics are related to the risk of plaque rupture, the most common cause of acute coronary syndromes. Specifically, the thinner the cap, the more likely it is to rupture. Shear stress at the edge or "shoulder" region of a plaque, inflammation at the endothelial surface of the cap, or internal degradation of the cap by enzymes known as metalloproteinases are other major determinants of the likelihood of plaque rupture. A ruptured plaque leads very quickly to thrombus formation. The complete occlusion of a coronary vessel by ruptured plaque manifests as an acute transmural or ST elevation myocardial infarction (ie, STEMI). Nonocclusive thrombus can cause unstable angina or non–ST elevation MI (ie, NSTEMI). Nonocclusive thrombus may not cause symptoms but, instead, may change plaque geometry, leading to rapid plaque growth. Studies have shown that an acute MI may be more likely to occur in an area that was previously not severely narrowed (ie, less than 50% luminal reduction by angiography) than in an area that was more severely narrowed (ie, more than 70% luminal reduction). Narrowing of a coronary artery by 70% or greater is more likely to cause exertional angina. The discordance between plaque severity and the development of acute MI indicates that MI is not simply a mechanical problem. Most patients who have classic angina by history have fixed atherosclerotic lesions of 70% or more in at least one major coronary artery [24]. However, a 70% stenosis viewed by two-dimensional angiography is associated with a reduction of approximately 90% in cross-sectional area. Angina is cause by a mismatch between myocardial oxygen supply and demand. Oxygen supply is determined by coronary perfusion pressure and coronary vascular resistance. Flow is autoregulated over a wide range of perfusion pressures, and therefore, most of the changes in flow are caused by changes in resistance (ie, vasodilation). However, the coronary bed, beyond a significant flow-limiting stenosis, is typically dilated maximally, so that small increases in demand (eg, increased heart rate and blood pressure during exercise) may result in myocardial ischemia. Demand is related to heart rate, systolic blood pressure, and wall tension. Wall tension is determined by ventricular pressure, cavity size, and wall thickness. Exercise and emotional stress have potent effects on these variables and, not coincidentally, are the common triggers for ischemic chest pain.

Risk Factors

Genetic and environmental risk factors influence the development of atherosclerotic heart disease. Research has been targeted at defining the role of these factors in the premature development of CAD. The recognition of risk factors is important especially because they may be modified to prevent disease. Landmark epidemiologic surveys like the Framingham Heart Study helped to define levels of risk for the individual risk factors. Treatment guidelines have been revised recently to include the important interactions between individual risk factors and age. Risk calculators (CHD event risk over 10 years) are available elsewhere [25,26].

The 27th Bethesda Conference[27] was designed to bring attention to specific patients who are at high-risk for the development of CAD events. The findings have been incorporated into the National Cholesterol Education Program (NCEP) Detection, Evaluation and Treatment of High Blood Cholesterol in Adults (adult treatment panel [ATP] III) [28]. The concepts of "risk" and "risk factor" are important in understanding and using the guidelines. The Bethesda Conference outlines four categories of risk based on observational studies and efficacy studies (clinical trials) (Table 2). Category 1 risk factors, for which interventions have been proven to reduce the risk of CHD events, include smoking, LDL cholesterol, high saturated fat diet, hypertension, LVH, and "thrombogenic factor," which are unnamed but reflect a reduction of risk with the use of aspirin. Category 2 risk factors, for which interventions are likely to lower CHD risk, include diabetes mellitus, physical inactivity, HDL cholesterol, elevated triglycerides, small, dense LDL particles, obesity, and postmenopausal status in women. Since the publication of these findings, diabetes has been reclassified as a CHD "risk equivalent" based on data suggesting that diabetic patients who do not have known CAD have similar survival to nondiabetic patients who have suffered a myocardial infarction. The ATP-III guidelines [28] focus attention on the "metabolic syndrome" that incorporates abdominal obesity, atherogenic dyslipidemia (elevated triglycerides, small LDL particles, low HDL cholesterol), elevated blood pressure, insulin resistance (with or without glucose intolerance), and prothrombotic and proinflammatory states. Patients who have this syndrome are now appropriately targeted for intensive lipid modification. HDL cholesterol, with the publication of the Veterans Affairs High-density Lipoprotein Intervention Trial (ie, VAHIT) [29], may now rightly be considered a category 1 risk factor because the intervention to raise HDL cholesterol level with gemfibrozil reduced the incidence of cardiovascular events. Although postmenopausal status correctly identifies the risk factor, hormone replacement therapy is now contraindicated for the treatment of women who have CAD or are at high risk for CAD for the purpose of reducing cardiovascular risk. Category 3 risk factors are those that are associated with an increased CAD risk that may, if modified, lower risk.

Table 2. Cardiovascular risk factors

Category 1: risk factors for which interventions have been proven to lower (cardiovascular disease) CVD risk:

      Cigarette smoking
      LDL cholesterol
      High fat/cholesterol diet
      Hypertension
      Left ventricular hypertrophy (LVH)
      Thrombogenic factors (as affected by aspirin)

Category 2: risk factors for which interventions are likely to lower CVD risk:

      Diabetes mellitus
      Physical Inactivity
      High-density lipoprotein (HDL) cholesterola
      Triglycerides
      Small, dense LDL particle size
      Obesity
      Postmenopausal status (women)

Category 3: risk factors associated with increased CVD risk that, if modified, might lower risk:

      Psychosocial factors
      Lipoprotein(a)
      Homocysteine
      Oxidative stress
      No alcohol consumption

Category 4: risk factors associated with increased risk but which cannot be modified:

      Age
      Male sex
      Low socioeconomic status
      Family history of early onset CVD

a May now be considered a category-1 risk factor; see text.
Adapted from Fuster V, Pearson TA, Co-Chairs. 27th Bethesda conference: matching the intensity of risk factor management with the hazard for coronary disease events. J Am Coll Cardiol 1996;27(5):957–1047.

These factors include the so-called putative or emerging risk factors such as depression, lipoprotein a, homocysteine, oxidative stress, and alcohol. Since 1997, this list should be expanded to include inflammatory markers (white blood cell count, high-sensitivity C-reactive protein [CRP] level, soluble adhesion molecules, and chlamydial infection), thrombotic risk factors (plasminogen activator inhibitor-1), and sleep apnea. Coronary calcification measured by electron beam CT [30] can be considered correctly a category 3 risk factor for now but may need to be reclassified (like diabetes) as a CAD risk equivalent because it functionally measures subclinical coronary artery plaque burden. Moderate alcohol consumption may reduce CAD risk. Category 4 risk factors, which are associated with increased risk but cannot be modified, include age, male sex, low socioeconomic status, and a family history of early onset CAD. A positive family history has been defined as a CAD risk factor in a male firstdegree relative younger than 55 years of age or in a female first-degree relative younger than 65 years of age. These factors are usually taken into consideration with the available risk scoring systems.

Clinical Feature

Diagnosis and History

A careful history is of paramount importance in the diagnosis of angina and can be as effective as exercise testing in predicting the extent of underlying coronary artery disease [31]. The discomfort of myocardial ischemia may be described variously by patients; many do not describe it as a pain, so it is often more effective to ask the patient to describe the discomfort. Some patients describe it as a squeezing, crushing, burning, or smothering sensation, whereas others describe a shortness of breath or simply a feeling of heaviness. Some patients may use a Levine's sign, a clenched fist in the middle of the chest, to describe the discomfort. Rarely is the patient able to point with one finger to the location; so when pain can be localized in this way, it is likely to be noncardiac in origin. A sharp pain is unlikely to have a cardiac origin, but the patient should be asked to characterize it further.

In some regions of the United States, ''sharp'' means severe rather than knifelike or piercing.

Angina, as described classically, begins and ends gradually, usually over 2 to 5 minutes, and is steady in character, although it can occasionally wax and wane. The anginal threshold may be lower in the morning. If ischemic pain continues for over 20 minutes, myocardial infarction is likely. The discomfort is midline and substernal; it often radiates to the shoulder, arm, hand or fingers, usually to the left. Radiation down the inside of the arm into the fingers supplied by the ulnar nerve is a classic sign. Pain also may radiate into the neck, the lower (but not the upper) jaw, or the intrascapular region. Occasionally, the patient may have pain only in a referred location and experience no chest discomfort at all. An ''anginal equivalent'' refers to a discomfort limited to the site typically noted in secondary radiation of pain. Dyspnea may be an anginal equivalent in older individuals but should be centrally located; the dyspnea of a pulmonary cause is not localized. Uncomfortable arm heaviness may represent angina. Gaseous distension, belching, nausea, and indigestion are common accompanying symptoms. Chest pain accompanied by severe diaphoresis is worrisome but is not always caused by cardiac ischemia.

The Canadian Cardiovascular Society (CCS) classification system [32] predicts the extent of CAD and risk of ischemic events. CCS class I angina occurs with strenuous, rapid, or prolonged exertion but not with ordinary physical activity. Class II is defined as a slight limitation of ordinary activity. Angina occurs on walking or climbing stairs rapidly, walking uphill, walking or stair climbing after meals, in cold or wind exposure, or under emotional stress. Class III angina has marked limitations of ordinary physical activity. Angina occurs on walking one or two blocks on a level surface and climbing one flight of stairs in normal conditions and at a normal pace. Class IV, the most severe, is the inability to carry on any physical activity without discomfort, and anginal symptoms may be present at rest.

A major feature of the history is the identification of precipitating and aggravating factors. The single most important diagnostic feature of the discomfort of myocardial ischemia is a predictable relationship to exertion, emotional stress, or other situations that increase myocardial oxygen demand or reduce supply. The cause of atypical pain, pain in an unusual location or of an unusual character, may be clarified by this relationship. Pain that is experienced at rest, if it is caused by ischemia, suggests unstable angina or myocardial infarction. Anxiety and mental stress are important and often overlooked provoking factors in many patients. Myocardial oxygen demand may be increased by anxiety to an extent and duration greater that that produced by exercise, resulting in prolonged pain. Angina is more likely to occur during cold or windy weather because of increased peripheral vascular resistance and consequently increased myocardial work. Sexual intercourse may represent the highest daily energy expenditure in sedentary elderly patients who have subclinical CAD. Sometimes, ischemic discomfort follows a heavy meal, perhaps caused by the shunting of blood to abdominal viscera and because of increased sympathetic tone. Nocturnal angina may be a consequence or manifestation of left ventricular failure or may represent unstable angina. Similarly, patients who describe breathlessness and chest pain with exertion may have angina as a consequence of transient left ventricular failure.

Because angina is caused by a discrepancy between oxygen supply and demand, the relief of pain is achieved by increasing coronary blood flow or decreasing oxygen demand, and angina begins to disappear within minutes thereafter. So-called walk-through angina is uncommon. Most people must stop or at least slow the activity responsible for precipitating the pain before it is relieved. However, it is common for people to resume their activities and walk farther the second time without symptoms; this is known as "preconditioning." A history of relief of pain by sublingual nitroglycerin is also useful. However, the patient must be told that the use of nitroglycerin in this way is a diagnostic trial and that the prescription of nitroglycerin does not necessarily mean coronary artery disease. The relief of chest pain by nitroglycerin is not specific for myocardial ischemia; the pain of esophageal spasm is commonly relieved by nitroglycerin. A placebo effect may relieve chest discomfort from other causes as well.

Physical Examination

Physical examination findings in patients who have angina are nonspecific. Particular attention is paid to uncovering circumstantial evidence that would support the diagnosis of coronary artery disease: high blood pressure, evidence of abnormal lipid metabolism such as tendon xanthomas or xanthelesma, fundoscopic changes reflecting long-standing hypertension or diabetes mellitus, or evidence of peripheral vascular disease. A complete cardiovascular examination should include measurement of bilateral blood pressures and auscultation of the carotid, abdominal aorta, and femoral arteries. Aortic stenosis should be excluded, with systolic murmurs (present in 70% of the elderly) confirmed by diminished and delayed pulses (pulsus parvus et tardus) in the carotids or left brachial artery. A focus on auscultation and the character and timing of murmurs will lead to an appropriate referral for echocardiography. If a patient has chest pain in the office, the blood pressure should be taken immediately because hypertension (ischemia) or hypotension (acute heart failure) can be important signs. Furthermore, the presence of a new mitral regurgitation murmur during chest pain may signal extensive ischemia.

Differential Diagnosis

A complete differential diagnosis of chest pain is outside the scope of this article but can be classified generally as cardiovascular causes and noncardiac causes. The cardiovascular causes include stable and unstable angina, myocardial infarction, pericarditis, aortic dissection (or enlarging aneurysm), pulmonary embolism, and pulmonary hypertension. Noncardiac causes include musculoskeletal disorders, esophageal and other gastrointestinal pain, neuropathic pain including herpes zoster, and anxiety.

Investigation

Laboratory Evaluation, Including Cardiac Biomarkers

The laboratory evaluation of patients presenting with new angina pectoris focuses on evaluating risk factors. Hypertensive patients should have an evaluation of renal function. Diabetic patients should have an assessment of the level of control of blood glucose (ie, hemoglobin A1c). Patients who have impaired glucose tolerance (fasting plasma glucose 100–126) or are suspected of having the metabolic syndrome (abdominal obesity, high triglycerides, hypertension, and low HDL cholesterol) should undergo an oral glucose tolerance test to screen for overt diabetes. The NCEP [28] recommends screening fasting lipid levels in all adults with a measurement of HDL cholesterol. Many practitioners are using advanced lipid testing (ie, LDL particle number and density), but there is no consensus on its use. Similarly, elevated levels of high-sensitivity CRP [33] and B-type natriuretic peptide [34] are associated with prognosis in patients who have angina pectoris but have not yet been incorporated into the guidelines. The measurement of cardiac troponin should be reserved for patients who have suspected acute coronary syndromes.

Electrocardiogram

A 12-lead ECG should be obtained as soon as possible in a patient suspected of having CAD or angina, but in many cases, results may be completely normal. The most reliable ECG sign of chronic ischemic heart disease is a pathologic Q wave, representing previous infarction. Nonspecific ST-T wave changes, abnormalities of conduction (except for LBBB), and arrhythmias do not help establish the diagnosis of myocardial ischemia. ST segment depression with a flat or downward sloping ST segment, however, is indicative of subendocardial ischemia. It is seldom present in the resting ECG of patients who have ischemic heart disease, unless they are experiencing angina at the time the tracing is being recorded. On the other hand, these transient ischemic changes are seen commonly when a patient who has ischemic heart disease is exercised to a point at which chest pain develops. Such ECG changes, appearing with exercise or pain and resolving with rest or with the resolution of pain, strongly indicate myocardial ischemia. Therefore, the necessity of repeating the ECG at rest or after the chest pain has resolved cannot be overemphasized. ST segment elevation during chest pain suggests myocardial infarction or variant angina.

T wave inversion in an ECG taken at rest is a nonspecific finding but can occur after infarction or as a specific transient finding in a patient who has angina. Thus, ECG changes noted during episodes of chest pain not only confirm the diagnosis of myocardial ischemia but also may indicate the extent and location of the ischemic myocardium. As a general rule, the more widespread the changes, the more myocardium is involved.

The differential diagnosis of Q waves on an ECG include previous myocardial infarction, healed myocarditis, an infiltrative myocardial disorder like amyloidosis or sarcoidosis, and pre-excitation (delta wave) from

Wolff-Parkinson-White syndrome. Similarly, ST segment elevation in the absence of chest pain is common in the resting ECG of healthy young adults and is caused by rapid or ''early'' repolarization of the ventricle. This pattern is noted usually in the mid-left chest leads (V2–V4) but has also been seen widely. ST segment elevation from pericarditis is diffuse, can be associated with PR segment depression, and has the other usual clinical features.

The presence of ST-T abnormalities in an otherwise healthy person is a nonspecific finding and should not be considered confirmation of CAD. There is a high association of left bundle branch block (LBBB) with organic heart disease, especially CAD. Right bundle branch block (RBBB), on the other hand, is present in 0.3% of normal people and is usually a benign, congenital condition. RBBB is rarely a manifestation of CAD.

Stress Testing

The American College of Cardiology (ACC)/American Heart Association (AHA) exercise testing guidelines were updated in 1997 [35]. Patients who have a high likelihood of having CAD by history should be referred directly for cardiac catheterization. Those with a low likelihood of CAD should not undergo exercise testing. (Table 3) shows the ACC/AHA criteria for determining the probability of underlying CAD by age, sex, and symptoms. Typical features of angina include the location and character of discomfort, timing of discomfort, and inciting and relieving factors. The ACC/AHA class I recommendation for exercise testing in the diagnosis of CAD is for adult patients who have an intermediate pretest probability of CAD (15%–85%).

Table 3. Pretest likelihood of coronary artery disease in symptomatic patients according to age and sex

	Nonanginal chest pain likelihood (%)		Angina			
			Atypical likelihood (%)		Typical likelihood (%)	
Age (y)	Men	Women	Men	Women	Men	Women
30–39	4	2	34	12	76	26
40–49	13	3	51	22	87	55
50–59	20	7	65	31	93	73
60–69	27	14	72	51	94	86

No data exists for patients <30 y or >69 y, but it can be assumed that prevalence of coronary artery disease increases with age. In a few cases, patients with ages at the extremes of the decades listed may have probabilities slightly outside the high or low range. High indicates 90%; intermediate 10%–90%; low, <10%; and very low, <5%. Data from Gibbons RJ, Abrams J, Chatterjee K, et al. ACC/AHA 2002 guideline update for the management of patients with chronic stable angina: a report of the American College of Cardiology/American Heart Association Task Force on Practice Guidelines (Committee to update the 1999 guidelines for the management of patients with chronic stable angina). 2002 American College of Cardiology and American Heart Association. Available at http://www.acc.org/clinical/guidelines/stable/stable.pdf. Accessed January 13, 2006.

For patients who are known to have CAD, the guidelines recommend stress testing for those who experience a significant change in clinical status. Absolute and relative contraindications to stress testing are outlined in Table 4 [35]. Unstable angina, decompensated heart failure, aortic stenosis, and uncontrolled hypertension are the most common reasons for canceling a test. The simplest and least expensive test is the exercise treadmill test [36].

Table 4. Absolute contraindications to exercise testing

Acute myocardial infarction (<2 d)

High-risk unstable angina

Decompensated heart failure

Uncontrolled cardiac arrhythmias with symptoms or

hemodynamic compromise

Advanced atrioventricular block

Acute myocarditis or pericarditis

Severe symptomatic aortic stenosis

Severe hypertrophic obstructive cardiomyopathy

Uncontrolled hypertension

Acute systemic illness (pulmonary embolism, aortic dissection)

Relative contraindications can be superseded if the benefits of exercise outweigh the risks. The appropriate timing of testing depends on the level of risk of unstable angina. In the absence of definitive evidence, the committee suggests systolic blood pressure greater than 200 mm Hg and/or diastolic blood pressure greater than 110 mm Hg.

Data from Gibbons RJ, Balady GJ, Beasley FW, et al. ACC/AHA guidelines for exercise testing: a report of the ACC/AHA task force on practice guidelines. J Am Coll Cardiol 1997;30:260–315.

Many European countries prefer bicycle stress testing; the routine use of bicycles in the United States is rare. Various protocols have been devised for graded, symptom-limited exercise testing, but all protocols have the same rationale. As cardiac work is increased, myocardial oxygen consumption increases and coronary blood flow must increase. If a fixed coronary obstruction limits changes in blood flow, the patient may experience chest discomfort, and ECG changes (ST segment depression) can occur. Figure 1 represents a simple algorithm for deciding what type of stress test to recommend. Baseline ECG abnormalities that preclude a simple exercise ECG include pre-excitation (Wolff-Parkinson-White syndrome), electronically paced ventricular rhythm, a resting ST depression greater than 1 mm, and complete left bundle branch block. These patients should be referred for imaging stress tests and their ability to exercise determined. The inability to perform 4 METs or metabolic equivalents of exercise is an independent, poor prognostic sign for long-term outcome. The Duke activity score [35] is useful for predicting exercise ability. The simple question ''Can you walk up a flight of stairs carrying laundry or groceries without stopping?'' is an excellent discriminator for exercise ability. If the answer is ''Yes,'' treadmill exercise is recommended; if the answer is ''No,'' a pharmacologic stress test with cardiac imaging is recommended. Cost-effectiveness analysis has shown that the choice between nuclear perfusion imaging and echocardiography imaging is so close that the most important factor is the relative expertise of the local laboratories [37].

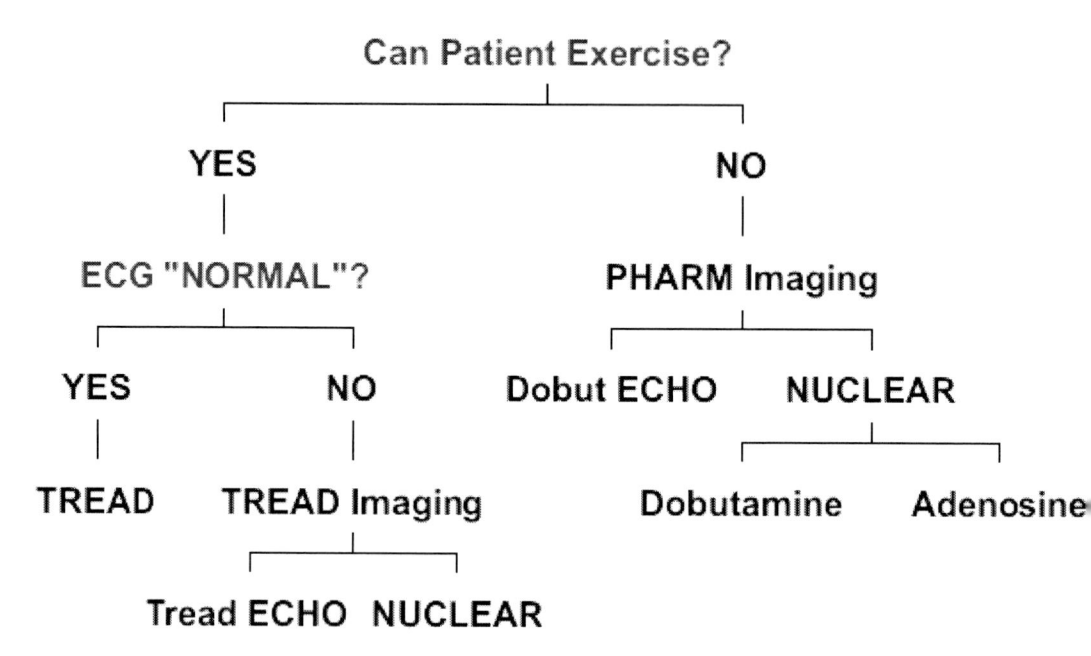

From Mark D. Kelemen etal Med Clin N Am 90 (2006) 391–416.

Figure 1. Algorithm for determining the appropriate stress test (see section ''Stress testing''). Dobut, dobutamine; ECHO, echocardiography.

Radioisotope Imaging

Radioisotope imaging can enhance the specificity of stress testing by evaluating myocardial function or flow [38]. Radioisotope imaging can be used in conjunction with either treadmill exercise testing or pharmacologic stress testing, using either dobutamine to increase cardiac work or adenosine or dipyridamole to alter coronary blood flow. Commonly used imaging modalities include radioisotope imaging with thallium-201 (201TI) or technetium- 99m (99mTc)–based agents (eg, 99mTc sestamibi). The usefulness of 201Tl as a perfusion tracer is based on its ability to function as an analog of ionic potassium. It is most efficiently extracted by healthy myocardial cells, and uptake is proportional to regional perfusion and myocardial viability. 99mTc sestamibi has a shorter half-life (6 hours) than 201Tl (73 hours), which allows a larger tracer dose to be administered. This and its higher emission energy make 99mTc an excellent agent for cardiac imaging. 99mTc sestamibi is particularly useful in obese patients and in patients who have large breasts (because of the possible attenuation of the radioisotopic images in the area of the anterior myocardium).

Both 201 Tl and 99mTc sestamibi can be used to assess regional myocardial blood flow, either by planar imaging or by single-photon emission CT (SPECT). Imaging usually occurs at two separate times: the stress scan is obtained very shortly after the patient has exercised or received a pharmacologic agent, and the rest scan is obtained either before or several hours after stress. The radioisotope is injected intravenously (IV) at the time of peak exercise (or at the time of peak infusion during a pharmacologic stress test), and scintigraphic images are obtained shortly thereafter, depicting regional myocardial perfusion at the time of peak stress. The rest scan is typically obtained later and shows redistribution of the isotope. Ischemia is indicated by the filling in of a cold spot defined on the stress images (ie, normalization or ''redistribution'' of a radioisotopic defect), and infarction is indicated by a persisting cold spot or one with only partial redistribution.

(Figure 2A) demonstrates the standard nomenclature for radioisotope imaging, and Figure 2B shows the typical coronary artery territories [39]. Radioisotope imaging with stress-gated blood pool scans (multiple gated acquisition [MUGA]) can also be used to assess myocardial ischemia. To allow for continuous imaging during exercise, stress MUGA is performed with the patient exercising on a semirecumbent bicycle. The rationale for this test is the fact that myocardium that becomes ischemic during graded exercise develops regional wall motion abnormalities that can be detected by sequential image analysis. This type of imaging labels the blood pool with a radioisotope and gates image acquisition to the ECG. Right and left ventricular volumes, regional left ventricular wall motion, and global and regional ejection fractions can be measured, both at rest and with stress.

Stress Echocardiography

Two-dimensional echocardiography can be used instead of radioisotope scanning to detect areas of regional myocardial dysfunction (as evidenced by a wall motion abnormality) with exercise or pharmacologic stress. Typically,baseline images are first obtained at rest to determine the adequacy of the echocardiographic images. If these images are technically inadequate (ie, because of obesity or obstructive lung disease), then IV contrast agents can be used or the patient should be referred for radioisotope imaging (most laboratories report a 5% failure rate).

If the images are technically adequate, the patient undergoes treadmill exercise stress, and then images are reacquired immediately, using special software to allow for the direct comparison of pre- and postexercise images. If pharmacologic stress testing with dobutamine is used, the doses of dobutamine are increased in a stepwise fashion and echocardiographic images are typically obtained each time the dose is increased. The safety of dobutamine stress echocardiography is comparable to that of a routine exercise stress test. Generally, SPECT is slightly more sensitive, and stress echo imaging is more specific for the diagnosis of CAD. Stress echocardiography may be preferred in some cases because some information is provided that is not obtained with radioisotopic scanning (ie, the presence of pericardial effusion, ventricular hypertrophy, or valve abnormalities); it also avoids exposure to radioactivity. The use of myocardial contrast echocardiography to add perfusion imaging to wall motion analysis is in development. Figure 3 demonstrates the standard nomenclature for two-dimensional echocardiography; the coronary artery territory is the same as in (Figure 2B).

Pharmacologic Stress Testing

Patients who are unable to exercise because of physical limitations can be evaluated after receiving IV administration of dipyridamole, adenosine, or dobutamine in conjunction with the imaging modality. Dipyridamole and adenosine dilate all coronary vessels, increasing flow to all areas of the heart.

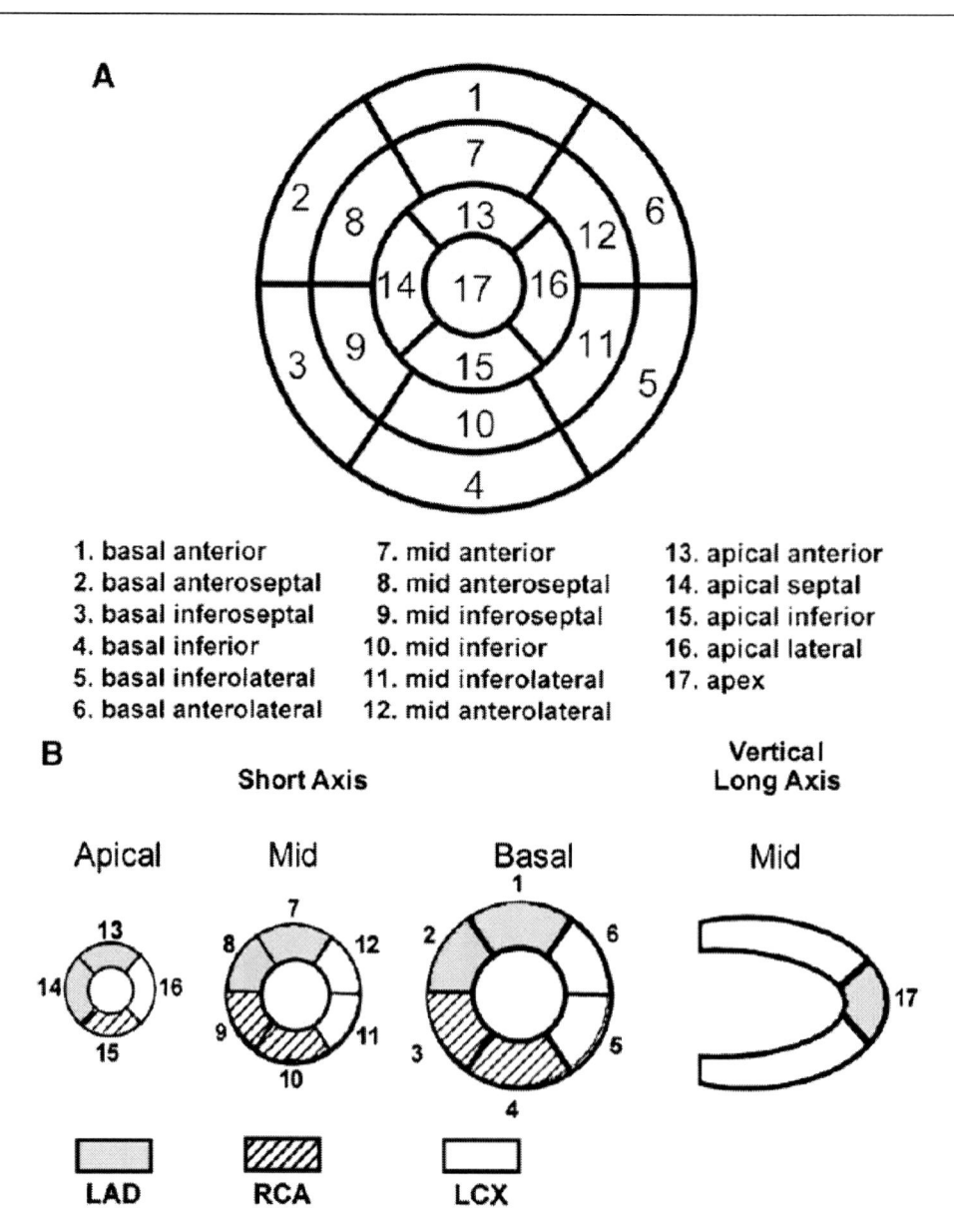

From Mark D. Kelemen etal Med Clin N Am 90 (2006) 391–416

Figure 2. (A) Left ventricular segmentation shows the standard nomenclature and segmentation used for SPECT myocardial perfusion imaging. The model divides the short-axis slices of the left ventricle into three major portions: apical, midventricular, and basal. The apex is a separate portion, which is analyzed from a vertical long-axis slice. The midventricular and basal shortaxis slices are divided into six segments, whereas the apical short-axis slices are divided into four segments. The apex on the vertical long-axis slice represents one more segment. (B) Coronary artery territories. Although the anatomy of coronary arteries may vary substantially in individual patients, the location of myocardial perfusion abnormalities on SPECT or echocardiography imaging allows for a general prediction of which coronary artery is likely to be diseased. Shown here is the standardized assignment of coronary artery territories of the left anterior descending coronary artery (LAD), the right coronary artery (RCA), and the left circumflex coronary artery (LCX). The prediction of disease in the RCA and LCX is often less accurate because of substantial variation in extent to myocardial territories.

The enhanced dilation of normal coronary arteries, compared with that which occurs in significantly narrowed vessels, augments differences in flow that usually are not apparent at rest. These agents are suitable for use with radioisotopic imaging modalities that may readily demonstrate this flow heterogeneity. Because these agents affect flow but not heart rate or contractility, they are used only in conjunction with radioisotopic imaging but not with echocardiography. After the administration of dipyridamole or adenosine followed by either 201Tl or 99mTc sestamibi (ie, the stress image), myocardial tissue supplied by a narrowed coronary artery typically demonstrates a perfusion defect that ''fills in'' during the rest image.

Because of its short duration of action, adenosine is preferred to dipyridamole for this test. For a number of technical reasons, they remain the stress test of choice for patients who have LBBB. Dobutamine is a b1 agonist that, at IV high dosages (20 mg/kg/min to 40 mg/kg/min), increases myocardial contractility and heart rate in a manner and extent similar to exercise. Heart rate may not be affected to the same extent as contractility, and IV atropine is often administered to increase the heart rate to the maximal predicted heart rate for the patient's age. Dobutamine may be used in conjunction with either echocardiography or radioisotopic imaging for the diagnosis of CAD. Mild side effects (nausea, flushing, and headache) are common with all of these agents and may occur in 75% of patients. Dipyridamole and adenosine can produce severe bronchospasm and should not be used in patients who have severe COPD. Adenosine causes chest pain in 50% of patients but has an exceedingly short half-life. Xanthine derivatives (eg, theophylline) and caffeine block adenosine receptors and should be avoided for 24 hours before a study.

Dobutamine can increase arteriovenous (AV) nodal conduction and should not be used in patients who have atrial flutter and only carefully in patients who have atrial fibrillation. Adenosine can cause transient AV block.

Diagnostic Use of Exercise Testing

A meta-analysis of 147 published studies has shown that the sensitivity and specificity of the exercise ECG for the detection of CAD (at least 50% stenosis angiographically) are 68% and 77%, respectively [40]. The sensitivity of the test increases with the severity of disease. The most common reasons for a false-positive exercise ECG are hypertension, cardiomyopathy, hyperventilation, and LVH. The goal of the standard exercise treadmill test is to reach 90% of the maximal predicted heart rate for age (estimated as 220 per age). The electrocardiographic criteria for a positive test are considered to be a downward sloping or horizontal ST segment depression of more that 1 mm for three consecutive beats. The sensitivity and specificity for the diagnosis of CAD (70% occlusion in at least 1 vessel) are listed in Table 3 for the primary stress testing modalities. If stricter ECG criteria (ie, 2 mm ST depression) are used, the sensitivity decreases with increased specificity. False-positive stress tests occur more commonly in women, patients who have mitral valve prolapse, and baseline ST-T wave changes. Some experts suggest that all women should undergo imaging stress tests because of the problem of false-positive tests; the cost implication of that recommendation would be substantial, and the negative predictive value of the test remains high.

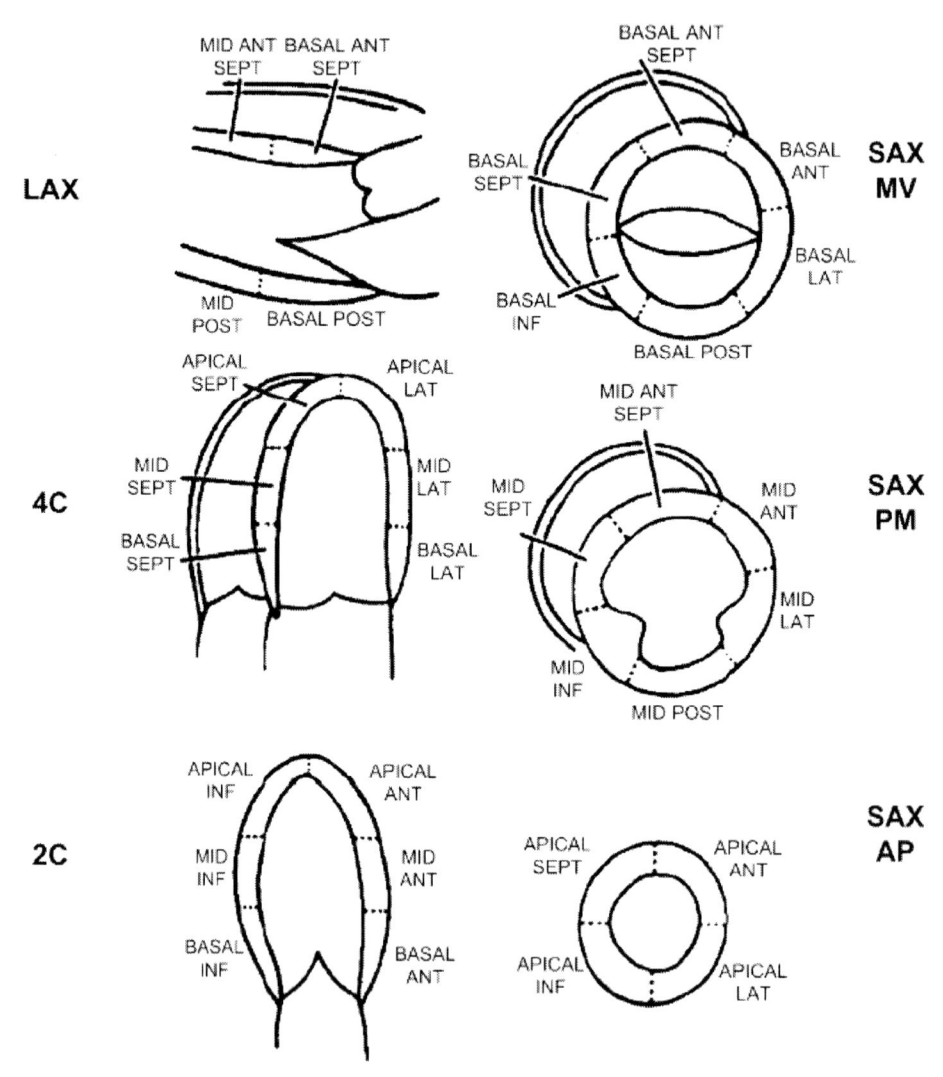

From Mark D. Kelemen etal Med Clin N Am 90 (2006) 391–416.

Figure 3. Regional wall segments showing the left ventricle divided into 16 segments for twodimensional echocardiography. These segments can be identified into a series of longitudinal views (LAX, 4C, 2C) or a series of short-axis views (SAM MV, SAX PM, SAX AP). The longitudinal and short-axis views overlap and complement each other. 2C, 2 chamber; 4C, 4 chamber; ANT, anterior; INF, inferior; LAT, lateral; LAX, long axis; POST, posterior; SAX AP, short-axis apex; SAX MV, short-axis mitral valve level; SAX PM, short-axis papillary muscle; SEPT, septum. (From Cerqueira MD, Weissman NJ, Dilsizian V, et al; for the American Heart.

Association Writing Group on Myocardial Segmentation and Registration for Cardiac Imaging. Standardized myocardial segmentation and nomenclature for tomographic imaging of the heart: a statement for healthcare professionals from the Cardiac Imaging Committee of the Council on Clinical Cardiology of the American Heart Association. Circulation 2002; 105(4):539–42.)

Stress test results predict prognosis as well. The factors that affect prognosis include the maximum amount of ST segment deviation during exercise, the presence or absence of angina, and the duration of exercise. The most extensive prognostic studies for abnormal stress tests have occurred in the field of radionuclide imaging, but the lessons carry over to treadmill and echo stress tests. The number, size, and location of abnormalities on stress myocardial perfusion studies reflect the location and extent of functionally significant coronary stenoses [41]. Echo and nuclear imaging can detect left ventricular dilation with stress, which suggests global, severe ischemia. Lung uptake of a radioactive tracer (201Tl or 99mTc sestamibi) indicates stress-induced left ventricular dysfunction and suggests multivessel CAD. Many studies have shown that high-risk abnormal stress tests are associated with an increased risk of cardiac events. Importantly, normal echo and nuclear stress tests are highly predictive of a benign prognosis. In a review of 16 studies involving almost 4000 patients over 2 years, a negative perfusion scan was associated with a 0.9% rate of cardiac death per year, similar to the general population [42].

Positron emission tomography (PET) increases the scope of cardiac evaluation from perfusion and function to metabolic substrate use [43]. Whereas SPECT measures relative blood flow, PET can measure absolute blood flow. The sensitivity and specificity of PET are over 90% [44], but the cost effectiveness of the strategy is unknown. PET must be performed with vasodilator stress. Combined with CT angiography (described below), PET offers the possibility of a single test describing left ventricular size and function, coronary anatomy and baseline and stress-induced flow characteristics, and myocardial metabolism in the resting and stressed states. Research in this field is just beginning.

Advanced Cardiac Imaging: CT and MRI

CT is a highly sensitive technique for detecting coronary artery calcium, and its clinical usefulness is being evaluated [30]. ECG gating allows data acquisition within 1 to 2 breath holds, making it a fast test with limited radiation exposure. Calcium is easy to distinguish, and coronary calcium is highly sensitive for atherosclerotic CAD. The calcium score is an index of calcium deposition in multiple arterial segments and is a good approximation of the overall plaque burden in the coronary tree. High calcium scores are associated with an increased risk of myocardial infarction [45] and offers improved discrimination over conventional risk factors in the identification of people with CAD [46]. Whether calcium scores are useful in the initial diagnosis of patients who have angina pectoris is unclear. Coronary CT angiography is a new technique using multislice CT and IV contrast with fast ECG gating and specialized software to reconstruct the coronary arteries. This technique is presently being used mostly in research studies, but it is available for clinical use in patients who have chest discomfort and equivocal stress test results or for patients who refuse cardiac catheterization to define the extent of CAD. The safety and efficacy of CT angiography in the initial emergency department evaluation of patients who presented with chest pain has been demonstrated [47]. MR coronary angiography also is under development and can detect the major coronary vessels. High-speed MRI techniques allow for the simultaneous assessment of myocardial perfusion with MRI contrast agents [38]. MR perfusion imaging with dipyridamole [48] or dobutamine [49] as the stress agent compares favorably with SPECT and echocardiography in the diagnosis of CAD.

Coronary Angiography and Revascularization Strategies

The 1999 ACC/AHA Guidelines for Coronary Angiography [50] outline the indications and contraindications for angiography. Class I indications for angiography include CCS class III or IV angina on medical treatment (angina at moderate exertion) and high-risk criteria on noninvasive testing, regardless of angina severity. High-risk stress tests are defined as more than 1 mm of ST segment depression, ischemia at a low workload (<5 METS), and ischemia involving a large territory of the LV myocardium. Class IIa recommendations include angina that improves with therapy but remains present; serial noninvasive testing showing progressively worsening abnormalities; patients who cannot tolerate medical therapy; patients who have angina who cannot be adequately risk stratified because of disability or illness; and individuals whose occupation involves the safety of others (pilots, bus drivers, and similar jobs) who have abnormal but not high-risk stress test results. There are no absolute contraindications to coronary arteriography. Relative contraindications include acute or chronic renal failure, active gastrointestinal bleeding, acute stroke, severe anemia, coagulopathy, unexplained fever or active untreated infection, severe uncontrolled hypertension, documented anaphylactoid reaction to angiographic contrast agents, and decompensated congestive heart failure. Renal insufficiency occurs in 0%to 5% of patients who do not have preexisting renal dysfunction and 10% to 40% of patients who have baseline renal insufficiency. Pretreatment with IV hydration (0.45% saline), N-acetylcysteine (600 mg twice daily), and limiting the use of IV contrast are the most effective means for mitigating renal dysfunction. In patients who are suspected of having iodine contrast allergy, pretreatment with corticosteroids and treatment with H1 and H2 histamine antagonists may reduce allergic complications. Major morbidity and mortality from coronary angiography is rare. In a survey of nearly 60,000 patients, the mortality from angiography was 0.11%; myocardial infarction occurred in 0.05% of patients; and stroke occurred in 0.07% of patients [51]. The most frequent major complication is vascular access complication (0.43%). Coronary revascularization can be performed with either percutaneous coronary intervention (PCI) or coronary artery bypass surgery (CABG). Currently, 80% of PCI procedures in the United States are performed with a drug-eluting coronary stent coated with sirolimus or paclitaxel [52]. Revascularization should be considered in patients who have limiting angina despite medications or high-risk features on clinical history, stress testing, or catheterization. Patients who have multivessel CAD, proximal left anterior descending or left main CAD, reduced LV function, or a large ischemic burden as found by stress testing should be referred for revascularization. Five-year rates of MI and death are similar between PCI and CABG [53], although CABG generally yields more complete revascularization and more complete resolution of symptoms. Recent data favor CABG in high-risk patients who have reduced ejection fraction and diabetes [54]. The choice of drug-eluting stents over bare metal stents is associated with lower rates of restenosis, reduced angina, and fewer repeat revascularizations [55].

Prognosis

Coronary artery disease is a chronic condition; however, certain patients are at an increased risk for death and nonfatal myocardial infarction in the short term (1 year). The four characteristics that best predict risk are reduced left ventricular ejection fraction, the extent and severity of CAD, a recent plaque rupture event (STEMI or non-STEMI), and noncardiac comorbidity. The Coronary Artery Surgery Study (CASS) [56] is the largest dataset of patients who underwent medical treatment for symptomatic CAD. In that study, patients who were able to perform less than 4 METS of work on a treadmill and had significant ST segment depression had an annual mortality of greater than 5% per year [56]. Those who were able to exercise for 10 METS and had no ischemic ECG changes had an annual mortality of less than 1% per year. Patients who present at a younger age and those who do not alter modifiable risk factors may have more aggressive disease. Unfortunately, we do not have an adequate means to predict which plaque is likely to rupture and cause events. Therefore, the ability of a stress test to predict MI is reduced because many of the plaques that cause events are not flow limiting.

Medical Treatment of Angina Pectoris

Medical management of angina pectoris falls into two categories: antianginal drugs [24,57,58], which may improve symptoms and exercise performance, and vasculoprotective agents [59–61], which modify the biology of atherosclerosis. A major advance in drug therapy has been the demonstration that long-acting antithrombotic agents and vigorous lipid lowering therapy can improve outcomes in selected patients who have CAD. Angina that occurs with exercise usually is caused by an increase in myocardial oxygen demand that cannot be met because of a fixed arterial obstruction. A decrease in or cessation of the work that produced angina usually results in a prompt reduction in myocardial oxygen demand. Therefore, rest or a decrease in the level of activity may relieve angina in 1 to 2 minutes. If anxiety is a contributing or provoking factor, myocardial work may take longer to decrease, and the episode of angina may be prolonged. Antianginal medications reduce angina and prolong exercise time but have not been demonstrated to improve the rate of mortality [57].

Antianginal Drugs

Nitrates

Traditionally, nitroglycerin has been an inexpensive mainstay of treatment of patients who have angina pectoris. Initially, these agents were believed to increase coronary blood flow by producing coronary artery dilation. Although nitrates may increase coronary blood flow in patients who have spasm or may increase collateral flow to obstructed vessels, evidence suggests that the mechanism of action of nitrates in most patients is not an increase in blood flow but a decrease in myocardial oxygen demand and peripheral vascular resistance. These compounds produce dilation of the venous circulation, resulting in reduced cardiac work and smaller left ventricular chamber size. Thus, the beneficial antianginal effect of nitrates is caused primarily by peripheral vasodilation.

Sublingual nitroglycerin is still the drug of choice for the relief and prevention of acute episodes of angina pectoris in most patients [52]. The initial dose should be small (0.4 mg) to minimize unpleasant side effects (flushing, headache, and light-headedness) in patients for whom higher dosages may be unnecessary. Patients should be taught that it is important that their pain be relieved as soon as possible, and they should be instructed to take nitroglycerin whenever such symptoms appear. Angina often produces discomfort and anxiety, which may increase heart rate and blood pressure and, hence, increased myocardial oxygen demand. If pain is not relieved by 2 to 3 tablets of nitroglycerin (the patient should wait for 3 minutes between doses) or if the use of nitroglycerin increases suddenly and dramatically, the patient should be instructed to call a physician or to go immediately to an emergency facility because of the danger of impending myocardial infarction.

Nitroglycerin may lose potency on storage; patients should be advised not to keep tablets longer than 3 to 4 months after opening the bottle, and if pain is not relieved and usual side effects are not experienced.

Prophylactic use of nitroglycerin is of particular value in patients who have angina in response to specific and reproducible stress, despite other therapies. It is important to teach the patient to use sublingual nitroglycerin correctly. The patient should cease the activity that caused angina, take sublingual nitroglycerin, and sit down to avoid the possible untoward effects of hypotension (increased in the standing position). The most common side effects are flushing and headache, both of which may diminish with increasing usage of the drug. Constant serum levels of nitrate predispose to the development of tolerance [62]. It appears that a 12- to 14-hour nitrate-free interval is needed for the drug to exercise its maximal effect [63]. Therefore, patients who develop increasing angina while using the transdermal patch may benefit by changing to an oral nitrate regimen or by removing the patch at night [47]. The side effects of all long-acting nitrates are similar to those produced by sublingual nitrates. Many patients have already experienced the headaches produced by sublingual nitroglycerin before being treated with a long-acting preparation. Phosphodiesterase type 5 inhibitors (ie, sildenafil, vardenafil, and tadalafil) and nitrates should not be used within 24 hours of one another because of the potential for serious hypotension [52]. Nitrates may increase oxidative stress and induce paradoxical vasoconstriction [64].

β-Blockers

In many respects B-blockade is an ideal approach to the treatment of angina. B-blockers reduce oxygen consumption by lowering heart rate, myocardial contractility, and systemic blood pressure. An added benefit for patients who have ischemic heart disease is that b blockade reduces the incidence of arrhythmias. The dosage of a b-blocker can be increased rapidly over hours or days until the desired effect is obtained. The heart rate is a useful guide to treatment; sinus bradycardia at a rate at rest between 50 and 60 beats per minute is a reasonable goal. However, the ideal dosage is one that not only results in mild sinus bradycardia at rest but also blocks an increase in heart rate with exercise. The dosage necessary to produce this effect and that necessary to relieve angina pectoris may vary considerably. Side effects of B-blockers have been overemphasized in recommending treatment of angina pectoris [65]. Erectile dysfunction occurs in 1% or less of the susceptible population. Asthma is still a relative contraindication, and selective b1 antagonists should be used. Patients who have chronic obstructive pulmonary disease or peripheral vascular disease commonly have no difficulties tolerating B-blockers.

Calcium Channel Blockers

Calcium channel blockers (CCB) dilate coronary and systemic arteries, reducing oxygen consumption and increasing coronary blood flow. They are indicated in the treatment of both stable and unstable angina and are also effective antihypertensive agents. Although there was early concern about short-acting calcium channel blockers [66], recent trials demonstrate no increased morbidity or mortality in patients receiving long-acting CCBs [67,68] for hypertension. The CCBs approved by the US Food and

Drug Administration for use in patients who have angina pectoris are amlodipine, diltiazem, nicardipine, long-acting nifedipine, and verapamil. The common side effects of the dihydropyridine calcium channel blockers (amlodipine, nicardipine, and nifedipine) are dizziness, flushing, headache, nausea, diarrhea, and, because of systemic vasodilation, peripheral edema. The major adverse effect is severe hypotension, which, in association with a reflex tachycardia, can actually intensify myocardial ischemia in some patients. Amlodipine is safe in patients who have left ventricular dysfunction. It only rarely affects AV conduction. Verapamil is prescribed more commonly for the treatment of hypertension or arrhythmias but is an effective antianginal. However, it has a more potent negative inotropic effect than other calcium channel blockers and significantly retards AV conduction. Therefore, it should not be used in patients who have compromised left ventricular function or with sinus bradycardia, sick sinus syndrome, or AV block. Diltiazem also significantly retards AV conduction, but it has less of a negative inotropic effect than verapamil and, in contrast to the dihydropyridines, is unlikely to cause hypotension or other vasodilatory side effects (eg, flushing, headache, edema).

Combination Therapy

None of the antianginal classes has been demonstrated to be significantly better in head-to-head trials. Combination therapy is often an underused strategy [24,57]. Some combinations (eg, β-blockers plus verapamil or possibly diltiazem) should be avoided because of concern about bradycardia. There are no data on the combinations of all three classes. In the initial evaluation of patients who have angina, cardiac catheterization may be recommended before reaching this level (catheter guidelines).

New Drugs with Novel Mechanisms of Action

Recently, new drugs based on novel mechanisms of action have emerged.[69]

Ranolazine

Ranolazine (approved recently by the US Food and Drug Administration) is a unique anti-ischaemic drug that does not significantly affect haemodynamic parameters.[70] It was originally believed to modify the use of substrate by the ischaemic myocardium from lipids to glucose, thereby increasing metabolic efficiency. However, recent studies suggest that it inhibits the late sodium current INA and the accumulation of intracellular sodium and congruent cellular calcium overload via the sodium/calcium exchanger. As opposed to treatment with calcium channel antagonists and B-blockers, the ranolazine-induced improvement in diastolic function occurs without a decrease in systolic function. Clinical studies of the anti-ischaemic effect of ranolazine monotherapy in patients with stable angina showed a significant increase in exercise duration and an improved 1 mm ST segment depression compared with atenolol. As an adjunct to standard doses of anti-ischaemia drugs (atenolol, amlodipine, diltiazem), ranolazine had an additional antianginal and anti-ischaemic effect, without causing significant haemodynamic changes. The ERICA study addressed the incremental benefit of adding ranolazine to maximal amlodipine regimen. Ranolazine significantly reduced the frequency of angina and glyceryl trinitrate (nitroglycerin) consumption compared with placebo. It also has another potentially favourable effect—namely, a dose-related reduction in haemoglobin A1C concentrations in diabetic patients. More comparative trials of ranolazine with other antianginal agents and studies of its effects on long-term morbidity and mortality are needed. So far, results indicate that ranolazine may serve as a useful alternative or adjunct to conventional antianginal treatment. Adverse effects include constipation, nausea, and dizziness. Postural hypotension due to a-adrenergic receptor blocking has also been reported. Increases in QT interval were observed but not associated torsade de points.

Trimetazidine

Trimetazidine is a pure metabolic agent that induces the myocardium to shift from free fatty acids to predominantly glucose utilisation in order to increase adenosine triphosphate (ATP) generation per unit oxygen consumption. Efficacy studies reported that trimetazidine reduced ischaemia during exercise stress tests, but there was no improvement in outcome. In a Cochrane meta-analysis of 23 studies including 1378 patients, trimetazidine was associated with a significant reduction in weekly angina episodes and improved exercise time to 1 mm ST segment depression compared to placebo.[71] In patients with stable angina who experienced concomitant erectile dysfunction, trimetazidine plus sildenafil was both safe and more effective in controlling episodes of ischaemia during sexual activity than nitrates alone. These data indicate that trimetazidine is safe and effective for the treatment of symptoms of stable angina, either as monotherapy or adjunctive treatment.

Nicorandil

Nicorandil exerts dual actions: it increases the opening of ATP gated K+ channels, thereby relaxing smooth muscle and contributing to coronary vasodilatation; and it has a nitratedonating moiety. Nicorandil may mimic the natural process of ischaemic preconditioning, which involves ATP-dependent potassium channels. Several small randomised trials of patients with stable angina have shown that nicorandil prolongs the time to onset of ST depression and exercise duration during stress testing and improves myocardial perfusion at rest and with exercise. In the IONA trial of 5126 patients, the administration of nicorandil in addition to standard treatments reduced the primary end point (coronary death, MI, or hospitalisation for angina) by 17% after a mean follow-up of 1.6 years. There was also a significant reduction in the incidence of acute coronary syndrome and all cardiovascular events.[72]

Ivabradine

Ivabradine inhibits the If channel in the sinus node, thereby causing bradycardia but without any negative inotropic effects. Double-blind trials showed that ivabradine treatment increased exercise time to 1 mm ST segment depression and limited angina compared to placebo, and had similar clinical effects to atenolol or amlodipine—namely, a two-third reduction in the number of anginal episodes and an increase in total exercise duration. Ivabradine offers clear therapeutic benefit for a whole range of patients with stable angina, including those with contraindication or intolerance to B-blockers; however, its effect on survival remains to be explored.[73]

Fasudil

Fasudil is an inhibitor of rho kinase, an intracellular signaling molecule involved in the vascular smooth muscle contractile response. In patients with stable angina, fasudil treatment led to a significantly greater time to >1 mm ST segment depression, but showed no difference from placebo in decreasing the time to angina, frequency of angina, or glyceryl trinitrate use.

Molsidomine

Molsidomine is a nitric oxide donating vasodilator. When compared with placebo, it reduced the incidence of anginal attacks and use of sublingual nitrates, and increased exercise capacity, in patients with stable angina. Higher doses provided better protection from angina, although hypotension was a side effect. These new drugs are not yet in routine clinical use; however, they may serve as useful alternatives or adjuncts to conventional antianginal treatment. Further studies and longer followup will determine their place in preventing death or MI.

Drugs to Prevent Myocardial Infarction and Death

There is considerable evidence that lifestyle changes and pharmacologic treatment may reduce the progression of atherosclerosis and stabilise plaque in patients with chronic stable angina. Therefore, risk factor modification should be the central component of management.[52] Suggested lifestyle changes include cessation of smoking, exercise and weight reduction, in addition to treatment of hypertension and glycaemic control in patients with diabetes. There are also numerous drugs available to improve prognosis by preventing MI and death. Aspirin at a dose of 75–325 mg per morbidity and mortality by 33% in patients with coronary artery disease. Most of the data, however day reduces cardiovascular, are derived from patients with acute coronary syndrome. Only one study reported a beneficial effect of aspirin in patients with chronic angina pectoris. Clopidogrel, a thienopyridine derivative, has been found to be more effective than aspirin in reducing cardiovascular events in patients with atherosclerotic vascular disease. However, a more recent study reported that clopidogrel combined with aspirin was not significantly more effective than aspirin alone in reducing the rate of MI, stroke, or death from cardiovascular causes in patients with stable cardiovascular disease or multiple cardiovascular risk factors.[74] Dipyridamole is often recommended as an adjunctive antiplatelet agent to aspirin in patients after a cerebrovascular event, but it can enhance exercise-induced myocardial ischaemia in patients with stable angina.

There is a plethora of evidence (which is beyond the scope of this review) to show that statins lower the rate of coronary events and mortality by 25–35% in patients with coronary artery disease.[75] Current guidelines recommend a target fasting low density lipoprotein cholesterol value of <100 mg/dl (< 2.59 mmol/l) in patients with stable angina. The most recent National Cholesterol Education Program directive (NCEP-ATP III) suggests a target of < 70 mg/dl (<1.81 mmol/l) for highrisk patients (those with diabetes, multivessel disease, multiple risk factors).

Two large clinical trials (EUROPA, HOPE) found angiotensin-converting enzyme (ACE) inhibitors effective in reducing morbidity and mortality in high-risk patients with cardiovascular disease. However, the PEACE trial failed to find a statistically significant reduction in clinical cardiovascular events. This discrepancy may be due to inclusion of a low-risk patient population in the PEACE trial. More recently, studies reported a consistent benefit of ACE inhibitors in high-, intermediate- and low-risk patients.[76] Omapatrilat, an ACE inhibitor and neutral endopeptidase, prolonged total exercise duration, time to onset of angina, and time to onset of ischaemic ST segment changes compared with placebo.

Those vasculoprotective drugs are essential in the treatment of patients with stable angina—every patient should receive an antiplatelet agent and a statin, and probably an ACE inhibitor as well. The European Society of Cardiology guidelines [77] recommend ACE inhibitors for patients with a co-existing history of MI, hypertension, left ventricular dysfunction, diabetes, or impaired renal function.

Pharmacotherapy of Unstable Angina

Medical therapy of unstable angina consists of antithrombotic and anti-ischemic agents. Antithrombotic agents include antiplatelet agents such as aspirin [84,85], thienopyridine derivatives [86,87], and glycoprotein IIbIIIa inhibitors [88]; anticoagulants such as heparin [89,90]; and direct thrombin inhibitors (hirudin and bivalirudin) [91].

Invasive versus Conservative Approach for Unstable Angina

Treating patients who have unstable angina involves one of two approaches: early invasive management, which consists of inpatient coronary angiography followed by percutaneous or surgical revascularization, and early conservative management, which consists of medical therapy followed by noninvasive stress testing [92].

Surgical Revascularisaton

Pharmacotherapy vs Revascularisation

Two meta-analyses of randomised trials comparing the efficacy of percutaneous coronary intervention (PCI) and medical treatment in patients with stable angina found similar MI and mortality rates in the two groups, though the patients undergoing PCI were less likely to have angina and more likely to require coronary artery bypass grafting (CABG).[78,79] The rates of subsequent revascularisation were similar as well. The authors concluded that PCI should be reserved for patients in whom symptoms are poorly controlled by medical treatment. The results of the ACIP trial indicate that patients who are asymptomatic or have minimal symptoms but demonstrable ischaemia may have a better outcome (lower mortality and MI) with revascularisation with either CABG or PCI compared with those managed medically. However, there are a number of important limitations in applying these results to current clinical practice. First, the patients tested represented only a small percentage of the total number screened and were not reflective of the general population. Second, most of the studies were conducted when the use of saphenous vein grafts rather than internal mammary artery grafts was prevalent. Third, the patients who underwent PCI did not receive the current antithrombotic regimens or drug-eluting stents that notably reduced the rate of restenosis and, therefore, revascularisation. Revascularisation with CABG was found to improve survival compared to medical management in selected patients with stable angina: patients with left main or three-vessel coronary disease; patients with two-vessel disease and significant lesions in the proximal left anterior descending artery; and patients with multivessel disease in the presence of left ventricular dysfunction or diabetes.

PCI vs CABG

A number of large randomised trials in the 1990s directly compared CABG with PCI. Their major finding was that survival was similar for the two modes of management, although PCI was associated with more repeated interventions. One important exception was patients with insulin-requiring diabetes, who had a significantly higher five year survival rate after CABG than after PCI (BARI trial). An observational analysis using a database of more 59 000 patients also showed a survival advantage for CABG in patients with left main triplevessel disease with proximal left anterior descending artery involvement.

It should be noted that similar to comparisons of PCI and pharmacotherapy, the early trials did not use stents or internal mammary artery grafts. These limitations were overcome in the ARTS I and SoS randomised trials comparing CABG with mostly arterial grafts to PCI with stent implantation. Outcomes were similar in the two groups, except for a much higher rate of target vessel revascularisation with PCI. The ARTS II registry indicated that the solution may lie in the use of drug-eluting stents. The rate of major adverse cardiac and cerebrovascular events in this study was similar to that of the CABG arm in the ARTS I trial and significantly lower than that of the PCI with bare metal stent arm. After adjusting for risk factors, the authors noted a lower rate of major cardiovascular and cerebrovascular events in the PCI arm of ARTS II than in the CABG arm of ARTS I. However, treatment assignment was not random.

Most of the patients included in these randomised trials were relatively low risk—fewer than 20% had left ventricular dysfunction and almost 70% had one- or two-vessel disease—and therefore were compatible with the patient group from whom CABG had not been found to be superior to PCI therapy.

CABG has an advantage over PCI, which does not detect unstable plaques or the lesions most likely to be the cause of subsequent cardiac events. The National Heart, Lung, and

Blood Institute Dynamic Registry reported that approximately 6% of patients after PCI have clinical plaque progression requiring non-target lesion repeat PCI by one year. A greater coronary artery disease burden confers a significantly higher risk of clinical plaque progression. Furthermore, PCI carries a risk of subacute and late stent thrombosis and a need for prolonged anti-aggregation treatment. A recent trial comparing PCI with CABG in patients with multivessel disease (ERACI III) reported a higher rate than expected of stent thrombosis (3.1% in 18 months). These data indicate that both revascularisation techniques are appropriate and comparable in outcome, except in patients with left main, three-vessel disease and in diabetics in whom CABG is currently preferred.

Other Treatments for Patients with Refractory Angina

Despite the increasing success of conventional medical treatment and the continued development and improvement of mechanical revascularisation approaches, a significant number of patients (5–10%) continue to have severe angina. For the many who are not candidates for revascularisation, there are currently several options.[80–82]

Enhanced External Balloon Counterpulsation (EECP)

EECP increases arterial blood pressure and retrograde aortic blood flow during diastole. Cuffs are wrapped around the patient's legs, and the compressed air applies sequential pressure (300 mm Hg) from the lower legs to lower and upper thighs in early diastole. The mechanisms underlying the benefits of this procedure in patients with angina are not clear, but may involve non-specific placebo effects and various haemodynamic factors that improve endothelial function and the release of growth factors which promote the formation of collaterals in the coronary circulation. This technique is contraindicated in patients with aortic regurgitation or peripheral vascular disease. In the MUST-EECP trial, patients undergoing active EECP showed a significant increase in time to >1 mm ST segment depression and a decrease in anginal episodes compared to the inactive group. Similar findings were noted in an analysis of multicentre registries. One recent study in patients with stable angina did not find a significant effect of EECP on myocardial perfusion. Although EECP is a valuable outpatient procedure, most of the studies conducted so far were small and uncontrolled. Therefore, EECP therapy should be limited at present to patients with debilitating angina who are not candidates for revascularisation and who remain symptomatic even with maximal antianginal pharmacotherapy.

Spinal Cord Stimulation

Spinal cord stimulation (SCS) is performed by placing a lead in the epidural space at the level of C7 through T1 and surgically implanting a pacemaker-sized generator in the left lower abdominal area. Patients receive 1 h of stimulation a day and can activate the device with a handled magnet to treat breakthrough pain. The beneficial effects of the technique on angina are explained by its suppression of the capacity of intrinsic cardiac neurons to generate activity during myocardial ischaemia, or its resolution of sympathetic activity, leading to improved myocardial blood flow. In patients with refractory angina, SCS increases the time to onset of ST segment depression and increases exercise capacity, thereby reducing the number of anginal attacks and the use of glyceryl trinitrate. The main reported adverse reactions were epidural haematoma and infection, occurring in about 1% of patients. In addition, SCS may interfere with the function of pacemakers and implantable defibrillators. So far, clinical trials have included only small samples, and none had a sham-controlled arm to prevent a placebo effect.

Laser Revascularisation

This technique involves the use of laser ablation to create transmural channels in the ischaemic myocardium in order to restore myocardial perfusion. It can be performed surgically, known as transmyocardial laser revascularisation (TMR), or percutaneously, known as percutaneous laser revascularisation (PMR). The mechanism whereby it alleviates anginal symptoms is unknown. Though the clinical improvement was originally attributed to better myocardial perfusion through open channels, more recent studies have shown that the channels fill with necrotic debris and close shortly after the procedure. Other proposed mechanisms include angiogenesis through the release of growth factors and denervation of pain fibres by laser.

Investigations of the use of TMR for refractory angina revealed an improvement in symptoms and exertion tolerance, but not in myocardial perfusion or mortality rate. In a study of 298 patients with refractory angina randomised to receive PMR or a sham procedure, no between-group differences were noted in exercise duration, exercise time to onset of chest pain, exercise time to the appearance of ST segment changes, or myocardial perfusion. Moreover, the laser treatment was associated with an increased rate of adverse clinical events at 30 days.[83] Two smaller randomised trials found similar results. The only sham-controlled trial to show benefit was conducted by Salem and colleagues, wherein more patients in the PMR group had a decrease of two or more anginal classes. Therefore, we conclude that PMR is not effective for the treatment of chronic angina. The benefit reported for TMR may be due to a placebo effect.

The SpiRiT trial randomised patients with refractory angina to SCS or PMR. There were no differences in angina-free exercise capacity, angina class, and quality of life between treatments. The patients receiving SCS had more adverse events in the first 12 months, mainly angina or SCS-system related.

Percutaneous in Situ Coronary Venous Arterialisation

Percutaneous in situ coronary venous arterialisation (PICVA) redirects arterial blood flow from the occluded artery into an adjacent coronary vein, thereby arterialising the vein and providing retroperfusion to the ischaemic myocardium.

Percutaneous in situ coronary artery bypass (PICAB) redirects the arterial blood flow from a diseased artery to an adjacent coronary vein, and then back to the artery after the lesion is bypassed. PICVA and PICAB hold enormous therapeutic potential for patients whose anatomic findings are incompatible with traditional revascularisation procedures. However, they must still be considered experimental owing to their high procedural complication rate.

Therapeutic Myocardial Angiogenesis with Growth Factors, Gene and Cell Therapy

The dearth of effective treatment strategies for "no option" patients, together with progress achieved in understanding the complex mechanisms inherent in the development of new blood vessels, has facilitated a new treatment strategy commonly termed therapeutic myocardial angiogenesis. Postembryonic angiogenic mechanisms involve growth factors—the most important are vascular endothelial growth factor (VEGF) and basic fibroblast growth factor (FGF). Because of this, supporters of therapeutic angiogenesis advocate the administration of angiogenic growth factor protein or gene packaged in either a plasmid or an adenovirus to promote the development of endogenous collateral vessels in ischaemic myocardium. The delivery strategy includes transcatheter delivery via an intracoronary route, direct intraoperative intramyocardial injection, and catheter-based transendocardial injection, all of which may be incorporated with a magnetic guidance catheter-based navigational system that can distinguish between healthy and infarcted myocardium. All trials so far of FGF or VEGF with a placebo-controlled arm have produced negative results in terms of symptomatic relief or improving myocardial perfusion.

Autologous stem cell transplantation from bone marrow or peripheral blood has recently emerged as a promising therapeutic approach for ischaemic cardiomyopathy syndromes. Clinical studies indicated improvements in myocardial perfusion and function, although most investigated the use of this technique in the acute phase after MI. Small studies of intramyocardial, transepicardial or intracoronary injection of unselected mononuclear bone marrow cells in patients with coronary artery disease not amenable to conventional revascularisation techniques yielded improvements in anginal symptoms, exercise capacity, regional tissue perfusion and left ventricular systolic function.

Conclusion

Angina pectoris is a clinical manifestation of myocardial ischemia. Complete evaluation consists of a review of risk factors, a careful history, and, typically, a provocative test (Figure 4). Patients who have high-risk features found by clinical history or by stress testing should be referred for coronary angiography and possible revascularization.

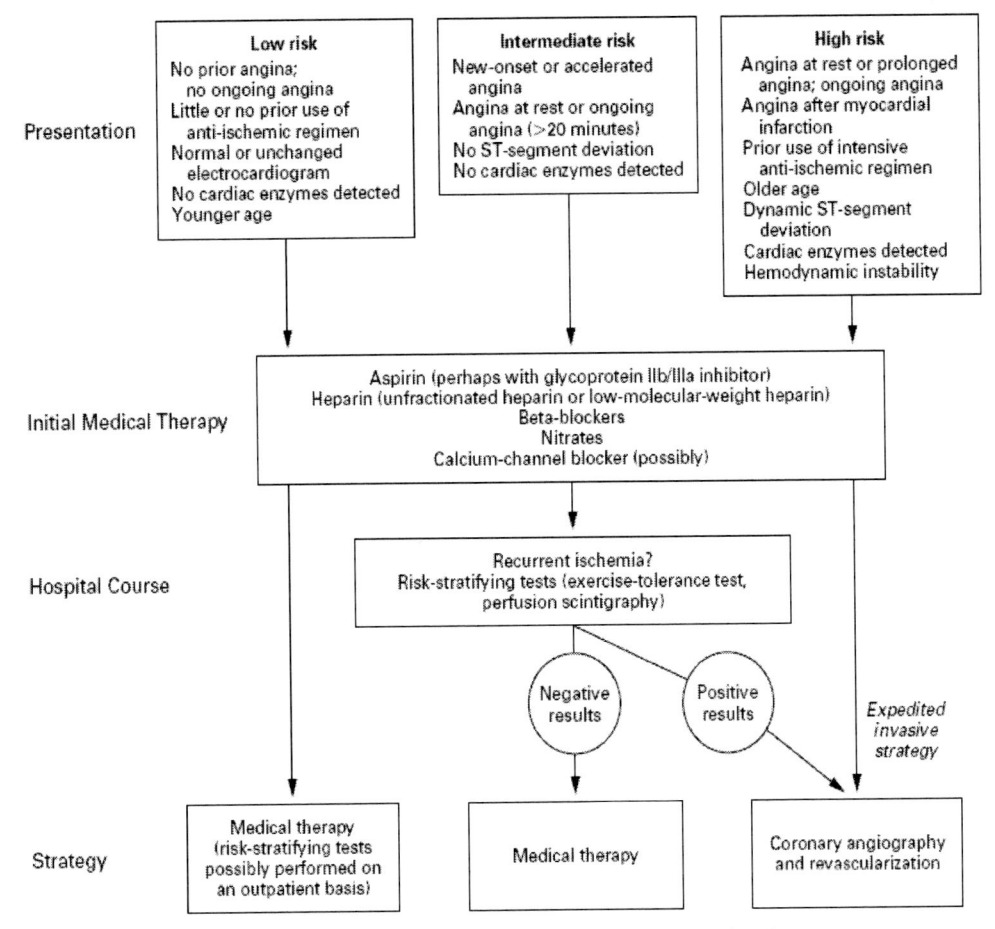

From YEREM Y EGHIAZARIANS etal N Engl J Med Volume 342 Number 2

Figure 4. Treatment Strategy for Patients Who Present with Angina pectoris.

However, none included a randomised control group. The idea of improving myocardial perfusion by bone marrow cell injection is intriguing, and prospective large, randomised clinical trials are warranted.

Symptoms of chronic stable angina can usually be managed with optimum doses of one of the available antianginal drugs alone or in combination. (Figure5) To slow the progression of atherosclerosis and reduce the incidence of MI and death, lifestyle modifications (smoking cessation, exercise, diet) together with pharmacologic treatment with aspirin, statins or ACE inhibitors are necessary. Several new drugs with a different mechanism of action provide new treatment options, though their precise indications, long-term impact and target population require further study. Patients who remain symptomatic despitemedical treatment and patients with high-risk anatomy should be considered for revascularisation. Revascularisation should be viewed as complementary to aggressive medical treatment, rather than as an opposing strategy. Selected patients who do not respond to medical treatment and are not candidates for revascularisation may be considered for treatment with neurostimulation and EECP. The use of laser revascularisation has decreased because of its invasiveness and concerns that the promising results may be due to a placebo effect. Angiogenic gene therapy and myocardial cell therapy via multiple routes are being investigated to enhance local myocardial perfusion and function.

Therapeutic opportunities for angina pectoris

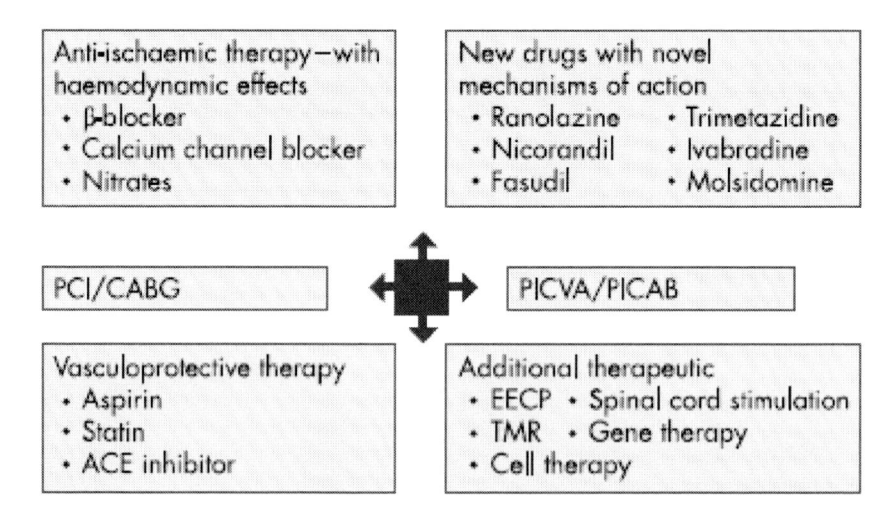

From Itsik Ben-Dor and Alexander Battler *Heart* 2007;93;868-874

Figure 5. Different modalities of treatment of stable angina. ACE,angiotensin-converting enzyme; CABG, coronary artery bypass grafting;EECP, enhanced external counter pulsation; PCAB, percutaneous in situ coronary artery bypass; PCVA, percutaneous in situ coronary venous arterialisation; PCI, percutaneous coronary intervention; TMR, transmyocardial laser revascularization.

References

[1]   Braunwald E. Unstable angina: a classification. *Circulation*. 1989;80: 410–414.
[2]   Theroux P, Fuster V. Acute coronary syndromes: unstable angina and non–Q-wave myocardial infarction. *Circulation*. 1998;97:1195–1206.
[3]   Sherman CT, Litvack F, Grundfest W, Lee M, Hickey A, Chaux A, Kass R, Blanche C, Matloff J, Morgenstern L, Ganz W, Swan HJC, Forrester J. Coronary angioscopy in patients with unstable angina pectoris. *N .Engl. J. Med.* 1986;315:913–919.
[4]   Ambrose JA, Winters SL, Arora R, Eng A, Riccio A, Gorlin R, Fuster V. Angiographic evolution of coronary artery morphology in unstable angina. *J. Am. Coll. Cardiol.* 1986;7:472– 478.
[5]   Hirsh PD, Hillis LD, Campbell WB, Firth BG, Willerson JT. Release of prostaglandins and thromboxane into the coronary circulation in patients with ischemic heart disease. *N. Engl. J. Med.* 1981;304:685– 691.
[6]   Merlini PA, Bauer KA, Oltrona L, Ardissino D, Cattaneo M, Belli C, Mannucci, PM, Rosenberg RD. Persistent activation of coagulation mechanism in unstable angina and myocardial infarction. *Circulation*. 1994;90:61– 68.

[7]   Theroux P, Ouimet H, McCans J, Latour JG, Joly P, Levy G, Pelletier E, Juneau M, Stasiak J, de Guise P, Pelletier GB, Rinzler D, Waters DD. Aspirin, heparin, or both to treat acute unstable angina. *N. Engl. J. Med.* 1988;319:1105–1111.

[8]   Cohen M, Demers C, Gurfinkel EP, Turpie AG, Fromell GJ, Goodman S, Langer A, Califf RM, Fox KA, Premmereur J, Bigonzi J. A comparison of low-molecular-weight heparin with unfractionated heparin for unstable coronary artery disease: the ESSENCE trial. *N. Engl. J. Med.* 1997;337: 447–452.

[9]   Balsano F, Rizzon P, Violi F, Scrutinio D, Cimminiello C, Aguglia F, Pasotti C, Rudelli G, the Studio della Ticlopidina nell'Angina Instabile Group. Antiplatelet treatment with ticlopidine in unstable angina: a controlled, multicenter clinical trial. *Circulation.* 1990;82:17–26.

[10] Braunwald E, Maseri A, Armstrong PW, Califf RM, Gibler WB, Hamm CW, Simoons ML, van de Werf F. Rationale and clinical evidence for the use of GP IIb/IIIa inhibitors in acute coronary syndromes. *Am. Heart J.* 1998;135:S56 –S66.

[11] Maseri A. Unstable angina. In: *Ischemic Heart Disease.* New York, NY:Churchill Livingstone; 1995:533–557.

[12] Epstein SE, Cannon RO III. Site of increased resistance to coronary flow in patients with angina pectoris and normal epicardial coronary arteries. *J. Am. Coll. Cardiol.* 1986;8:459–461.

[13] Diver DJ, Bier JD, Ferreira PE, Sharaf BL, McCabe C, Thompson B, Chaitman B, Williams DO, Braunwald E. Clinical and arteriographic characterization of patients with unstable angina without critical coronary arterial narrowing. *Am. J. Cardiol.* 1994;74:531–537.

[14] Kaski JC, Chester MR, Chen L, Katritsis D. Rapid angiographic progression of coronary artery disease in patients with angina pectoris: the role of complex stenosis morphology. *Circulation.* 1995;92:2058 –2065.

[15] Mehta JL, Saldeen TGP, Rand K. Interactive role of infection, inflammation and traditional risk factors in atherosclerosis and coronary artery disease. *J. Am. Coll Cardiol.* 1998;31:1217–1225.

[16] van der Wal AC, Becker AE, van der Loos CM, Das PK. Site of intimal rupture or erosion of thrombosed coronary atherosclerotic plaques is characterized by an inflammatory process irrespective of the dominant plaque morphology. *Circulation.* 1994;89:36–44.

[17] Liuzzo G, Biasucci LM, Gallimore JR, Grillo RL, Rebuzzi AG, Pepys MB, Maseri A. The prognostic value of C-reactive protein and serum amyloid A protein in severe unstable angina. *N. Engl. J. Med.* 1994;331: 417–424.

[18] Morrow DA, Rifai N, Antman EM, Weiner DL, McCabe CH, Cannon CP, Braunwald E. C-reactive protein is a potent predictor of mortality independently and in combination with troponin T in acute coronary syndromes. *J. Am. Coll. Cardiol.* 1998;31:1460 –1465.

[19] Ridker PM. Inflammation, infection, and cardiovascular risk: how good is the clinical evidence? *Circulation.* 1998;97:1671–1674.

[20] Pasceri V, Cammarota G, Patti G, Cuoco L, Gasbarrani A, Grillo RL, Fedeli G, Gasbarrini G, Maseri A. Association of virulent *Helicobacter pylori* strains with ischemic heart disease. *Circulation*. 1998;97: 1675–1679.

[21] Leibovitz E, Hertz Y, Liberman E, Sclarovsky S, Berliner S. Increased adhesiveness of white blood cells in patients with unstable angina: additional evidence for an involvement of the immune-inflammatory system. *Clin. Cardiol*. 1997;20:1017–1019.

[22] Gurfinkel E, Bozovich G, Daroca A, Beck E, Mautner B. Randomised trial of roxithromycin in non-Q-wave coronary syndromes: ROXIS Pilot Study. *Lancet*. 1997;350:404–407.

[23] Gupta S, Leatham EW, Carrington D, Mendall MA, Kaski JC, Camm AJ. Elevated *Chlamydia pneumoniae* antibodies, cardiovascular events, and azithromycin in male survivors of acute myocardial infarction. *Circulation*. 1997;96:404–407.

[24] Gibbons RJ, Abrams J, Chatterjee K, et al. ACC/AHA/ACP-ASIM guidelines for the management of patients with chronic stable angina: a report of the American College of Cardiology/ American Heart Association Task Force on Practice Guidelines (Committee on Management of Patients With Chronic Stable Angina). *J. Am. Coll. Cardiol* .1999;33(7):2092–197.

[25] Grundy SM. Primary prevention of coronary heart disease: integrating risk assessment with intervention. *Circulation* 1999;100(9):988–98.

[26] Grundy SM. Coronary calcium as a risk factor: role in global risk assessment. *J. Am.Coll .Cardiol* .2001;37(6):1512–5.

[27] Fuster V, Pearson TA, Co-Chairs. 27th Bethesda conference: matching the intensity of risk factor management with the hazard for coronary disease events. *J. Am. Coll. Cardiol*. 1996; 27(5):957–1047.

[28] National Cholesterol Education Program (NCEP) Expert Panel on High Blood Cholesterol. Detection, evaluation, and treatment of high blood cholesterol in adults: adult treatment panel III [third report]. Washington, DC: National Heart, Lung and Blood Institute; 2001. Bethesda (MD), NIH Publication #01–3670.Available at:http://www.nhlbi.nih.gov/guidelines/cholesterol/index.htm. Accessed January 3, 2006.

[29] Boden WE. High-density lipoprotein cholesterol as an independent risk factor in cardiovascular disease: assessing the data from Framingham to the Veterans Affairs high-density lipoprotein intervention trial. *Am. J. Cardiol*. 2000;86(12, Suppl 1):19–22.

[30] O'Rourke RA, et al. American College of Cardiology/American Heart Association expert consensus document on electron-beamcomputed tomography for the diagnosis and prognosis of coronary artery disease. *J. Am. Coll. Cardiol*. 2000;36(1):326–40.

[31] Sandler G. The importance of the history in the medical clinic and the cost of unnecessary tests. *Am. Heart J*. 1980;100:980.

[32] Campeau L. Grading of angina pectoris [letter]. Circulation 1976;54(3):522–3.

[33] Zouridakis E, et al. Markers of inflammation and rapid coronary artery disease progression in patients with stable angina pectoris. *Circulation* 2004;110:1747–53.

[34] Kragelund C, et al. N-Terminal pro-B-type natriuretic peptide and long-term mortality in stable coronary heart disease. *N. Engl. J. Med*. 2005;352(7):666–75.

[35] Gibbons RJ, et al. ACC/AHA guidelines for exercise testing: a report of the American College of Cardiology/American Heart Association Task Force on Practice Guidelines (Committee on Exercise Testing). *J. Am. Coll. Cardiol.* 1997;30(1):260–311.

[36] Lee TH, Boucher CA. Noninvasive tests in patients with stable coronary artery disease. *N .Engl .J. Med.* 2001;344(24):1840–5.

[37] Hlatky M, Mark D. Economics and cardiovascular disease, in heart disease: a textbook of cardiovascular medicine. 6th edition. Philadelphia: WB Saunders; 2001. p. 19–26.

[38] Beller G. Relative merits of cardiovascular diagnostic techniques. In: Braunwald E, Zipes DP, Libby P, editors. Heart disease: a textbook of cardiovascular medicine. 6th edition. Philadelphia: WB Saunders; 2001. p. 422–41.

[39] Wackers F. SPECT detection of coronary artery disease. In: Narula VDaJ, editor. Atlas of nuclear cardiology. Philadelphia: *Current Medicine*; 2003. p. 63–77.

[40] Gianrossi R, Detrano R, Mulvihill D, et al. Exercise-induced ST depression in the diagnosis of coronary artery disease. A meta-analysis. *Circulation* 1989;80:87–98.

[41] Ritchie JL, et al. Guidelines for clinical use of cardiac radionuclide imaging: report of the American College of Cardiology/American Heart Association Task Force on Assessment of Diagnostic and Therapeutic Cardiovascular Procedures (Committee on Radionuclide Imaging), developed in collaboration with the American Society of Nuclear Cardiology. *J. Am. Coll. Cardiol.* 1995;25(2):521–47.

[42] Brown KA. Prognostic value of thallium-201 myocardial perfusion imaging: a diagnostic tool comes of age. *Circulation* 1991;83(2):363–81.

[43] Dilsizian V. SPECT and PET techniques. In: Narula VDaJ, editor. Atlas of nuclear cardiology. Philadelphia: *Current Medicine*; 2003. p. 19–46.

[44] Schelbert HR. Measurements of myocardial metabolism in patients with ischemic heart disease. *Am. J. Cardiol.* 1998;82(Suppl 1):K61–7.

[45] Raggi P, et al. Identification of patients at increased risk of first unheralded acute myocardial infarction by electron-beam computed tomography. *Circulation* 2000;101(8):850–5.

[46] Guerci AD, et al. Comparison of electron beam computed tomography scanning and conventional risk factor assessment for the prediction of angiographic coronary artery disease. *J. Am. Coll. Cardiol.* 1998;32(3):673–9.

[47] White C, Kuo O, Kelemen MD, et al. Chest pain evaluation in the emergency room: can multi-detector CT provide a comprehensive evaluation? *AJR Am. J. Roentgenol.* 2005;185:533–40.

[48] Mathejssen N, et al. Comparison of ultrafast dipyridamole magnetic resonance imaging with dipyridamole sestamibi SPECTfor detection of perfusion abnormalities in patients with onevessel coronary artery disease: assessment by quantitative model fitting. *Magn. Reson. Med.* 1996;35:221.

[49] Nagel E, et al. Noninvasive diagnosis of ischemia-induced wall motion abnormalities with the use of high-dose dobutamine stress MRI: comparison with dobutamine stress echocardiography. *Circulation* 1999;99:763.

[50] Scanlon PJ, et al. ACC/AHA guidelines for coronary angiography: a report of the American College of Cardiology/American Heart Association Task Force on practice guidelines (Committee on Coronary Angiography), developed in collaboration with the

Society for Cardiac Angiography and Interventions. *J. Am. Coll. Cardiol.* 1999;33(6):1756–824.

[51] Noto TJ Jr, et al. Cardiac catheterization 1990: a report of the Registry of the Society for Cardiac Angiography and Interventions. *Cathet. Cardiovasc. Diagn.* 1991;24(2):75–83.

[52] Abrams J. Chronic stable angina. *N. Engl. J. Med.* 2005;352(24):2524–33.

[53] Hoffman SN, et al. A meta-analysis of randomized controlled trials comparing coronary artery bypass graft with percutaneous transluminal coronary angioplasty: one- to eight-year outcomes. *J. Am. Coll. Cardiol.* 2003;41(8):1293–304.

[54] Hannan EL, et al. Long-term outcomes of coronary-artery bypass grafting versus stent implantation. *N .Engl. J. Med.* 2005;352(21):2174–83.

[55] Al Suwaidi J, et al. Impact of coronary artery stents on mortality and nonfatal myocardial infarction: meta-analysis of randomized trials comparing a strategy of routine stenting with that of balloon angioplasty. *Am. Heart J.* 2004;147:815–22.

[56] Weiner DA, Ryan TJ, McCabe CH, et al. Prognostic importance of a clinical profile and exercise test in medically treated patients with coronary artery disease. *J.Am.Coll. Cardiol.* 1984; 3:772–9.

[57] Thadani U. Treatment of stable angina. Curr Opin Cardiol 1999;14:349–58.

[58] Heidenreich PA, et al. Meta-analysis of trials comparing [beta]-blockers, calcium antagonists, and nitrates for stable angina. *JAMA* 1999;281(20):1927–36.

[59] Heart Outcomes Prevention Evaluation Study Investigators. Effects of an angiotensinconverting- enzyme inhibitor, ramipril, on cardiovascular events in high-risk patients. *N. Engl. J. Med.* 2000;342(3):145–53

[60] Nissen SE, et al. Effect of intensive compared with moderate lipid-lowering therapy on progression of coronary atherosclerosis: a randomized controlled trial. *JAMA* 2004;291(9): 1071–80.

[61] Cannon CP, et al. Intensive versus moderate lipid lowering with statins after acute coronary syndromes. *N. Engl .J. Med.* 2004;350(15):1495–504.

[62] Gori T, Parker J. The puzzle of nitrate tolerance: pieces smaller than we thought? *Circulation* 2002;106:2404–8.

[63] Gori T, Parker J. Nitrate tolerance: a unifying hypothesis. *Circulation* 2002;106:2510–3.

[64] Munzel T, et al. Evidence for enhanced vascular superoxide anion production in nitrate tolerance: a novel mechanism underlying tolerance and cross-tolerance. *J. Clin. Invest.* 1995;95: 187–94.

[65] Ko DT, et al. [beta]-Blocker therapy and symptoms of depression, fatigue, and sexual dysfunction. *JAMA* 2002;288(3):351–7.

[66] Chaitman BR, et al. Anti-ischemic effects and long-term survival during ranolazine monotherapy in patients with chronic severe angina. *J. Am. Coll. Cardiol.* 2004;43(8): 1375–82.

[67] Blood Pressure Lowering Treatment Trialists. Effects of different blood-pressure-lowering regimens on major cardiovascular events: results of prospectively-designed overviews of randomised trials. *Lancet* 2003;362(9395):1527–35.

[68] The ALLHAT Officers and Coordinators for the ALLHAT Collaborative Research Group. Major Outcomes in high-risk hypertensive patients randomized to angiotensin-converting enzyme inhibitor or calcium channel blocker vs diuretic: the Antihypertensive and Lipid- Lowering Treatment to Prevent Heart Attack trial (ALLHAT). *JAMA* 2002;288(23): 2981–97.

[69] Chaitman BR. Pharmacological approaches to the symptomatic treatment of chronic stable angina: a historical perspective and future directions. *Can. J. Cardiol.* 2005;21:1031–4.

[70] Siddiqui MA, Keam SJ. Ranolazine: a review of its use in chronic stable angina pectoris. *Drugs* 2006;66:693–710.

[71] Ciapponi A, Pizarro R, Harrison J. Trimetazidine for stable angina. Cochrane Database *Syst. Rev.* 2005;19:CD003614.

[72] IONA Study Group. Effect of nicorandil on coronary events in patients with stable angina: the impact of nicorandil in angina (IONA) randomised trial. *Lancet* 2002;359:1269–75.

[73] Borer JS. Therapeutic effects of I(f) blockade: evidence and perspective. *Pharmacol. Res.* 2006;53:440–5.

[74] Bhatt DL, Fox KA, Hacke W, et al. Clopidogrel and aspirin versus aspirin alone for the prevention of atherothrombotic events. *N Engl J Med* 2006;354:1706–17.

[75] Opie LH, Commerford PJ, Gersh BJ. Controversies in stable coronary artery disease. *Lancet* 2006;367:69–7.

[76] Deckers JW, Goedhart DM, Boersma E, et al. Treatment benefit by *perindopril in patients with stable coronary artery disease at different levels of risk. Eur. Heart. J.* 2006;27:796–801.

[77] Fox K, Garcia MA, Ardissino D, et al. Guidelines on the management of stable angina pectoris: executive summary: The Task Force on the Management of Stable Angina Pectoris of the European Society of Cardiology. *Eur. Heart J.* 2006;27:1341–81.

[78] Bucher HC, Hengstler P, Schindler C, et al. Percutaneous transluminal coronary angioplasty versus medical treatment for non-acute coronary heart disease: meta-analysis of randomised controlled trials. *BMJ* 2000;321:73–7.

[79] Katritsis DG, Ioannidis JP. Percutaneous coronary intervention versus conservative therapy in nonacute coronary artery disease: a meta-analysis. *Circulation* 2005;111:2906–12.

[80] Yang EH, Barsness GW, Gersh BJ, et al. Current and future treatment strategies for refractory angina. *Mayo. Clin. Proc.* 2004;79:1284–92.

[81] Kim MC, Kini A, Sharma SK. Refractory angina pectoris: mechanism and therapeutic options. *J Am Coll Cardiol* 2002;39:923–34.

[82] DeJongste MJ, Tio RA, Foreman RD. Chronic therapeutically refractory angina pectoris. *Heart* 2004;90:225–30.

[83] Leon MB, Kornowski R, Downey WE, et al. A blinded, randomized, placebocontrolled trial of percutaneous laser myocardial revascularization to improve angina symptoms in patients with severe coronary disease. *J. Am. Coll .Cardiol .*2005;46:1812–9.

[84] LewisHDJr, Davis JW, Archibald DG, et al. Protective effects of aspirin against acute myocardial infarction and death in men with unstable angina: results of a Veterans Administration Cooperative Study. *N Engl J Med* 1983;309:396–403

[85] Cairns JA, Gent M, Singer J, et al. Aspirin, sulfinpyrazone, or both in unstable angina. Results of a Canadian multicenter trial. *N. Engl.J. Med.* 1985;313:1369–75.

[86] Love BB, Biller J, Gent M. Adverse haematological effects of ticlopidine: prevention, recognition and management. *Drug Saf.* 1998;19:89–98.

[87] Yusuf S, Zhao F, Mehta SR, et al. Clopidogrel in Unstable Angina to Prevent Recurrent Events Trial Investigators. Effects of clopidogrel in addition to aspirin in patients with acute coronary syndromes without ST-segment elevation. *N. Engl. J. Med.* 2001;345:494–502.

[88] Cannon CP, Weintraub WS, Demopoulos LA, et al. Comparison of early invasive and conservative strategies in patients with unstable coronary syndromes treated with the glycoprotein IIb/IIIa inhibitor tirofiban. *N. Engl. J. Med.* 2001;344:1879–87.

[89] Oler A, Whooley MA, Oler J, et al. Adding heparin to aspirin reduces the incidence of myocardial infarction and death in patients with unstable angina, a meta-analysis. *JAMA* 1996; 276:811–5.

[90] Petersen JL, Mahaffey KW, Hasselblad V, et al. Efficacy and bleeding complications among patients randomized to enoxaparin or unfractionated heparin for antithrombin therapy in non-ST-Segment elevation acute coronary syndromes: a systematic overview. *JAMA* 2004;292:89–96.

[91] Kong DF, Topol EJ, Bittl JA, et al. Clinical outcomes of bivalirudin for ischemic heart disease. *N Engl J Med* 1999;100:2049–53.

[92] Braunwald E, Antman EM, Beasley JW, et al. American College of Cardiology /American Heart Association Committee on the Management of Patients With Unstable Angina. ACC/AHA 2002 guideline update for the management of patients with unstable angina and non-ST-segment elevation myocardial infarction: a report of the American College of Cardiology/American Heart Association Task Force on Practice Guidelines (Committee on the Management of Patients With Unstable Angina). 2002. Available at: http://www. acc.org/clinical/guidelines/unstable /incorporated/ index.htm. Accessed May 1, 2005.

In: Angina Pectoris: Etiology, Pathogenesis and Treatment
Editors: A. P. Gallo, M. L. Jones

ISBN: 978-1-60456-674-1
© 2008 Nova Science Publishers, Inc.

Chapter II

Endothelial Dysfunction in Stable Angina Pectoris: Potential Therapeutic Implications

*Dimitris Tousoulis, Nikolaos Papageorgiou, Marietta Charakida,
Gerasimos Siasos, and Christodoulos Stefanadis*
Cardiology Unit, Athens University Medical School
Hippokration Hospital, Athens, Greece

Abstract

In patients with stable angina, endothelial function has been found to be impaired and closely related from the early steps of atheromatosis. In this article we will review the association of stable angina pectoris and endothelial dysfunction, focusing on classical and novel risk factors that predispose to endothelial dysfunction, while suggesting potential therapeutic approaches of improving vascular endothelium status. Classical risk factors include hypercholesterolemia-dyslipidemia, diabetes mellitus, hypertension, cigarette smoking, while novel risk factors refer to inflammation-infection, hyperhomocysteinemia and genetics. Classical therapeutic approaches such as statin treatment and angiotensin converting enzyme inhibitors (ACE-I) treatment are nowadays accompanied by novel therapies including insulin sensitizers and antioxidant vitamins and others still under investigation such as folic acid supplementation.

Introduction

Vascular endothelium is a unique organ responsible for the secretion of a large number of substances. Novel data reported that endothelium plays a key role in the atherosclerotic process. Specifically, endothelial function represents a defensive mechanism against the development of atheromatous plaque. On the other hand, endothelial dysfunction is a major factor of atherogenesis. It has been found, that many factors encourage the development of atheromatous plaque by affecting nitric oxide bioavailability (NO) resulting to several clinical manifestations such as stable angina [1, 2]. Classical risk factors such as hypercholesterolemia-dyslipidemia, hypertension, smoking, diabetes mellitus along with novel risk factors such as hyperhomocysteinemia, infections and genetics represent important factors predisposing to endothelial dysfunction.

Endothelial Dysfunction Related to Nitric Oxide Bioavailability

Endothelium has numerous properties including inhibition of the following mechanisms: platelet aggregation, inflammation, thrombosis, leukocyte adhesion as well smooth muscle (cells) contraction (critical processes at the early stages of atherosclerosis) (Figure 1) [1, 2].

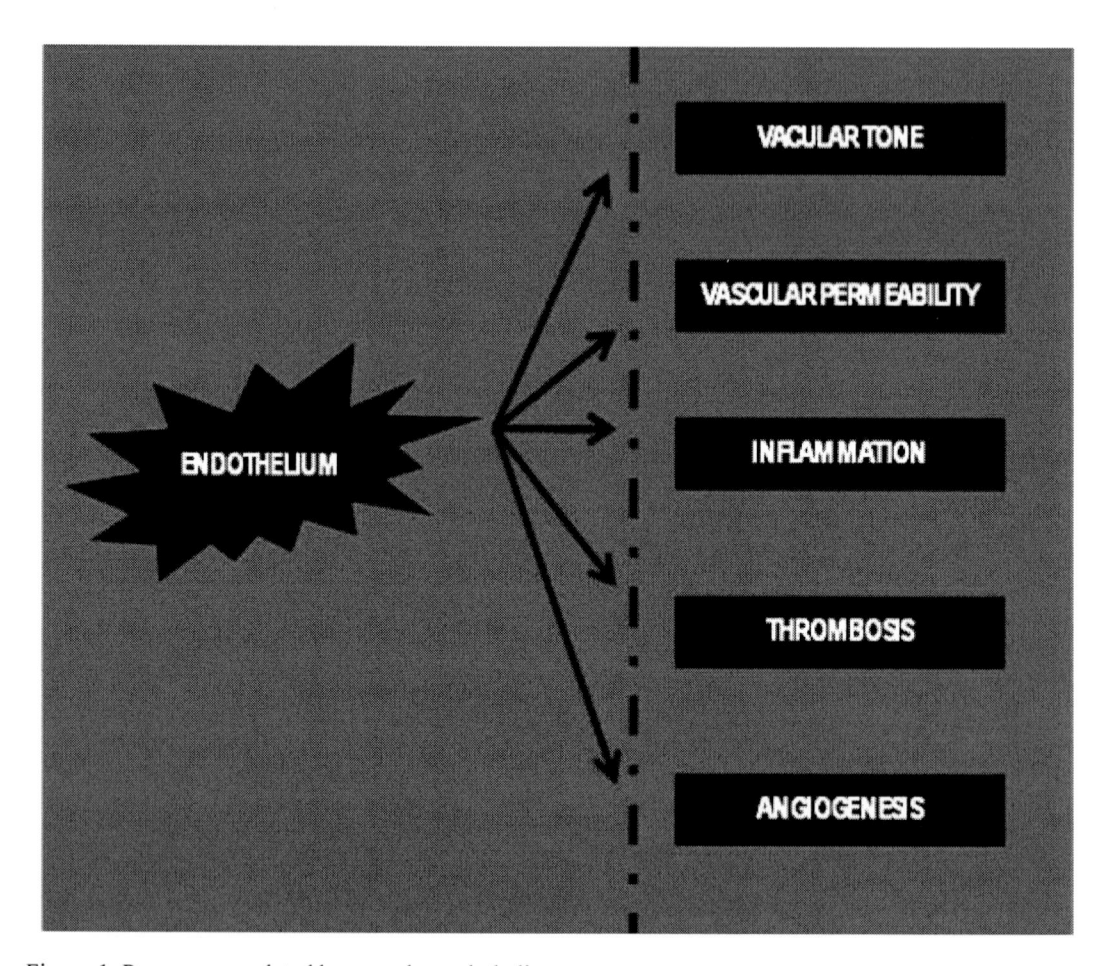

Figure 1. Processes regulated by vascular endothelium.

Endothelial dysfunction is characterized from downregulation of the protective effects of endothelium. Mechanisms which take part in the decreased vasodilatory response during endothelial dysfunction are the decreased NO production and the increased oxidative stress. Furthermore, elevation of both adhesion molecules levels and cytokines as well as plasminogen activator inhibitor (PAI-1) production take part in the inflammatory response leading in a pre-thrombotic state. Vasoactive peptides such as angiotensin II, endothelin-1, asymmetrical dimethylarginine (ADMA) act in a specific way which participates in the overall process of endothelial dysfunction [1-4]. Impaired endothelial function and decreased NO bioavailability in human endothelium, plays a critical role in the development and progression of atherosclerosis and coronary artery disease [5]. Several risk factors for coronary artery disease (CAD) may facilitate the development of atherosclerosis by decreasing NO bioavailability in vascular endothelium. Modern therapeutic approaches are focused on the stimulation of its synthesis by endothelial cells and the prevention of its reaction with reactive oxygen species [6].

Pathophysiology of the Atheromatous Disease

It has been proposed that the atherosclerotic plaque develops as a response to injury of the vascular endothelium [7]. In states of injury in vascular endothelium, platelets and monocytes aggregate in the sites of injury. Dysfunction of vascular endothelial cells is thought to induce pathologic reactions of cell groups mediated by the expression of adhesion molecules [8]. Simultaneously, peripheral monocytes invade the sub-endothelial tissue through the spaces between endothelial cells and subsequently differentiate into macrophages. When large amounts of low-density lipoprotein (LDL) exist, denatured LDL modified by oxidation or other reactions on the vascular wall is taken up by macrophages via scavenger receptors, leading to the formation of foam cells and the accumulation of cholesterol esters [8-10]. Furthermore, as the macrophages accumulate large amounts of lipid, they form droplets or foam cells (the principal cells in the fatty streak and the initial lesion of atherosclerosis) [8]. It is worth to mention that, in their early stages of atherosclerosis, plaques are primarily composed of foam cells derived from macrophages. In addition, smooth muscle proliferation also occurs in the intima. Macrophage-derived foam cells in the sub endothelium secrete growth factors that chemotactically attract smooth muscle cells to migrate into the intima from the media, proliferate and create a series of conditions that result in the formation of the intimal lesion [7, 8]. As the lesion progresses, fibrosis, lipid deposition, necrosis, and calcification may ensue to yield the plaque.

The Role of Endothelial Dysfunction in Atheromatosis

Injury or activation of the endothelium changes its normal regulatory functions and results in abnormal endothelial cell function which is characterized by an imbalance of endothelium derived relaxing and contracting factors. In atherogenesis, endothelial injury appears to play a key role in early events (Figure 2) [7, 8]. It precedes any structural vascular alterations and potentially triggers the initiation and progression of atherosclerotic lesions. Several studies performed both in experimental models of atherosclerosis and in humans, have demonstrated that, in states of dysfunctional endothelium, the release of nitric oxide is impaired [11, 12]. Debility of the endothelium to elicit NO-mediated vasodilation may be due to either decreased formation or accelerated degradation of NO. Accumulating evidence suggests that increased vascular production of reactive oxygen species plays an important role in endothelial dysfunction and accounts for a large proportion of reduced NO bioavailability [11, 13]. Enhanced low-density lipoprotein (LDL) cholesterol and particularly oxidized LDL plays also important role in endothelial dysfunction. A direct effect on protein kinase C and G proteins appears to be the link with nitric oxide signalling pathway [13, 14]. Several other factors may also affect endothelial nitric oxide synthase (eNOS) function at post-translational level. Experimental evidence suggests that hypercholesterolemia can contribute to decreased NO production by upregulating caveolin abundance and promoting caveolin-eNOS interaction [14, 15]. Moreover, protein kinase Akt dependent phosphorylation of eNOS also plays a critical role in eNOS activation and endothelial function [11-13]. Finally, abundance of endogenous eNOS inhibitors, such as asymmetric dimethylarginine may also alter eNOS activity at post-translational level [16, 17].

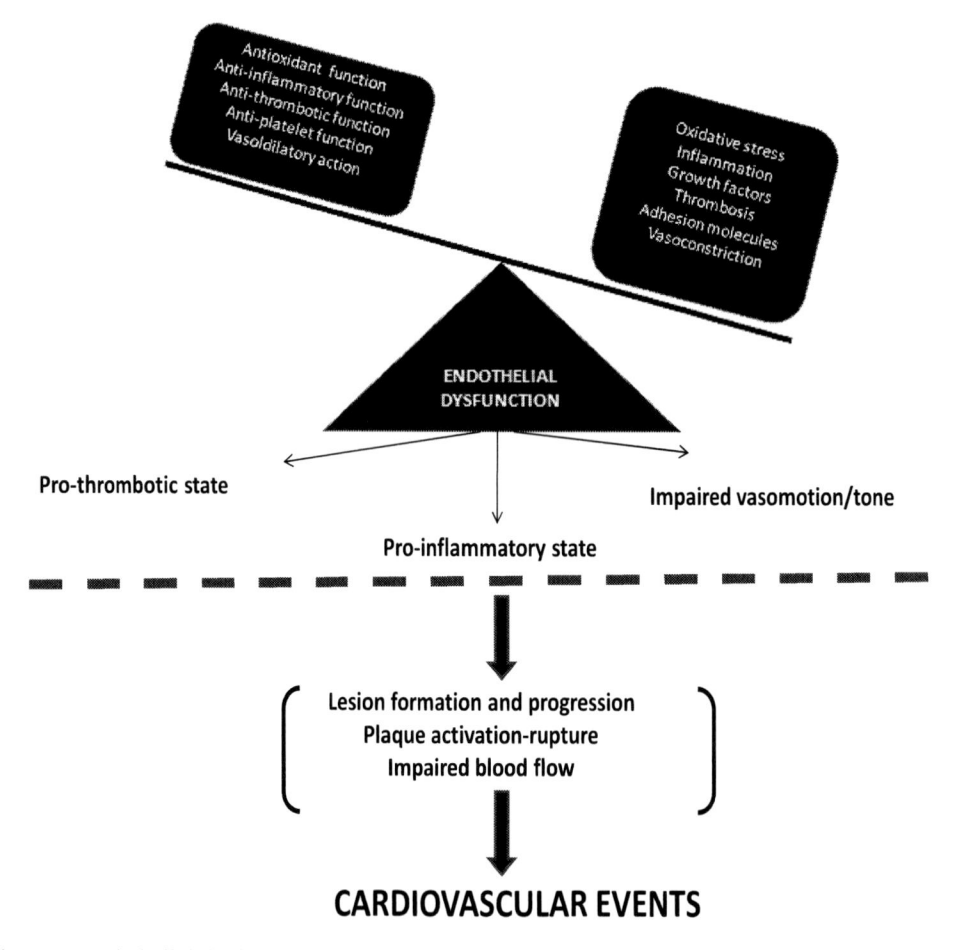

Figure 2. Endothelial dysfunction and cardiovascular events.

Risk Factors for Endothelial Dysfunction

Hypercholesterolemia-Dyslipidemia

It has been found that high levels of cholesterol represent a major factor for coronary artery disease (CAD) [18, 19]. Low density lipoprotein cholesterol (LDL) and specifically oxidized-LDL (ox-LDL) induces inflammatory processes in the vasculature and promotes local production of oxygen free radicals, enhancing local mechanisms which lead in endothelial dysfunction [18-22]. It is worth to mention that endothelial function as this was estimated with ultrasonic techniques including flow-mediated dilation (FMD) is impaired in children with familiar hypercholesterolemia [20].

Diabetes Mellitus

Increased leukocytes-endothelial cells aggregation and vascular permeability found in young individuals with diabetes mellitus may be responsible for endothelial dysfunction, via several mechanisms such as activation of protein kinase C, reduction of cellular nicotinamide adenine dinucleotide phosphate (NADP), insulin resistance (including vasodilatory effects) and increased reactive oxygen species [23-27]. Asymmetric dimethylarginine (ADMA) plays a pivotal role in diabetic endothelial dysfunction [28, 29]. Although, the extension of vascular disorder is associated both with diabetes duration and LDL levels, changes during adolescent life affect strongly the development of vascular dysfunction in young diabetic subjects [23, 30].

Hypertension

Peripheral endothelial dysfunction has been reported in several studies focusing on hypertension. In hypertensive patients, the levels of the vasoconstrictive angiotensin II and endothelin-1 are elevated. Hypertension is also associated with mild inflammation and increased oxidative stress which reduces endothelial NO bioavailability [31-33]. Endothelial dysfunction can be observed in children with secondary hypertension and this can be explained in part due to elevated ADMA levels [29, 34]. Family history and genetic factors also have been accused for the pathogenesis of endothelial dysfunction and hypertension in young individuals.

Cigarette Smoking

Active cigarette smoking is a well known risk factor for atherosclerosis. It is associated with dose-dependent injury of the endothelium-dependent dilation in healthy subjects [35-37]. Moreover, passive smoking has been also correlated with a dose-related injury of endothelium-dependent dilation in healthy young individuals supporting the previous knowledge of being an important risk factor for cardiovascular events [38-40]. Although, a specific mechanism for endothelial dysfunction is not explicit, several mechanisms have been proposed such as inflammation, increased ADMA levels, increased oxidative stress, platelet activation and the direct detrimental effects of smoke compound on endothelial cells. These represent mechanisms which are able to reduce endothelial NO and disturb the normal vasodilatory function [41-44].

Inflammation-Infection

Recent studies have shown that infections and systemic inflammation play a critical role in the beginning and development of cardiovascular disease [45-47]. A number of different mechanisms have been accused for the inflammatory response in the vasculature. It has been found that viral and bacterial infections contribute to the development and progress of atherosclerosis inducing the expression of cytokines and adhesion molecules, migration and differentiation of smooth muscle cells, while inhibiting the apoptosis and increasing lipid accumulation [48, 49].

Hyperhomocysteinemia

Hyperhomocysteinemia represents a novel cardiovascular risk factor that leads to endothelial dysfunction, while folic acid supplementation appears to be able to reduce homocysteine levels and result in an improvement of the impaired endothelial function [50, 51]. Data suggest that homocysteine reduces NO bioavailability by increasing the oxidative status [50, 52, 53]. It is now commonly accepted that homocysteine may cause ADMA accumulation by inhibition of the enzyme dimethylarginine dimethylaminohydrolase (DDAH) [54]. Experimental studies in humans have confirmed that hyperhomocysteinemia may lead to endothelial dysfunction through the accumulation of ADMA [55, 56]. Nevertheless, scientific data referring to the impact of hyperhomocysteinemia on endothelial function remain unclear [57]. Several mechanisms have been proposed to enlighten the role of hyperhomocysteinemia and some of them such as the previous may explain the increased cardiovascular risk of patients with hyperhomocysteinemia. This is of special importance for some specific groups of patients who often face increased homocysteine levels [58].

Genetics

The impact of genetic factors on endothelial function is reported to be of a great importance. Atherosclerosis is a multi-gene disease in which polymorphisms of genes that regulate endothelial biology seem to affect vascular function strongly in response to environmental risk factors [59-61]. Several polymorphisms have been identified to be associated with endothelial function and cardiovascular disease including those of renin-angiotensin system, pro-inflammatory cytokines and chemokines, NADPH oxidase and bradykinin receptor among many important polymorphisms [62-69].

Endothelium-Derived Vasodilators and Vasoconstrictors

The normal endothelium regulates vascular tone and structure and exerts anticoagulant, anti-platelet, and anti-inflammatory properties. The maintenance of vascular tone is accomplished by the release of numerous dilator and constrictor substances. A major vasodilator released by the endothelium is NO, originally identified as endothelium-derived relaxing factor (EDRF) [11, 12]. Nitric oxide is a freely diffusible. The actions of the endogenously released NO in mammals were first described in experiments using isolated blood vessels. Stimulation of rabbit aorta with acetylcholine (ACH) showed a resulting relaxation that was dependent on the presence of the endothelium. This endothelium dependent relaxation was in turn mediated by the release of a labile factor, identified as endothelial derived relaxing factor or EDRF [11, 12, 16]. The identity of EDRF was finally shown to be indistinguishable from NO. Nitric oxide is established as the active metabolite which mediates the smooth muscle relaxant effects of nitroglycerin and other anti-anginal organic nitrates [16, 70]. Other endothelium-derived vasodilators include prostacyclin and bradykinin [11, 12, 71]. Prostacyclin acts synergistically with NO to inhibit platelet aggregation. Bradykinin stimulates release of NO, prostacyclin, and endothelium-derived hyperpolarizing factor [11, 12, 71]. Endothelial cells produce various prostaglandin molecules according to their tissue type, with prostacyclin and thromboxane A2 being the most important in the vasculature. They are derived from arachidonic acid, which is mobilised by plasma membrane by phospholipase A2 and metabolised by cyclo-oxygenase (COX) [72, 73]. Once produced, prostacyclin increases cyclic 3', 5'-adenosine monophosphate (cAMP) in smooth muscle cells and platelets. [72-74].

There is also an additional pathway that is involved in smooth muscle hyperpolarization. This was attributed to a non-characterized endothelial factor called endothelium-derived hyperpolarizing factor (EDHF) [75, 76]. Endothelium-derived hyperpolarizing factor causes hyperpolarization following the activation of potassium channels of the vascular smooth muscle cells. However it seems that EDHF-mediated responses are also associated with an increase in calcium in endothelial cells. Thus, substances that increase endothelial calcium enhance EDHF responses, while a decrease in extracellular calcium concentration attenuates EDHF responses [75-77]. The endothelium also produces vasoconstrictor substances, such as endothelin and angiotensin II. Angiotensin II not only acts as a vasoconstrictor but is also pro-oxidant and stimulates production of endothelin [78]. Endothelin and angiotensin II promote proliferation of smooth muscle cells and thereby contribute to the formation of plaque [71]. Activated macrophages and vascular smooth muscle cells produce large amounts of endothelin [79]. When a blunted endothelium exists, it affects the balance between vasoconstriction and vasodilation and initiates a number of processes that promote or exacerbate atherosclerosis. These include increased endothelial permeability, platelet aggregation, leukocyte adhesion, and generation of cytokines [80]. Angiotensin II is a peptide that has vasoconstrictor, prothrombotic, oxidant and atherogenic properties. The activation of AT1 receptors on endothelial cells leads to secretion of NO and prostaglandin while stimulation of smooth muscle receptors leads to vasoconstriction, generation of reactive oxygen species and endothelin-1 release [81,82]. Endothelin-1 (ET-1) is synthesised from its precursor, big ET-1. Endothelin-1 is produced in response to different factors such as hypoxia, hyperoxia, pressure, low shear stress, catecholamines [83, 84]. By acting on vascular smooth muscle receptors ET-a and ET-B, ET-1 causes vasoconstriction while the same isoform, by acting on the ET-B receptors of endothelial cells, induces vasorelaxation [85]. It is worth to mention that the coronary constrictor effects of endothelin can be partially blocked by calcium antagonists [86, 87].

Endothelial Function and Stable Angina. The Prognostic Role of Endothelial Function

Evaluation of endothelial function in patients has recently emerged as a useful tool for the identification and estimation of atherosclerosis. In the setting of cardiovascular disease (CVD) risk factors, the endothelium loses its normal regulatory functions. Clinical syndromes such as stable angina relate in part, to a loss of endothelial control. Studies have demonstrated that the severity of endothelial dysfunction is associated with the risk for an initial or recurrent cardiovascular event [88, 89]. Both invasive and not invasive studies of endothelial function have shown a significant correlation between the coronary and vascular bed. Studies have shown that endothelial dysfunction is present in patients who have risk factors but not overt atherosclerosis [88, 90, 91].

Estimation of endothelial function as a test for assessing vascular status, seems to be a useful diagnostic tool and a new target on which to focus to improve cardiovascular outcome. Studies performed at the time of cardiac catheterization clearly demonstrated a direct association between endothelial dysfunction and cardiovascular events. On the other hand the peripheral endothelial assessment gave also similar results regarding to the previous association, but a little bit conflicting (Table 1). Moreover studies using invasive forearm venous occlusion plethysmography highlighted the prognostic importance of endothelial dysfunction [92, 93]. Other groups using non invasive methods shared similar findings while others failed to do so.

Nitric oxide bioavailability is determined in humans by several invasive and non-invasive techniques [94]. Intra-arterial (or even intracoronary) infusions of vasoactive agents inducing NO-mediated vasodilation are critical in evaluating endothelial function in humans. Methods like these are invasive, with all the negative consequences that arise. This is the reason why non-invasive techniques such as the non invasive evaluation of flow-mediated dilation (FMD) in the brachial artery by ultrasound are used in large scale nowadays. Data suggest that endothelial function is a useful prognostic marker in coronary artery disease patients, such as those suffering from stable angina [95, 96]. In these patients, it has been reported that endothelial dysfunction is an independent prognostic factor [95]. Moreover, evidence suggests that a low brachial artery FMD appears to be an independent predictor of cardiovascular risk in patients with peripheral arterial disease [97].

Table 1. Association of endothelial dysfunction and stable angina pectoris. Prognostic significance of endothelial function in coronary/peripheral circulation and clinical outcome.

Study	Population	Duration	Circulation type	Predictive value	Endpoint
Al Suwaidi [154]	CAD (157 subjects)	28 months	coronary	+	Cardiac death, MI, CHF, CABG and PCI
Schachinger [155]	CAD (147 subjects)	7.7 years	coronary	+	MI, UA, ischemic stroke, CABG, PTCA, peripheral bypass
Hollenberg [156]	Heart transplantation (73 subjects)	32 months	coronary	+	Cardiac death Cardiac allograft vasculopathy
Targonski [157]	Without CAD (503 subjects)	90 months		+	Cerebrovascular events
Schindler [158]	Normal coronary angiograms (130 subjects)	45 months	coronary	+	CVD death, UA, MI, PTCA, CABG, stroke, peripheral bypass
Heitzer [93]	CAD (281 subjects)	4.5 years	peripheral	+	CVD, stroke, MI, CABG, PTCA, peripheral bypass
Perticone [92]	Hypertension (225 subjects)	32 months	peripheral	+	CVD death, MI, stroke, TIA, UA, CABG, PTCA, PVD
Modena [159]	Hypertensive postmenopausal women (400 subjects)	67 months	peripheral	+	CVD event

Table 1. (Continued)

Study	Population	Duration	Circulation type	Predictive value	Endpoint
Chan [160]	CAD (152 subjects)	34 months	peripheral	+	CVD death, MI, Coronary revascularisation, UA, Stroke, TIA, Carotid endarterectomy
Fathi [161]	Patients at risk of coronary events (444 subjects)	24 months	peripheral	–	Cardiovascular death, MI, Stroke, Revascularization

CAD: Coronary artery disease, MI: myocardial infarction, CHF: Congestive heart failure, CVD: cardiovascular disease, PTCA: percutaneous transluminal coronary angioplasty, PVD: peripheral vascular disease, CABG: coronary artery bypass graft surgery, UA: unstable angina, PCI: percutaneous coronary intervention , TIA: transient ischemic attack, +: independent predictor, – : not independent predictor of events.

Further to the predictive role of evaluating endothelial function in diseased populations, FMD seems to be also a useful tool in assessing cardiovascular risk in the general population as well, since it predicts the development of coronary artery disease independently from the classic risk factors for atherosclerosis [98]. Screening of endothelial function with non-invasive techniques may contribute to the early identification of atherosclerosis in general population, thus regulating in a manner future clinical outcomes.

Therapeutic Approaches Targeting Vascular Endothelium in Stable Angina

Several drug categories have been used in treating cardiovascular disease such as stable angina with beneficial effects, while showing a unique effect by improving vascular endothelium. Classical therapeutic approaches such as statin treatment and angiotensin converting enzyme inhibitors (ACE-I) treatment are nowadays accompanied by novel therapies including insulin sensitizers and antioxidant vitamins and others still under investigation such as folic acid supplementation which we will review in the following paragraph.

Statins (3-Hydroxy-3- Methyl Glutaryl Co Enzyme A Reductase, HMG-Coa Inhibitors)

These are agents which reduce cholesterol levels and are widely used in primary and secondary prevention of cardiovascular disease. Beyond cholesterol lowering statins act directly on vascular endothelium targeting thrombotic and inflammatory processes [99-102]. This is a fact evaluated in several studies which have shown that the beneficial effects on vascular endothelium are prior to cholesterol lowering. Furthermore, it has been shown that statins are able to improve endothelial function both by increasing the expression and action of endothelial nitric oxide synthase (eNOS) and through the antioxidant effects that they exert [103, 104].

Statins increase the expression of eNOS, thus activating protein kinase Akt which is an important regulator of cellular processes. It has been shown that such an activation inhibits apoptosis and leads directly to an increase in production of NO. Statins play a key role in regulating eNOS through their capability to inhibit the action of proteins such as Rho (Table 2) [105, 106]. Another mechanism through which statins may affect endothelium is through their antioxidant effects. They attenuate angiotensin II–induced free radical production in vascular smooth muscle cells by inhibiting Rac1-mediated NAD(P)H oxidase activity and downregulating angiotensin AT_1-receptor expression [107]. Referring to the fact that NO is scavenged by the detrimental effects of reactive oxygen species (ROS), the previous data indicate that the antioxidant effects of statins may further contribute to their ability to improve endothelial function.

Table 2. Studies focusing on the effects of statins on endothelial function

Study	Population type/ Number	Drug/dose	Duration	Endothelium
Treasure [104]	CAD (23 subjects)	Lovastatin (80 mg /day)	6 months	+
Dupuis [162]	Hyperlipidemics, MI (55 subjects)	Pravastatin (40 mg / day)	6 weeks	+
Mullen [163]	Diabetics (38 subjects)	Atorvastatin (40 mg / day)	6 weeks	+
Marchesi [164]	Postmenopausal women, hypercholesterolemics (30 subjects)	Atorvastatin (10 mg / day)	8 weeks	+
van Venrooij [165]	Diabetics, hyperlipidemics (87 subjects)	Atorvastatin (80 mg / day)	30 weeks	-

Table 2. (Continued)

Study	Population type/ Number	Drug/dose	Duration	Endothelium
Beishuizen [166]	Diabetics (250 subjects)	Simvastatin (20 mg / day)	2 years	-
Dupuis [167]	After ACS (50 subjects)	Pravastatin (40 mg / day) or Atorvastatin (80 mg / day)	4 weeks	+
Kayikcioglu [168]	Cardiac syndrome X (38 subjects)	Pravastatin (40 mg / day)	3 weeks	+
Taneva [169]	Hyperlipidemics (33 subjects)	Atorvastatin (80 mg / day)	6 weeks	+

+: positive effect, -: no effect, CAD: coronary artery disease, MI: myocardial infarction, ACS: acute coronary syndromes.

ACE-I (Angiotensin Converting Enzyme Inhibitors)

These are agents which are used widely in the management of hypertension. It is well known that the levels of angiotensin converting enzyme in plasma reflects only a small percent of the total amount, as its' largest amount exists on the surface of vascular endothelium [108]. It has been found that ACE inhibitors affect vascular endothelium through several mechanisms. A reduction in the production of angiotensin II results in regression of endothelial dysfunction via reduced expression of NAD(P)H oxidase and decreased production of oxygen free radicals, while leading to an aggregation of bradykinin to the B2 receptors of endothelium [109, 110].

Furthermore, studies have shown that ACE-inhibitors contribute to an increase of NO production and prostacyclin (PGI2) from the vascular endothelium. It is worth to mention that long-term administration of ACE-inhibitors induces the activation of B1 receptors [111]. Thus, both diminished angiotensin II production and accumulation of bradykinin lead to improvement of endothelial cell function and vascular tone and such an effect may beneficial not only for normotensive patients but also for patients with established vascular disease as well [112]. Numerous scientific data reported beneficial effects of this drug class on endothelial function of patients including diabetics, hypertensives and coronary artery disease patients including those suffering from chronic stable angina (Table 3).

Table 3. Studies focusing on the effects of ACE-inhibitors and endothelial function

Study	Population type/ Number	Drug/dose	Duration	Endotheli um
McFarlane [170]	Diabetics type I (20 subjects)	Perindopril (4mg/ day)	12 weeks	-
Kovacs [171]	Post MI patients (50 subjects)	Enalapril or Quinapril (10mg/day)	12 weeks	+
Mancini [172]	Normotensives with CAD (105 subjects)	Quinapril (40mg/ day)	6 months	+
Trevelyan [173]	CAD patients waiting for CABG (49 subjects)	Losartan (50 mg/ day) Or Enalapril (20mg/ day)	2 months	+
Mullen [174]	Diabetics type I (91 subjects)	Enalapril (20mg/ day)	6 months	-
O'Driscoll [175]	Diabetics type II (10 subjects)	Enalapril (20mg/ day)	4 weeks	+

+: posititive effect, -: no effect , CAD: coronary artery disease, CABG: coronary artery bypass grafting, MI: myocardial infarction.

Insulin (Sensitizers)

Studies have demonstrated that insulin resistance and endothelial dysfunction co-exist [113]. Insulin-induced vasodilation is partially mediated by NO release and obese individuals who face an insulin resistance appear to have impaired endothelial fuction [113]. Thus, agents that increase insulin sensitivity may act beneficially by improving endothelial function. The beneficial effects of such drugs on endothelium are held by elevating NO bioavailability as well as by inhibiting the expression of adhesion molecules in activated endothelial cells and by reducing monocyte/macrophage homing to atherosclerotic plaques [114, 115]. Several clinical trials have demonstrated the beneficial effects of insulin sensitizers on vascular endothelium, in diabetics and non diabetics [116, 117]. It is worth to mention that studies evaluating forearm blood flow (FBF) by venous occlusion plethysmography in healthy male volunteers have shown an increase in peripheral blood flow, after a single oral dose of troglitazone [118].

L-arginine

L-arginine is an amino acid which is the substance for eNOS and a precursor for NO synthesis [2, 119]. Data have reported that several factors are responsible for the inhibition of NO production such as ADMA. On that basis it seems that L-arginine could act antergically [120, 121]. Studies have shown that L-arginine could be beneficial for endothelial function both in short-term and long-term administration [122, 123]. Moreover, it has been found that L-arginine exerts antioxidant and antiapoptotic effects [2]. Among numerous actions of L-arginine, smooth muscle cells relaxation, inhibition of the adhesion molecules expression and chemotactic peptides, inhibition of platelet aggregation as well as endothelin-1 expression seem to be critical [2]. Despite the positive results where L-arginine seems to improve NO bioavailability in human vasculature, it is still unclear whether chronic administration of L-arginine has any effect on clinical outcome in patients with CAD. It is commonly accepted that L-arginine may be useful at a clinical level in those conditions associated with L-arginine deficiency. It is important to have in mind that L-arginine may even be harmful if supplemented in patients with a high degree of eNOS uncoupling or in the presence of eNOS co-factor tetrahydrobiopterin deficiency [124]. It should be also mentioned that other approaches such as the inhibition of arginase (the enzyme responsible for intracellular catabolism of L-arginine) [125] may be more effective in improving intracellular L-arginine bioavailability, than exogenous L-arginine administration. Furthermore, endothelial nitric oxide synthase functional status may be better regulated by modifying enzymes implicated in ADMA metabolism, such as dimethylarginine dimethylaminohydrolase or protein arginine methyltransferases [126, 127].

Antioxidant Vitamins

It is well known that oxidative stress leads to endothelial dysfunction, reducing and inhibiting NO synthesis [128, 129]. Vitamins such as C and E have been found to improve impaired endothelium-dependent vasodilation in the brachial artery of patients with risk factors for atherosclerosis such as diabetes mellitus, hypertension and patients with advanced atherosclerosis. [130, 131]. Thus, it is possible that antioxidant vitamins could be beneficial in populations with elevated oxidative stress. Even though, a combination of antioxidant vitamins could be beneficial, adversely long-term effects may occur, such as an inhibition of endogenous antioxidant mechanisms, resulting in an imbalance between oxidant and antioxidants [132]. Despite the previous positive results, recent studies suggested that administration of vitamin E may prevent the beneficial effects of statins [133] . Indeed, our observations have shown that [134] the beneficial effect of atorvastatin on endothelial function and inflammation is negatively affected by co-administration of vitamin E.

Tetrahydrobiopterin (BH4)

Tetrahydrobiopterin is an essential substance for NO formation. It is an important regulator of eNOS activity implicated in eNOS uncoupling [135]. Intracellular oxidation of BH4 induced by reactive oxygen species such as superoxide anions or peroxynitrite [136] leads to eNOS uncoupling, turning this enzyme to a source of superoxide anions instead of NO [137]. It has been proposed that BH4 is oxidized to BH2, leading to eNOS uncoupling, decreased NO production and increased oxidative inactivation, which is partly responsible for the impaired endothelial function [137]. Evidence suggests that blood vessel function is improved by the addition of BH4 to vessel rings from animals with atherosclerosis, diabetes or hypertension [138]. In humans, BH4 administration augments NO-mediated effects on forearm blood flow in smokers , or subjects with diabetes, hypercholesterolemia, and hypertension [139-141]. Previous data have shown that co-administration of BH4 increased the Ach-induced coronary blood flow in subjects who had diminished coronary blood flow responses to acetylcholine (ACh) at baseline, [142]. On the contrary, BH4 had no effect on subjects with normal coronary blood flow at baseline.

Folic Acid Treatment (Folate)

Plasma levels of homocysteine and folate are related to cardiovascular risk and endothelial function [143, 144]. Homocysteine leads to an intracellular increase of oxidative stress status in vascular endothelium, leading to both the increased oxidative inactivation of NO, the formation of ONOO, and the decreased NO production [144]. Clinical trials have reported that lowering homocysteine with folic acid may retard progression of atherosclerosis [145], but these findings were not evaluated by more recent studies [146]. Even though, folic acid treatment may be beneficial in patients with elevated homocysteine levels [147], benefits in other patient groups have been inconsistent [148]. Studies recruiting patient with stroke [147] myocardial infarction [149], or stable CAD [150] have shown that folic acid treatment had no effect on clinical outcome. Folic acid treatment seems to improve endothelial function in patients with advanced atherosclerosis that are discordant with changes in plasma homocysteine [151]. 5-methyl-tetrahydrofolate (5-MTHF), the circulating metabolite of folic acid, appears to be strongly associated with endothelial function, independently from homocysteine levels [152], suggesting a direct effect of this molecule on vascular function. Interventional studies focusing on the effects of 5-MTHF showed that its infusion leads to an improvement of flow mediated dilatation in patients with coronary artery disease [144]. In addition, 5-MTHF has a rapid, direct effect on the human vascular endothelium, by improving NO bioavailability in human vessels [153].

Conclusion

It is a fact that vascular endothelium plays an important role in the development and progress of atherosclerosis. Several studies have shown that impaired endothelial function affects directly atherogenesis and its clinical manifestations such as stable angina. A number of factors have been found to be associated with endothelial dysfunction, while there are still others under investigation. Classical and new treatments have a beneficial impact on endothelial function, although some of these strategies are under investigation. Thus, it is necessary for further randomized clinical trials in order to evaluate the potential beneficial effects of the existing therapeutic approaches.

References

[1]   Libby, P. and Theroux, P. Pathophysiology of Coronary Artery Disease. *Circulation.* 2005;111:3481-3488.

[2]   Tousoulis, D., Antoniades, C., Tentolouris, C., Goumas, G., Stefanadis, C., and Toutouzas, P. L-Arginine in cardiovascular disease: Dream or reality? *Vascular Medicine.* 2002;7:203–211.

[3]   Endemann, D. and Schiffrin, E. Endothelial Dysfunction. *J Am Soc Nephrol.* 2004;15:1983–1992.

[4]   Glasser, S., Selwyn, A., and Ganz, P. Atherosclerosis: Risk factors and the vascular endothelium. *Am Heart J.* 1996;131:379-84.

[5]   Forstermann, U. and Munzel, T. Endothelial nitric oxide synthase in vascular disease: from marvel to menace. *Circulation.* 2006;113(13): 1708-14.

[6]   Laursen, J.B., Somers, M., Kurz, S., et al. Endothelial regulation of vasomotion in apoE-deficient mice: implications for interactions between peroxynitrite and tetrahydrobiopterin. *Circulation.* 2001;103(9):1282-8.

[7]   Ross, R. The pathogenesis of atherosclerosis. In: Braunwald E,ed. Heart disease: a textbook of cardiovascular medicine. 3rd ed.Philadelphia: *WB Saunders*, 19881146-52.

[8]   Yamada, N. Plaque Formation and Its Rupture. *Internal Medicine,* 2000 (April);39:335-336.

[9]   Penny, W.J., Chesebro, J.H., Heras, M., and Fuster, V. Antithrombotic therapy for patients with cardiac disease. *Curr Probl Cardiol.* 1988;13:425-513.

[10]   Fuster, V., Steele, P.M. and Chesebro, J.H. Role of platelets and thrombosis in coronary atherosclerotic disease and sudden death. *J Am Coll Cardiol.* 1985;5:175B-84B.

[11]   Davignon, J. and Ganz, P. Role of Endothelial Dysfunction in Atherosclerosis. *Circulation.* 2004;109 [suppl III]:III-27–III-32.

[12]   Furchgott, R. and Vanhoutte, P. Endothelium-derived relaxing and contracting factors *FASEB J.* 1989;3:2007-2018.

[13]   Landmesser, U., Hornig, B. and Drexler, H. Endothelial Function: A Critical Determinant in Atherosclerosis? *Circulation,* 2004;109;II-27-II-33

[14]   Feletou, M. and Vanhoutte, P. Endothelial dysfunction: a multifaceted disorder. *Am J Physiol Heart Circ Physiol.* 2006;291: H985–H1002.

[15]   Romano, M., Mezzetti, A., Marulli, C., et al. Fluvastatin reduces soluble P-selectin and ICAM-1 levels in hypercholesterolemic patients: role of nitric oxide. *J Invest Med.* 2000;48:183–189.

[16]   Yang, Z. and Ming, X. Recent Advances in Understanding Endothelial Dysfunction in Atherosclerosis. *CM & R.* 2006 ;4(1): 53-65.

[17]   Goligorsky, M. Endothelial cell dysfunction: can't live with it, how to live without it. *Am J Physiol Renal Physiol.* 2005;288: F871–F880.

[18]   The multiple risk factor intervention trial (MRFIT). A national study of primary prevention of coronary heart disease. *JAMA.* 1976;235:825-827.

[19]   Sorensen, K.E., Celermajer, D.S., Georgakopoulos, D., et al. Impairment of endothelium-dependent dilation is an early event in children with familial hypercholesterolemia and is related to the lipoprotein(a) level. *J Clin Invest.* 1994;93:50-55.

[20]   de Jongh, S., Lilien, M.R., Bakker, H.D., et al. Family history of cardiovascular events and endothelial dysfunction in children with familial hypercholesterolemia. *Atherosclerosis.* 2002;163:193-197.

[21]   Balligand, J.L. New mechanisms of LDL-cholesterol induced endothelial dysfunction; correction by statins. *Bull Mem Acad R Med Belg.* 2002;157(10-12):427-31; discussion 431-4.

[22]   Vakkilainen, J., Makimattila, S., Seppala-Lindroos, A., et al. Endothelial dysfunction in men with smallLDLparticles. *Circulation.* 2000 Aug 15;102(7):716-21.

[23]   Varughese, G.I. The impact of diabetes mellitus on endothelial dysfunction. *South Med J.* 2007 Feb;100(2):128-9.

[24]   Rask-Madsen, C. and King, G.L. Mechanisms of Disease: endothelial dysfunction in insulin resistance and diabetes. *Nat Clin Pract Endocrinol Metab.* 2007 Jan;3(1):46-56.

[25]   Avogaro, A., Fadini, G.P., Gallo, A., Pagnin, E., and de Kreutzenberg, S. Endothelial dysfunction in type 2 diabetes mellitus. *Nutr Metab Cardiovasc Dis.* 2006 Mar;16 Suppl 1:S39-45.

[26]   Neri, S., Signorelli, S.S., Torrisi, B., et al. Effects of antioxidant supplementation on postprandial oxidative stress and endothelial dysfunction: a single-blind, 15-day clinical trial in patients with untreated type 2 diabetes, subjects with impaired glucose tolerance, and healthy controls. *Clin Ther.* 2005 Nov;27(11):1764-73.asc Dis. 2006 Mar;16 Suppl 1:S39-45.

[27]   Hink, U., Tsilimingas, N., Wendt, M., and Munzel, T. Mechanisms underlying endothelial dysfunction in diabetes mellitus: therapeutic implications. *Treat Endocrinol.* 2003;2(5):293-304.

[28]   Chan, N.N. and Chan, J.C. Asymmetric dimethylarginine (ADMA): a potential link between endothelial dysfunction and cardiovascular diseases in insulin resistance syndrome? *Diabetologia.* 2002 Dec;45(12):1609-16.

[29]   Cooke, J.P. Does ADMA cause endothelial dysfunction? *Arterioscler Thromb Vasc Biol.* 2000 Sep;20(9):2032-7.

[30]   Elhadd, T.A., Khan, F., Kirk, G., et al. Influence of puberty on endothelial dysfunction and oxidative stress in young patients with type 1 diabetes. *Diabetes Care.* 1998;21:1990-1996.

[31]   Vaziri ND, Rodriguez-Iturbe B.Mechanisms of disease: oxidative stress and inflammation in the pathogenesis of hypertension. Nat Clin Pract Nephrol. 2006 Oct;2(10):582-93.

[32] Savoia, C. and Schiffrin, E.L. Inflammation in hypertension. *Curr Opin Nephrol Hypertens.* 2006 Mar;15(2):152-8.

[33] Cottone, S., Mule, G., Nardi, E., et al.C-reactive protein and intercellular adhesion molecule-1 are stronger predictors of oxidant stress than blood pressure in established hypertension. *J Hypertens.* 2007 Feb;25(2):423-8.

[34] McCarty, M.F.Vascular endothelium is the organ chiefly responsible for the catabolism of plasma asymmetric dimethylarginine--an explanation for the elevation of plasma ADMA in disorders characterized by endothelial dysfunction. *Med Hypotheses.* 2004;63(4):699-708.

[35] Celermajer, D.S., Sorensen, K.E., Georgakopoulos, D., et al. Cigarette smoking is associated with dose-related and potentially reversible impairment of endothelium-dependent dilation in healthy young adults. *Circulation.* 1993;88:2149-2155.

[36] Tanriverdi, H., Evrengul, H., Kuru, O., et al.Cigarette smoking induced oxidative stress may impair endothelial function and coronary blood flow in angiographically normal coronary arteries. *Circ J.* 2006 May;70(5):593-9.

[37] Noma, K., Goto, C., Nishioka, K., et al. .Smoking, endothelial function, and Rho-kinase in humans. *Arterioscler Thromb Vasc Biol.* 2005 Dec;25(12):2630-5.

[38] Holay, M.P., Paunikar, N.P., Joshi, P.P., Sahasrabhojney, V.S., and Tankhiwale, S.R. Effect of passive smoking on endothelial function in: healthy adults. *J Assoc Physicians India.* 2004 Feb;52:114-7.

[39] Woo, K.S., Chook, P., Leong, H.C., Huang, X.S., and Celermajer, D.S. The impact of heavy passive smoking on arterial endothelial function in modernized *Chinese. J Am Coll Cardiol.* 2000 Oct;36(4):1228-32.

[40] Davis, J.W., Shelton, L., Watanabe, I.S., and Arnold, J. Passive smoking affects endothelium and platelets. *Arch Intern Med.* 1989 Feb;149(2):386-9.

[41] Davis, J.W. Some acute effects of smoking on endothelial cells and platelets. *Adv Exp Med Biol.* 1990;273:107-18.

[42] Blann, A.D., Kirkpatrick, U., Devine, C., Naser, S., and McCollum, C.N. The influence of acute smoking on leucocytes, platelets and the endothelium. *Atherosclerosis.* 1998 Nov;141(1):133-9.

[43] Miller, E.A., Pankow, J.S., Millikan, R.C., et al. Glutathione-S-transferase genotypes, smoking, and their association with markers of inflammation, hemostasis, and endothelial function: the atherosclerosis risk in communities (ARIC) study. *Atherosclerosis.* 2003 Dec;171(2):265-72.

[44] Morrow, J.D., Frei, B., Longmire, A.W., et al. Increase in circulating products of lipid peroxidation (F2-isoprostanes) in smokers. Smoking as a cause of oxidative damage. *N Engl J Med.* 1995;332:1198-1203.

[45] Prasad, A., Zhu, J., Halcox, J.P., Waclawiw, M.A., Epstein, S.E., and Quyyumi, A.A. Predisposition to atherosclerosis by infections: role of endothelial dysfunction. *Circulation.* 2002 Jul 9;106(2):184-90.

[46] Gabrielli, M., Santarelli, L. and Gasbarrini, A. Role for chronic infections in atherosclerosis? *Circulation.* 2002 Aug 13;106(7):e32;

[47] Mayr, M., Kiechl, S., Willeit, J., Wick, G., and Xu, Q. Infections, immunity, and atherosclerosis: associations of antibodies to Chlamydia pneumoniae, Helicobacter

pylori, and cytomegalovirus with immune reactions to heat-shock protein 60 and carotid or femoral atherosclerosis. *Circulation.* 2000 Aug 22;102(8):833-9.

[48] Jacob, H.S., Visser, M., Key, N.S., Goodman, J.L., Moldow, C.F., and Vercellotti, G.M. Herpes virus infection of endothelium: new insights into atherosclerosis. *Trans Am Clin Climatol Assoc.* 1992;103:95-104.

[49] Chiu, B., Viira, E., Tucker, W., and Fong, I.W. Chlamydia pneumoniae, cytomegalovirus, and herpes simplex virus in atherosclerosis of the carotid artery. *Circulation.* 1997 Oct 7;96(7):2144-8.

[50] Virdis, A., Ghiadoni, L., Cardinal, H., et al. Mechanisms responsible for endothelial dysfunction induced by fasting hyperhomocystinemia in normotensive subjects and patients with essential hypertension. *J Am Coll Cardiol.* 38: 1106–1115, 2001

[51] Bennett-Richards, K., Kattenhorn, M., Donald, A., et al. Does oral folic acid lower total homocysteine levels and improve endothelial function in children with chronic renal failure? *Circulation,* 2002;105: 1810–1815.

[52] Virdis, A., Iglarz, M., Neves, M.F., Touyz, R.M., Rozen, R., and Schiffrin, E.L. Effect of hyperhomocystinemia and hypertension on endothelial function in methylenetetrahydrofolate reductase-deficient mice. *Arterioscler Thromb Vasc Biol.* 2003;23: 1352–1357.

[53] Zhang, X., Li, H., Jin, H., Ebin, Z., Brodsky, S., and Goligorsky, M.S. Effects of homocysteine on endothelial nitric oxide production. *Am J Physiol Renal Physiol.* 2000;279: F671–F678.

[54] Stuhlinger, M.C., Tsao, P.S., Her, J.H., Kimoto, M., Balint, R.F., and Cooke, J.P. Homocysteine impairs the nitric oxide synthase pathway: Role of asymmetric dimethylarginine. *Circulation,* 2001;104: 2569– 2575.

[55] Stuhlinger, M.C., Oka, R.K., Graf, E.E., et al. Endothelial dysfunction induced by hyperhomocyst(e)inemia: Role of asymmetric dimethylarginine. *Circulation,* 2003;108: 933–938.

[56] Boger, R.H., Lentz, S.R., Bode-Boger, S.M., Knapp, H.R., and Haynes, W.G. Elevation of asymmetrical dimethylarginine may mediate endothelial dysfunction during experimental hyperhomocyst(e)inaemia in humans. *Clin Sci.* (Lond) 2001;100: 161–167.

[57] Wanby, P., Brattstrom, L., Brudin, L., Hultberg, B., and Teerlink, T. Asymmetric dimethylarginine and total homocysteine in plasma after methionine loading. *Scand J Lab Invest.* 2003;63: 347–357.

[58] Mallamaci, F., Zoccali, C., Tripepi, G., et al. Hyperhomocysteinemia predicts cardiovascular outcomes in hemodialysis patients. *Kidney Int.* 2002;61: 609–614.

[59] Lee, W.H., Hwang, T.H., Oh, G.T., Kwon, S.U., Choi, Y.H., and Park, J.E. Genetic factors associated with endothelial dysfunction affect the early onset of coronary artery disease in Korean males. *Vasc Med.* 2001;6(2):103-8.

[60] Channon, K.M. and Guzik, T.J. Mechanisms of superoxide production in human blood vessels: relationship to endothelial dysfunction, clinical and genetic risk factors. *J Physiol Pharmacol.* 2002 Dec;53(4 Pt 1):515-24.

[61]   Loscalzo, J., Voetsch, B., Liao, R., and Leopold, J. Genetic determinants of vascular oxidant stress and endothelial dysfunction. *Congest Heart Fail.* 2005 Mar-Apr;11(2):73-9.

[62]   Imamura, A., Okumura, K., Matsui, H., et al. Endothelial nitric oxide synthase and methylenetetrahydrofolate reductase gene polymorphisms are associated with endothelial dysfunction in young, healthy men. *Can J Cardiol.* 2004 Oct;20(12):1229-34.

[63]   Antoniades, C., Tousoulis, D., Vasiliadou, C., et al. Genetic polymorphism on endothelial nitric oxide synthase affects endothelial activation and inflammatory response during the acute phase of myocardial infarction. *J Am Coll Cardiol.* 2005 Sep 20;46(6):1101-9.

[64]   Antoniades, C., Tousoulis, D. and Stefanadis, C. Letter regarding article by Becker, et al, "Hyperhomocysteinemia, a cardiac metabolic disease: role of nitric oxide and the p22phox subunit of NADPH oxidase". *Circulation.* 2005 Oct 11;112(15):e266.

[65]   Antoniades C, Tousoulis D, Vasiliadou C, Stefanadi E, Marinou K, and Stefanadis C. Genetic polymorphisms of platelet glycoprotein Ia and the risk for premature myocardial infarction: effects on the release of sCD40L during the acute phase of premature myocardial infarction. *J Am Coll Cardiol.* 2006 May 16;47(10):1959-66.

[66]   Kretowski, A., McFann, K., Hokanson, J.E., et al. Polymorphisms of the renin-angiotensin system genes predict progression of subclinical coronary atherosclerosis. *Diabetes.* 2007 Mar;56(3):863-71.

[67]   Georges, J.L., Rupprecht, H.J., Blankenberg, S., et al; AtheroGene Group. Impact of pathogen burden in patients with coronary artery disease in relation to systemic inflammation and variation in genes encoding cytokines. *Am J Cardiol.* 2003 Sep 1;92(5):515-21.

[68]   Libby, P. and Galis, Z.S. Cytokines regulate genes involved in atherogenesis. Ann N Y Acad Sci. 1995 Jan 17;748:158-68; discussion 168-70.

[69]   Zalba, G., San Jose, G., Moreno, M.U., Fortuno, A., and Diez, J. NADPH oxidase-mediated oxidative stress: genetic studies of the p22(phox) gene in hypertension. *Antioxid Redox Signal.* 2005 Sep-Oct;7(9-10):1327-36.

[70]   Ku, D.D. Nitric oxide- and nitric oxide donor-induced relaxation. *Methods Enzymol.* 1996;269:107-19.

[71]   Drexler, H. Factors involved in the maintenance of endothelial function. *Am J Cardiol.* 1998;82:3S–4S.

[72]   Campbell, W.B. and Falck, J.R. Arachidonic acid metabolites as endothelium-derived hyperpolarizing factors. *Hypertension.* 2007 Mar;49(3):590-6.

[73]   Köhler, R. and Hoyer, J. The endothelium-derived hyperpolarizing factor: insights from genetic animal models. *Kidney Int.* 2007 Jul;72(2):145-50.

[74]   Vane, J.R. and Botting, R.M. Formation by the endothelium of prostacyclin, nitric oxide and endothelin. *J Lipid Mediat.* 1993 Mar-Apr;6(1-3):395-404.

[75]   Suzuki, H., Chen, G. and Yamamoto, Y. Endothelium-derived hyperpolarizing factor (EDHF). *Jpn Circ J.* 1992 Feb;56(2):170-4.

[76]   Cohen, R.A. The endothelium-derived hyperpolarizing factor puzzle: a mechanism without a mediator? *Circulation.* 2005 Feb 15;111(6):724-7.

[77] Hyslop, S. and de Nucci, G. The mechanisms and significance of the coupled release of endothelium-derived relaxing factor (EDRF) and prostacyclin (PGI2) from endothelial cells. *Wien Klin Wochenschr.* 1991;103(14):422-34.

[78] Sowers, J.R. Hypertension, angiotensin II, and oxidative stress. *N Engl J Med.* 2002;346:1999–2001.

[79] Kinlay, S., Behrendt, D., Wainstain, M., et al. The role of endothelin-1 in the constriction of human atherosclerotic coronary arteries. *Circulation.* 2001;104:1114–1118.

[80] Ross, R. Atherosclerosis: an inflammatory disease. *N Engl J Med.* 1999; 340:115–126.

[81] Schulman, I.H., Zhou, M.S. and Raij, L. Interaction between nitric oxide and angiotensin II in the endothelium: role in atherosclerosis and hypertension. *J Hypertens Suppl.* 2006 Mar;24(1):S45-50.

[82] Watanabe, T., Barker, T.A. and Berk, B.C. Angiotensin II and the endothelium: diverse signals and effects. *Hypertension.* 2005 Feb;45(2):163-9.

[83] Coessens, B.C. Endothelin: an endothelium-derived vasoactive peptide. *J Reconstr Microsurg.* 1994 Nov;10(6):405-10.

[84] Le Monnier de Gouville, A.C., Lippton, H.L., Cavero, I., Summer, W.R., and Hyman, A.L. Endothelin--a new family of endothelium-derived peptides with widespread biological properties. *Life Sci.* 1989;45(17):1499-513.

[85] Karwatowska-Prokopczuk, E. and Wennmalm, A. Endothelium-derived constricting factor(s): the last novelty--endothelin. *Clin Physiol.* 1990 Mar;10(2):113-21. Review.

[86] Nava, E. and Lüscher, T.F. Endothelium-derived vasoactive factors in hypertension: nitric oxide and endothelin.J Hypertens Suppl. 1995 Aug;13(2):S39-48.

[87] Taddei, S., Virdis, A., Ghiadoni, L., and Salvetti, A.Vascular effects of endothelin-1 in essential hypertension: relationship with cyclooxygenase-derived endothelium-dependent contracting factors and nitric oxide. *J Cardiovasc Pharmacol.* 2000;35(4 Suppl 2):S37-40.

[88] Widlansky, M., Gokce, N., Keaney, J., and Vita, J. The Clinical Implications of Endothelial Dysfunction. *J Am Coll Cardiol.* 2003;42:1149–60.

[89] McGorisk, C. and Treasure, C. Endothelial dysfunction in coronary artery disease. *Curr Opin Cardiol.* 1996;11:341-350.

[90] Anderson, T.J., Uehata, A., Gerhard, M.D., et al. Close relation of endothelial function in the human coronary artery and peripheral circulations. *J Am Coll Cardiol.* 1995;26:1235-1241.

[91] Celermajer, D.S., Sorenson, K.E., Gooch, V.M., et al. Non-invasive detection of endothelial dysfunction in children and adults at risk of atherosclerosis. *Lancet.* 1992;340: 1111-1115.

[92] Perticone, F., Ceravolo, R., Pujia, A., Ventura, G., Iacopino, S., Scozzafava, A., et al. Prognostic significance of endothelial dysfunction in hypertensive patients. Circulation 2001;104:191-6.

[93] Heitzer, T., Schlinzig, T., Krohn, K., Meinertz, T., and Munzel, T. Endothelial dysfunction, oxidative stress, and risk of cardiovascular events in patients with coronary artery disease. *Circulation*, 2001;104:2673-8.

[94]   Tousoulis, D., Antoniades, C. and Stefanadis C. Evaluating endothelial function in humans: a guide to invasive and non-invasive techniques. *Heart.* 2005;91(4): 553-8.

[95]   Halcox, J., Schenke, W., Zalos, G., et al. Prognostic value of coronary vascular endothelial dysfunction. *Circulation.* 2002; 106(6): 653-8.

[96]   Chan, L., Shaw, A., Busfield, F., et al. Carotid artery intimal medial thickness, brachial artery flow-mediated vasodilation and cardiovascular risk factors in diabetic and non-diabetic indigenous Australians. *Atherosclerosis.* 2005; 180(2): 319-26.

[97]   Brevetti, G., Silvestro, A., Schiano, V.M. and Chiariello, M. Endothelial dysfunction and cardiovascular risk prediction in peripheral arterial disease: additive value of flow-mediated dilation to ankle-brachial pressure index. *Circulation.* 2003; 108(17): 2093-8.

[98]   Shimbo, D., Grahame-Clarke, C., Miyake, Y., et al. The association between endothelial dysfunction and cardiovascular outcomes in a population-based multi-ethnic cohort. *Atherosclerosis,* (2006).

[99]   Li, D. and Mehta, J.L. 3-Hydroxy-3-methylglutaryl coenzyme A reductase inhibitors protect against oxidized low-density lipoprotein-induced endothelial dysfunction. *Endothelium.* 2003;10:17–21.

[100] Mehta, J.L. Pleiotropic effects of statins: How important are they in the prevention of vascular disease? *Endothelium.* 2003;10:3–4.

[101] Tousoulis, D., Antoniades, C., Bosinakou, E., et al. Effects of atorvastatin on reactive hyperemia and inflammatory process in patients with congestive heart failure. *Atherosclerosis.* 2005;178:359–363.

[102] Tousoulis, D., Antoniades, C., Bosinakou, E., et al. Effects of atorvastatin on reactive hyperaemia and the thrombosis-fibrinolysis system in patients with heart failure. *Heart.* 2005;91:27–31.

[103] O'Driscoll, G., Green, D. and Taylor, R.R. Simvastatin, an HMG coenzyme A reductase inhibitor, improves endothelial function within 1 month. *Circulation.* 1997; 95:1126–1131.

[104] Treasure, C.B, Klein, J.L., Weintraub, W.S., et al. Beneficial effects of cholesterol-lowering therapy on the coronary endothelium in patients with coronary artery disease. *New England Journal of Medicine.* 1995;332:481–487.

[105] Kureishi, Y., Luo, Z., Shiojima, I., et al. The HMG-CoA reductase inhibitor simvastatin activates the protein kinase Akt and promotes angiogenesis in normocholesterolemic animals. *Nature Medicine.* 2000;6:1004–1010.

[106] Laufs, U. and Liao, J.K. Post-transcriptional regulation of endothelial nitric oxide synthase mRNA stability by Rho GTPase. *Journal of Biological Chemistry.* 1998;273:24266–24271.

[107] Wassmann, S., Laufs, U., Baumer, A., et al. Inhibition of geranylgeranylation reduces angiotensin II-mediated free radical production in vascular smooth muscle cells: involvement of angiotensin AT1 receptor expression and Rac1 GTPase. *Mol Pharmacol.* 2001; 59(3): 646-54.

[108] Zhuo, J.L., Froomes, P., Casley, D., et al. Perindopril chronically inhibits angiotensin converting enzyme in both the endothelium and adventitia of the internal mammary artery in patients with ischemic heart disease. *Circulation.*1997;96:174–182.

[109] Nickenig G. and Harrison D.G. The AT(1)-type angiotensin receptor in oxidative stress and atherogenesis: Part I: Oxidative stress and atherogenesis. *Circulation.* 2002;105:393–396.

[110] Faggiotto, A. and Paoletti, R. State-of-the-Art lecture. Statins and blockers of the renin-angiotensin system: Vascular protection beyond their primary mode of action. *Hypertension.* 1999;34:987–996.

[111] Marin-Castano, M.E., Schanstra, J.P., Neau, E., et al. Induction of functional bradykinin b(1)-receptors in normotensive rats and mice under chronic angiotensin-converting enzyme inhibitor treatment. *Circulation.* 2002;105:627–632.

[112] Mancini, G., Henry, G., Macaya, C., et al. Angiotensin-converting enzyme inhibition with quinapril improves endothelial vasomotor dysfunction in patients with coronary artery disease. The TREND (Trial on Reversing ENdothelial Dysfunction) Study. *Circulation,* 1996; 94(3): 258-65.

[113] Steinberg, H.O., Chaker, H., Leaming, R., Johnson, A., Brechtel G., and Baron, A.D. Obesity/insulin resistance is associated with endothelial dysfunction. Implications for the syndrome of insulin resistance. *Journal of Clinical Investigation.* 1996;97:2601–2610.

[114] Jackson, S.M., Parhami, F., Xi, X.P., et al. Peroxisome proliferator-activated receptor activators target human endothelial cells to inhibit leukocyte-endothelial cell interaction. *Arteriosclerosis, Thrombosis, and Vascular Biology.* 1999;19:2094–2104.

[115] Pasceri, V., Wu, H.D., Willerson, J.T., and Yeh, E.T. Modulation of vascular inflammation in vitro and in vivo by peroxisome proliferator-activated receptor-gamma activators. *Circulation.* 2000;101:235–238.

[116] Caballero, A., Saouaf, R., Lim, S., et al. The effects of troglitazone, an insulin-sensitizing agent, on the endothelial function in early and late type 2 diabetes: a placebo-controlled randomized clinical trial. *Metabolism,* 2003; 52(2): 173-80.

[117] Watanabe, Y., Sunayama, S., Shimada, K. et al. Troglitazone improves endothelial dysfunction in patients with insulin resistance. *J Atheroscler Thromb.* 2000; 7(3): 159-63.

[118] Fujishima, S., Ohya, Y., Nakamura, Y., et al. Troglitazone, an insulin sensitizer, increases forearm blood flow in humans. *Am J Hypertens.* 1998; 11(9): 1134-7.

[119] Tentolouris, C., Tousoulis, D., Goumas, G., Stefanadis, C., Davies, G., and Toutouzas P. L-Arginine in coronary atherosclerosis. *International Journal of Cardiology.* 2000;75:123–128.

[120] Channon K.M. and Guzik T.J. Mechanisms of superoxide production in human blood vessels: Relationship to endothelial dysfunction, clinical and genetic risk factors. *Journal of Physiology and Pharmacology.* 2002;53:515–524.

[121] Boger R.H. Asymmetric dimethylarginine (ADMA): A novel risk marker in cardiovascular medicine and beyond. *Annals of Medicine.* 2006;38:126–136.

[122] Tousoulis, D., Xenakis, C., Tentolouris, C., et al. Effects of vitamin C on intracoronary L-arginine dependent coronary vasodilatation in patients with stable angina. *Heart.* 2005;91:1319–1323.

[123] Lerman, A, Burnett, J.C. Jr., Higano, S.T, McKinley, L.J, and Holmes, D.R. Jr. Long-term L-arginine supplementation improves small-vessel coronary endothelial function in humans. *Circulation.* 1998;97:2123–2128.

[124] Loscalzo, J. Adverse effects of supplemental L-arginine in atherosclerosis: consequences of methylation stress in a complex catabolism? *Arterioscler Thromb Vasc Biol.* 1998; 23(1): 3-5.

[125] Berkowitz, D. E., R. White, D. Li, et al. Arginase Reciprocally Regulates Nitric Oxide Synthase Activity and Contributes to Endothelial Dysfunction in Aging Blood Vessels. *Circulation.* 2003;108(16): 2000-2006.

[126] Jacobi, J., K. Sydow, G. von Degenfeld, et al. Overexpression of Dimethylarginine Dimethylaminohydrolase Reduces Tissue Asymmetric Dimethylarginine Levels and Enhances Angiogenesis. *Circulation.* 2005; 111(11): 1431-1438.

[127] Vallance P. and Leiper J. Cardiovascular Biology of the Asymmetric Dimethylarginine:Dimethylarginine Dimethylaminohydrolase Pathway. *Arterioscler Thromb Vasc Biol.* 2004;24(6): 1023-1030.

[128] Ohara, Y., Peterson, T.E and Harrison, D.G. Hypercholesterolemia increases endothelial superoxide anion production. *Journal of Clinical Investigation.* 1993;91:2546–2551.

[129] Antoniades, C., Tousoulis, D., Tentolouris, C., et al. Effects of antioxidant vitamins C and E on endothelial function and thrombosis/fibrinolysis system in smokers. *Thrombosis and Haemostasis.* 2003;89:990–995.

[130] Toutouzas, P.C., Tousoulis, D. and Davies, G.J. Nitric oxide synthesis in atherosclerosis. *European Heart Journal.* 1998;19:1504–1511.

[131] Tousoulis, D., Antoniades, C., Tentolouris, C., et al. Effects of combined administration of vitamins C and E on reactive hyperemia and inflammatory process in chronic smokers. *Atherosclerosis.* 2003;170:261.

[132] Jialal, I. and Devaraj, S. Antioxidants and atherosclerosis: Don't throw out the baby with the bath water. *Circulation.* 2003;107:926–928.

[133] Brown, B, Zhao X, Chait A., et al. Simvastatin and niacin, antioxidant vitamins, or the combination for the prevention of coronary disease. *N Engl J Med.* 2001; 345(22):1583-92.

[134] Tousoulis, D., Antoniades, C., Vassiliadou, C., Toutouza, M., Pitsavos, C., Tentolouris, C., Trikas, A., and Stefanadis, C. Effects of combined administration of low dose atorvastatin and vitamin E on inflammatory markers and endothelial function in patients with heart failure. *Eur J Heart Fail.* 2003 ;7(7): 1126-32.

[135] Alp, N.J. and Channon K.M. Regulation of endothelial nitric oxide synthase by tetrahydrobiopterin in vascular disease. *Arteriosclerosis, Thrombosis, and Vascular Biology.* 2004;24:413–420.

[136] Kuzkaya, N., N. Weissmann, D. G. Harrison and S. Dikalov (2003). "Interactions of peroxynitrite, tetrahydrobiopterin, ascorbic acid, and thiols: implications for uncoupling endothelial nitric-oxide synthase." *J Biol Chem.* 278(25), 22546-54.

[137] Channon, K. M. and T. J. Guzik (2002). "Mechanisms of superoxide production in human blood vessels: relationship to endothelial dysfunction, clinical and genetic risk factors." *J Physiol Pharmacol.* 53(4 Pt 1), 515-24.

[138] Channon K.M. Tetrahydrobiopterin regulator of endothelial nitric oxide synthase in vascular disease. *Trends In Cardiovascular Medicine*. 2004;14:323– 327.

[139] Heitzer, T., Brockhoff, C., Mayer, B., et al. Tetrahydrobiopterin improves endothelium dependent vasodilation in chronic smokers: Evidence for a dysfunctional nitric oxide synthase. *Circulation Research*. 2000;86:36–41.

[140] Nystrom, T., Nygren, A. and Sjoholm, A. Tetrahydrobiopterin increases insulin sensitivity in patients with type 2 diabetes and coronary heart disease. 665 *American Journal of Physiology Endocrinology and Metabolism*. 2004;287:919– 925.

[141] Fukuda, Y., Teragawa, H., Matsuda, K., Yamagata, T., Matsuura H., and Chayama, K. Tetrahydrobiopterin restores endothelial function of coronary arteries in patients with hypercholesterolaemia. *Heart*. 2002;87:264–269.

[142] Setoguchi, S., M. Mohri, H. Shimokawa and A. Takeshita . Tetrahydrobiopterin improves endothelial dysfunction in coronary microcirculation in patients without epicardial coronary artery disease. *J Am Coll Cardiol*. (2001); 38(2): 493-8.

[143] Wald, D. S., M. Law and J. K. Morris. Homocysteine and cardiovascular disease: evidence on causality from a meta-analysis. *BMJ*, (2002);325(7374): 1202.

[144] Doshi, S. N., I. F. McDowell, S. J. Moat, et al. Folate improves endothelial function in coronary artery disease: an effect mediated by reduction of intracellular superoxide? *Arterioscler Thromb Vasc Biol*. (2001)21(7): 1196-202.

[145] Schnyder, G., M. Roffi, R. Pin, et al. Decreased rate of coronary restenosis after lowering of plasma homocysteine levels. *N Engl J Med*. (2001); 345(22): 1593-600.

[146] Lange, H., H. Suryapranata, G. De Luca, et al. Folate therapy and in-stent restenosis after coronary stenting. *N Engl J Med*. (2001); 350(26): 2673-81.

[147] Toole, J. F., M. R. Malinow, L. E. Chambless, et al. "Lowering Homocysteine in Patients With Ischemic Stroke to Prevent Recurrent Stroke, Myocardial Infarction, and Death: The Vitamin Intervention for Stroke Prevention (VISP) Randomized Controlled Trial." *JAMA*. (2004) ;291(5): 565-575.

[148] Liem, A., G. H. Reynierse-Buitenwerf, A. H. Zwinderman, J. W. Jukema, and D. J. van Veldhuisen. Secondary prevention with folic acid: effects on clinical outcomes. *J Am Coll Cardiol*. 2003; 41(12): 2105-13.

[149] Bonaa, K. H., I. Njolstad, P. M. Ueland, et al. Homocysteine Lowering and Cardiovascular Events after Acute Myocardial Infarction. *N Engl J Med*. 2006; 354(15): 1578-1588.

[150] The-Heart-Outcomes-Prevention-Evaluation-(HOPE)-2 Investigators. Homocysteine Lowering with Folic Acid and B Vitamins in Vascular Disease. *N Engl J Med*. 2006; 354(15): 1567-1577.

[151] Vermeulen, E. G., C. D. Stehouwer, J. W. Twisk, M., et al. Effect of homocysteine-lowering treatment with folic acid plus vitamin B6 on progression of subclinical atherosclerosis: a randomised, placebo-controlled trial. *Lancet*. 2000; 355(9203): 517-22.

[152] Spijkerman, A. M., Y. M. Smulders, P. J. Kostense, et al. S-adenosylmethionine and 5-methyltetrahydrofolate are associated with endothelial function after controlling for confounding by homocysteine: the Hoorn Study. *Arterioscler Thromb Vasc Biol*. (2005); 25(4): 778-84.

[153] Antoniades, C., C. Shirodaria, P. Leeson, et al. 5-methyl-tetrahydrofolate rapidly improves endothelial function and superoxide production in human atherosclerosis: Effects on tetrahydrobiopterin-dependent eNOS coupling. *J Am Coll Cardiol.* 2006; 47(4A): 356.

[154] Suwaidi, J.A., Hamasaki, S., Higano, S.T., Nishimura, R.A., Holmes, D.R. Jr., and Lerman, A. Long-term follow-up of patients with mild coronary artery disease and endothelial dysfunction. *Circulation,* 2000;101:948-54.

[155] Schachinger, V., Britten, M.B. and Zeiher, A.M. Prognostic impact of coronary vasodilator dysfunction on adverse long-term outcome of coronary heart disease. *Circulation,* 2000;101:1899-906.

[156] Hollenberg, S.M., Klein, L.W., Parrillo, J.E., Scherer, M., Burns, D., Tamburro, P., et al. Coronary endothelial dysfunction after heart transplantation predicts allograft vasculopathy and cardiac death. *Circulation,* 2001;104:3091-6.

[157] Targonski, P.V., Bonetti, P.O., Pumper, G.M., Higano, S.T., Holmes, D.R. Jr., and Lerman, A. Coronary endothelial dysfunction is associated with an increased risk of cerebrovascular events. *Circulation,* 2003;107:2805-9.

[158] Schindler, T.H., Hornig, B., Buser, P.T., Olschewski, M., Magosaki, N., Pfisterer, M., et al. Prognostic value of abnormal vasoreactivity of epicardial coronary arteries to sympathetic stimulation in patients with normal coronary angiograms. *Arterioscler.Thromb.Vasc.Biol.* 2003;23:495-501.

[159] Modena, M.G., Bonetti L, Coppi F, Bursi F, and Rossi R. Prognostic role of reversible endothelial dysfunction in hypertensive postmenopausal women. *J Am Coll.Cardiol.* 2002;40:505-10.

[160] Chan, S.Y., Mancini, G.B., Kuramoto, L., Schulzer, M., Frohlich, J., and Ignaszewski, A. The prognostic importance of endothelial dysfunction and carotid atheroma burden in patients with coronary artery disease. *J Am Coll.Cardiol.* 2003;42:1037-43.

[161] Fathi, R, Haluska, B, Isbel, N, Short, L, and Marwick, T.H. The relative importance of vascular structure and function in predicting cardiovascular events. *J Am Coll.Cardiol.* 2004;43:616-23.

[162] Dupuis, J, Tardif, J.C., Cernacek, P, and Theroux, P. Cholesterol reduction rapidly improves endothelial function after acute coronary syndromes. The RECIFE (reduction of cholesterol in ischemia and function of the endothelium) trial. *Circulation.* 1999;99(25):3227-33.

[163] Mullen, M.J., Wright, D., Donald, A.E., Thorne, S., Thomson, H., and Deanfield, J.E. Atorvastatin but not L-arginine improves endothelial function in type I diabetes mellitus: a double-blind study. *J Am Coll Cardiol.* 2000;36(2):410-6.

[164] Marchesi, S., Lupattelli, G., Siepi, D., et al. Short-term atorvastatin treatment improves endothelial function in hypercholesterolemic women. *J Cardiovasc Pharmacol.* 2000;36(5):617-21.

[165] van Venrooij, F.V., van de Ree, M.A., Bots, M.L., Stolk, R.P., Huisman, M.V., Banga, J.D.; and DALI Study Group. Aggressive lipid lowering does not improve endothelial function in type 2 diabetes: the Diabetes Atorvastatin Lipid Intervention (DALI) Study: a randomized, double-blind, placebo-controlled trial. *Diabetes Care.* 2002;25(7):1211-6.

[166] Beishuizen, E.D., Tamsma, J.T., Jukema, J.W., et al. The effect of statin therapy on endothelial function in type 2 diabetes without manifest cardiovascular disease. *Diabetes Care*. 2005;28(7):1668-74.

[167] Dupuis J, Tardif J.C., Rouleau J.L., et al. Intensity of lipid lowering with statins and brachial artery vascular endothelium reactivity after acute coronary syndromes (from the BRAVER trial) *Am J Cardiol*. 2005;96(9):1207-13.

[168] Kayikcioglu M, Payzin S, Yavuzgil O, Kultursay H, Can L.H., and Soydan I. Benefits of statin treatment in cardiac syndrome-X1. *Eur Heart J*. 2003;24(22):1999-2005.

[169] Taneva E, Borucki K, Wiens L, et al. Early effects on endothelial function of atorvastatin 40 mg twice daily and its withdrawal. *Am J Cardiol*. 2006;97(7):1002-6.

[170] McFarlane R, McCredie R.J, Bonney M.A et al. Angiotensin converting enzyme inhibition and arterial endothelial function in adults with type 1 diabetes mellitus. *Diabetic Medicine,* 1999;16:62–66.

[171] Kovacs I, Toth J, Tarjan J, Koller A. Correlation of flow mediated dilation with inflammatory markers in patients with impaired cardiac function. Beneficial effects of inhibition of ACE. *Eur J Heart Fail*. 2006;8(5):451-9.

[172] Mancini G.B, Henry G.C, Macaya C et al. Angiotensin-converting enzyme inhibition with quinapril improves endothelial vasomotor dysfunction in patients with coronary artery disease. The TREND (Trial on Reversing ENdothelial Dysfunction) Study. *Circulation*. 1996;94:258–265.

[173] Trevelyan J, Needham E.W, Morris A, Mattu R.K. Comparison of the effect of enalapril and losartan in conjunction with surgical coronary revascularization versus revascularisation alone on systemic endothelial function. *Heart*. 2005;91:1053–1057.

[174] Mullen M.J, Clarkson P, Donald A.F, et al. Effect of enalapril on endothelial function in young insulin-dependent diabetic patients: A randomized, double-blind study. *Journal of the American College of Cardiology*. 1998;31:1330–1335.

[175] O'Driscoll G, Green D, Rankin J, Stanton K, Taylor R. Improvement in endothelial function by angiotensin converting enzyme inhibition in insulin-dependent diabetes mellitus. *Journal of Clinical Investigation*. 1997;100:678–684.

In: Angina Pectoris: Etiology, Pathogenesis and Treatment ISBN: 978-1-60456-674-1
Editors: A. P. Gallo, M. L. Jones © 2008 Nova Science Publishers, Inc.

Chapter III

Kounis Syndrome (Allergic Angina and Allergic Myocardial Infarction)

Nicholas G. Kounis[1,*], Taxiarchis Kourelis[3], George Hahalis[2,†],
Akrivi Manola[3] and Theoharis C. Theoharides[3,‡]

[1] Department of Medical Sciences, School of Health Sciences, Patras Highest Institute of Education and Technology, Patras, Greece

[2] Department of Cardiology, Catheterization Laboratory, University of Patras Medical School, Rion, Patras, Greece

[3] Department of Pharmacology and Experimental Therapeutics, Tufts University School of Medicine, Boston, MA USA

Summary

Background

The concurrence of acute coronary syndromes with hypersensitivity reactions as well as anaphylactic or anaphylactoid insults is increasingly in clinical practice and there are several reports associating mast cell activation with acute cardiovascular events.

[*] Department of Medical Sciences, School of Health Sciences, Patras Highest Institute of Education and Technology, Queen Olgas Square, 7 Aratou Street, Patras 26221, Greece Phone: +30 2610 279579, Fax: +30 2610 279579, E-mail: ngkounis@otenet.gr

[†] Department of Cardiology, Catheterization Laboratory, University of Patras Medical School , Rion, Patras, Greece, Phone: + 30 2610 999111, Fax: +2610 279579, E-mail: ghahalis@otenet.gr

[‡] Department of Pharmacology and Experimental Therapeutics, Tufts University School of Medicine, 136 Harrison Avenue, Boston, MA 02111, USA, Phone: (617) 636-6866 Fax: (617) 636-2456, E-mail: theoharis.theoharides@tufts.edu

Definition

Kounis syndrome is the coincidental occurrence of acute coronary syndromes with hypersensitivity reactions involving activation of interrelated and interacting inflammatory cells and including allergic or hypersensitivity and anaphylactic or anaphylactoid insults. It is caused by inflammatory mediators such as histamine, neutral proteases, arachidonic acid products, platelet activating factor and a variety of cytokines and chemokines released during the hypersensitivity insult. All these inflammatory cells participate in a vicious inflammatory cycle and via multidirectional signals mast cells can enhance T cell activation, T cells can mediate mast cell proliferation and activation, inducible macrophage protein-1α can activate mast cells, mast cells can activate macrophages, and T cells can regulate macrophage activity.Clinical and experimental findings show that there is a common pathway between allergic and non allergic coronary events, because the same mediators from the same cells are present in both hypersensitivity episodes and acute coronary syndromes.

Variants

Type I variant: includes patients with normal coronary arteries without predisposing factors for coronary artery disease in whom the acute release of inflammatory mediators can induce either coronary artery spasm without increase of cardiac enzymes and troponins or coronary artery spasm progressing to acute myocardial infarction with raised cardiac enzymes and troponins

Type II variant: includes patients with culprit but quiescent pre-existing atheromatous disease in whom the acute release of inflammatory mediators can induce either coronary artery spasm with normal cardiac enzymes and troponins or plaque erosion or rupture manifesting as acute myocardial infarction.

Cardiac Actions of Main Mediators

Tryptase and chymase actions: Activate the zymogen forms of metalloproteinases such as interstitial collagenase, gelatinase, and stromelysin and can promote plaque disruption or rupture.

Furthermore, chymase converts angiotensin I to angiotensin II and angiotensin II receptors are found in the medial muscle cells of human coronary arteries. Thus, angiotensin II generated by chymase could act synergistically with histamine and aggravate the local spasm of the infarcted coronary artery.

Leukotrienes are powerful arterial vasoconstrictors and their biosynthesis is enhanced in the acute phase of unstable angina. Thromboxane is a potent mediator of platelet aggregation with vasoconstricting properties. Platelet activating factor: In myocardial ischemia acts as proadhesive signalling molecule or via activation of leucocytes and platelets to release other mediators. In experimental anaphylaxis reproduces the electrical and mechanical effects observed in allergic reactions such as ST changes and arrhythmias acting either through the release of leukotrienes or as a direct vasoconstrictor.

Histamine can induce: coronary vasoconstriction, intimal thickening, inflammatory cell modulation, platelet activation, proinflammatory cytokine production, p-selectine upregulation, sensitization of nerve ending in coronary plaques, tissue factor expression.

Clinical and Therapeutic Implications

Today, concern has been raised that intracoronary stents could be associated with in stent thrombosis, paradoxical coronary vasoconstriction and hypersensitivity reactions. Components of currently used DES have been reported to induce either separately or synergistically hypersensitivity reactions and in some occasions hypersensitivity cardiac events. Stent-activated intracoronary mast cells could release histamine, arachidonic acid metabolites, proteolytic enzymes such as tryptase and chymase, as well as a variety of cytokines -chemokines and platelet activating factor leading to local inflammation and thrombosis. These events may be more common than suspected because it is hard to document them, unless they become systemic, in which case they manifest as the Kounis syndrome. Recognition of this problem may lead to better vigilance, as well as new stent with mast cell blocking molecules that may also be disease modifying.

So far, attempts have been made to counteract the actions of the inflammatory mediators by using mediator antagonists, inhibitors of mediator biosynthesis and mediator receptor blockers. However, in the medical armamentarium there are drugs and natural molecules that are capable to stabilize and protect mast cell surface which could prevent also acute thrombotic events , at least in some instances. This has already been achieved experimentally.

Abreviations

CRH = corticotropin-releasing hormone
CSF = colony stimulating factor
CGRP = calcitonin gene related peptide
CTMC = connective tissue mast cells
EGF = endothelial growth factor
b-FGF = fibroblast growth factor
GM-CSF = granulocyte monocyte-colony
INFγ = Interferon-γ
MCP = monocyte chemotactic protein

MIF = macrophage inflammatory factor
MIP = monocyte inflammatory peptide
NGF = nerve growth factor
PACAP = Pituitary adenylate cyclase activating peptide
PAR = Protease activated receptor
SCF = Stem cell factor
TGF-β = transforming growth factor-β
TNF-α = tumor necrosis factor-α
VEGF = vascular endothelial growth factor

1. Definition

Kounis syndrome is the concurrence of acute coronary syndromes with conditions associated with mast cell activation, involving interrelated and interacting inflammatory cells, and including allergic or hypersensitivity and anaphylactic or anaphylactoid insults. It is caused by inflammatory mediators such as histamine, neutral proteases, arachidonic acid products, platelet activating factor and a variety of cytokines and chemokines released during the activation process.

Mast cells enter the circulation from bone marrow as mononuclear cell precursors that both express messenger ribonucleic acid (mRNA) for stem cell factor and have SCF receptors on their cell membrane. They migrate into the tissues, including the brain which does not suffer from allergic reactions because IgE does not cross the blood-brain barrier, where the differentiate and mature. This takes several days to weeks.

On the other hand, basophils developing in bone marrow from granulocyte precursors and entering the circulation only when fully mature. They are not normally found in extravascular tissues compartments, only migrating there during late-phase allergic responses.

2. Historical Background

Although, the coincidental occurrence of acute coronary syndromes with allergic or hypersensitivity as well as with anaphylactic or anaphylactoid reactions is increasingly encountered in clinical practice it was only until 1950 when several reports associating mast cell activation with acute cardiovascular events started to appear in the medical literature (Table 1).

Table 1. Historical background of Kounis syndrome

1950	Pfister CW, et al.	Acute myocardial infarction during a prolonged allergic reaction to penicillin. Am Heart J 1950; 40: 945
1965	Zosin P, et al.	Allergic myocardial infarction. Romanian Medical Review 1965;19: 26
1991	Kounis NG, et al.	Histamine-induced coronary artery spasm: the syndrome of allergic angina. Br J Clin Pract 1991; 45: 121
1995	Constantinides P.	"Allergic reactions can promote plaque disruption" Circulation 1995; 92: 1083
1996	Kounis NG, et al.	Allergic angina and allergic myocardial infarction. Circulation 1996; 94: 1789
1998	Braunwald E.	"Allergic reactions with mediators such as histamine or leukotrienes acting on coronary smooth muscle can induce vasospastic angina" Circulation 1998;98: 2219
2003	Zavras GM, et al.	Kounis syndrome secondary to allergic reaction. Int J Clin Pract 2003; 57: 62
2006	Kounis NG.	Kounis syndrome. Int J Cardiol 2006; 119: 7
2006	Kounis NG, et al.	Hypersensitivity to DES: a manifestation of Kounis syndrome? J Am Coll Cardiol 2006; 48: 592
2007	Kounis NG, et al.	Coronary stents, Hypersensitivity and the Kounis Syndrome. J Interv Cardiol 2007; 20: 314
2008	Tavil Y, et al.	Kounis syndrome secondary to amoxicillin/clavulanic acid use. Int J Cardiol 2008 Feb 20; 124: e4

In 1991, Kounis and Zavras [1] described the "syndrome of allergic angina" as the coincidental occurrence of chest pain and allergic reactions accompanied by clinical and laboratory findings of classical angina pectoris caused by inflammatory mediators released during the allergic insult Allergic angina can progress to acute myocardial infarction which was named "allergic myocardial infarction" [2-4]. Following this clinical description, Constantinides [5], in 1995, raised the possibility that "even ordinary allergic reactions could promote plaque disruption". In 1998, Braunwald [6], in an editorial, noted that vasospastic angina can be induced by "allergic reactions with mediators such as histamine or leukotrienes acting on coronary vascular smooth muscle".

Today, allergic angina and allergic myocardial infarction are referred as "Kounis syndrome" [7-13] and are cited in major cardiovascular textbooks [14], as a new cause of coronary artery spasm.

3. Kounis Syndrome Variants

There are two variants of this syndrome that have been described recently [15]. Type I variant includes patients with normal coronary arteries without predisposing factors for coronary artery disease in whom the acute allergic insult induces either coronary artery spasm with normal cardiac enzymes and troponins or coronary artery spasm progressing to acute myocardial infarction with raised cardiac enzymes and troponins. This variant might represent a manifestation of endothelial dysfunction or microvascular angina. Type II variant includes patients with culprit but quiescent pre-existing atheromatous disease in whom acute allergic episode can induce plaque erosion or rupture manifesting as an acute myocardial infarction. Kounis syndrome is regarded as magnificent natural paradigm and nature's own experiment [7-13] which may shed light on potential therapeutic strategies that may apply to the area of interference with plaque erosion or rupture and primary as well as secondary prevention of acute coronary and cerebrovascular events.

4. Mast Cell Activation-Degranulation

Mast cells are derived from a distinct precursor in the bone marrow and mature under local tissue micro environmental factors [16, 17]. These cells are found in most parts of the human body, including heart and vessels, and are involved in allergic and anaphylactic reactions through activation-degranulation. This activation-degranulation is taking place via the following mechanisms:

1) IgE mediated cross linking of Fce receptor I (i.e. the high affinity IgE receptors) [18],
2) by histamine-releasing factors secreted by neighbouring macrophages [19] or T-lymphocytes [20] and
3) by anaphylatoxin components of the complement system (C3a, C5a) [21], by many neuropeptides and bacterial products through Toll-like receptors [22] and by drugs such as opioids [23] or analgesics such as high doses of acetylsalicylic acid [24]. Endothelin also activates cardiac mast cells and this is regarded as a potential mechanism responsible for myocardial remodeling [25].

Upon their activation, mast cells release the contents of their granules by two separate mechanisms which may operate individually or in parallel:

1) a rapid process of anaphylactic degranulation [26],
2) a slow process of piecemeal degranulation or intra-granular activation or differential or selective release [27]. During the latter, mast cells appear to undergo ultra structural alterations of their electron dense granules indicative of secretion but without overt degranulation. Such subtle mast cell activation may be associated with the ability of mast cells to release some mediators selectively such us eicosanoids [28] and interleukin-6 [29]. In fact, it has been shown that interleukin-1 can stimulate human mast cells to release interleukin-6, without degranulation, through unique process utilizing 40-80 nm vesicles unrelated to secretory granules [30].

Mast cells are an additional source of renin and constitute a unique extrarenal renin-angiotensin system [31]. Furthermore, preformed angiotensin II and gene expression of the renin-angiotensin system have been detected in human mast cells [32].

In anaphylaetic degranulation several vasoconstricting and collagen degrading compounds are released locally and in the peripheral circulation. These compounds include preformed mediators such as, histamine, neutral proteases (tryptase, chymase, cathepsin-D), platelet activating factor and newly synthesized mediators such us an array of cytokines and chemokines and others by the metabolism of arachidonic acid through activation of a phospholipase. The latter include leukotrienes by the lipoxygenase pathway and prostaglandins such as thromboxane by cycloxygenase pathway. These mediators have been incriminated, in many clinical and experimental studies to induce, coronary artery spasm and/or acute myocardial infarction.

Cardiac mast cell-derived histamine can (Table 2 and Table 3) constrict the coronary arteries [33] and sensitize nerve endings [34] localized close to adventitial mast cells in atherosclerotic coronary arteries [35]. Apart from being powerful coronary vasoconstrictor, histamine can activate platelets and potentiates the aggregatory response of other agonists including adrenaline, 5-hydroxytryptamine, and thrombin [36-38]; it modulates the activity of inflammatory cells such as neutrophils [39], monocytes [40], and eosinophils [41]. Moreover, histamine induces proinflammatory cytokine production from endothelial cells [42], upregulates P-selectin on the endothelial cell surface [43, 44], and induces intimal thickening in a mouse model of thrombosis [45]. Cardiac histamine and interleukin-6 can be released by acute stress and this may help explain stress-related coronary inflammation [46, 47]. Stress and corticotropin-releasing hormone activate human mast cells to release vascular endothelial growth factor selectively [48, 49].

Table 2. Histamine: Effects of H1, H2, H3 and H4 receptors

	H1-receptors	H2-receptors	H3-receptors	H4-receptors
Coronary arteries	Mediate contraction	Mediate relaxation	Inhibit endogenous norepinephrine release and enhance the degree of shock during anaphylaxis	Control chemotaxis of mast cells and eosinophils and the release of Interleukin-I6
Sinus node-Atria	Do not affect the rate. Do not affect inotropic action. Do not affect chronotropic action.	Increase sinus rate stimulation. Positive inotropic action. Positive chronotropic action.		
Ventricles	Do not affect inotropic action. Do not affect chronotropic action. Do not affect auromatically.	Positive inotropic action. Positive chronotropic action. Increase automatically.		
AV conduction	Slow AV conduction	Attenuate the response to sympathetic stimulation		

Table 3. Cardiac effects of histamine

- Coronary vasoconstriction
- Activates platelets and potentiates the aggregatory response of agonists e.g. adrenaline, 5-hydroxytryptamine, and thrombin
- Intimal thickening
- Inflammatory cell modulation
- Modulates the activity of neutrophils, monocytes, and eosinophils
- Platelet activation
- Proinflammatory cytokine production
- P-selectine upregulation
- Sensitizites nerve endings in coronary plaques
- Tissue factor expression

A novel action of histamine is the induction of tissue factor expression and activity in human aortic endothelial cells and human vascular smooth muscle cells [50]. Tissue factor is a key enzyme in the activation of coagulation. It binds activated factor VII, which in turn activates factor X leading to thrombin formation. Elevated tissue factor antigen and activity have been detected in plasma and in atherectomy specimens of patients with unstable angina

[51] denoting that tissue factor is involved in the initiation and propagation of acute coronary syndromes. This effect of histamine is completely abolished by H1 receptor antagonists [50].

Table 4. Cardiac actions of proteases, leukotrienes, thromboxane, platelet activating factor

Tryptase

1. Activates the zymogen forms of metalloproteinases such as interstitial collagenase, gelatinase, and stromelysin and can promote plaque disruption or rupture.
2. Degrates the pericellular matrix components fibronectin and vitronectin and neuropeptides, such as vasoactive intestinal peptide (VIP) and calcitonin gene related peptide (CGRP)
3. Activates neighboring cells by cleaving and activating protease-activated receptor (PAR)-2, and thrombin receptors
4. Tryptase can degrade HDL

Chymase

1. Converts angiotensin I to angiotensin II and angiotensin II receptors are found in the medial muscle cells of human coronary arteries. Thus, angiotensin II generated by chymase could act synergistically with histamine and aggravate the local spasm of the infarcted coronary artery. Chymase also can remove cholesterol from HDL
2. Activates MMP-1,-2,-9 and plays a major role in the physiologic degradation of fibronectin and thrombin
3. Releases latent TGF-β1 from the extracellular matrix
4. Inhibits smooth muscle growth
5. Induces apoptosis of arterial smooth muscle cells and endothelial cells

Cathepsin D

1. Elastolytic, angiotensin II-forming protease
2. Degrates both fibronectin and VE-cadherin which are necessary for adhesion of endothelial cells to their basement membrane and to each other

Leukotrienes

Powerful arterial vasoconstrictors and their biosynthesis is enhanced in the acute phase of unstable angina.

Thromboxane

A potent mediator of platelet aggregetion with vasoconstricting properies.

Platelet Activating Factor

In myocardial ischemia acts as proadhesive signalling molecule or vial activation of leucocytes and platelets to release other mediators. In experimental anaphylaxix reproduces the electrical and mechanical efforts observed in allergic reactions such as ST changes and arrhythmias acting either through the release of leukotrienes or as a direct vasoconstrictor.

Tryptase and chymase (Table 4) effectively activate the zymogen forms of metalloproteinases such as interstitial collagenase, gelatinase and stromelysin found in atheromatous plaques and play an important role in atheromatous plaque erosion or rupture [52]. Chymase converts angiotensin I to angiontensin II and angiotensin II receptors are found in the medial muscle cells of human coronary arteries. Thus, the angiotensin II generated by chymase released from mast cells could act synergistically with histamine and aggravate the local spasm of the infarcted coronary artery [53]. Platelet activating factor (PAF) has been implicated in acute myocardial ischemia either as proadhesive signaling molecule or through activation of leucocytes and platelets to release other mediators [54]. Leukotrienes are powerful arterial vasoconstrictors and enhance leukotriene biosynthesis has been detected during the acute phase of unstable angina [55]. Thromboxane is a potent mediator of platelet aggregation and has vasoconstricting properties [56]. Moreover, during experimental anaphylaxis, PAF reproduces the mechanical and electrical changes observed during allergic reactions such as ischemic S-T segment changes and arrhythmias [57, 58]. During these experiments, PAF acted either through the release of leukotrienes and thromboxane [59] or directly producing vasoconstriction [60].

Mast cells are important for allergic reactions [61], but also in immunity [62-64] and inflammatory conditions [65- 67]. Mast cells develop from CD 34+,c-kit+ progenitor cells that arise from hematopoietic stem cells in the bone marrow [68]. These progenitor cells express the receptor c-kit for Stem Cell Factor (SCF), which has growth, differentiate and chemoattractant properties for mast cells. Mast cell progenitors have also been described in the peripheral blood [69, 70]. Mast cells mature in tissues depending on microenvironmental conditions. In addition to SCF, mast cell chemoattractants include, nerve growth factor (NGF) [71], RANTES (Regulated on Activation, Normal T Cell Expressed and Secreted) (CCL5) and MCP 1(Mast Cell Protein) (CCL2) [72, 73]. Several cytokines play an important role in mast cell differentiation and proliferation. IL-3 directly stimulates proliferation of uncommitted progenitors and directly promotes granule assembly [74]. IL-4 possesses mast cell growth factor activity [75], can promote phenotype switching to connective tissue-type mast cells [76], and enhances expression of neuropeptide receptors [77]. Mature mast cells vary considerably [78] in their cytokine [79] and proteolytic enzyme content. However, the phenotypic expression of mast cells does not appear to be fixed [75, 80]. In fact, brain mast cells in normal rodents lack c-kit receptor [81] and FcεRI proteins [82].

Mast cells are located perivascularly [83] in close proximity to neurons [84-90], in particular close to CRH-positive neurons in the rat median eminence [91].

5. Mast Cell Triggers

Mast cells are well known to be stimulated by IgE and antigen through aggregation of their specific receptors (FcεR1) [92, 93]. However there are numerous additional mast cell triggers (Table 5). These include immunoglobulin free light chains [94-96], anaphylatoxins, cytokines, hormones, neuropeptides, toxins and a number of drugs [67, 90, 97-102]. Neuropeptide triggers include substance P(SP) [103-105], neurotensin (NT) [106], nerve growth factor (NGF) [84, 107], which is released under stress [108], hemokinin [109], and pituitary adenylate cyclase activating polypeptide (PACAP) [110, 111], SCF and IL-6 have been shown to induce IL-6 release without degranulation. IL-33 is a recently identified member of the IL-1 family of molecules that can induce cytokine production in human mast cells even in the absence of FceRI aggregation [112]. IL-33 induced IL-6 and IL-1b production by P815 mastocytoma and bone marrow mast cells(BMMC).Stimulation of BMMC with IL-33 for 24 h significantly increased TNF-α and MCP-1 secretion, as well as IL-2 secretion and PGD-2 [113, 114]. IL-33 induced IL-13 production by mouse mast cells independently of IgE-FcεRI signals [115]. IL-33 enhanced the survival of naive human umbilical cord blood mast cells(HUCBMC) and promoted their adhesion to fibronectin; it

Table 5. Mast cell triggers

I. Natural

A. Immunologic
Anaphylatoxins (C3a, C5a)
CGRP
IgG 1 + IgE
IL-1
IL-33
Immunoglobulin – free light chains
PAF
PGE 2
Superallergens
MCP -1,-2,-3
MIP-1 Table 1. Mast cell Triggers

B. Neuropeptides /Neurotransmitters
Acetylcholine
Adrenomedullin
Bombesin
PACAP
Somatostatin
S P
VIP

C. Growth Factors
NGF
SCF
Lymphopoietin

D. Hormones
CRH
Ucn

E. Infectious
LPS (TLR 4)
Peptidoglycan (TLR 2)
Viral antigens (TLR 3,5,7,9)

F. Toxins
Fire ants
Jelly fish
Snake venoms
Wasps

G. Vascular
Adenosine
Endothelin
Oxidized LDL
Reactive oxygen species
Thrombin

II. Drugs
Adenosine
Contrast media
Curare
Ibuprofen (high doses)
Morphine

also induced IL-8 and IL-13 production in naïve HUCBMCs, and enhanced production of these cytokines in IgE/anti-IgE-stimulated HUCBMCs [112]. IL-33 also acts both alone and in concert with thymic stromal lymphopoietin (TSL) to accelerate the in vitro maturation of CD34(+) mast cell precursors and induce the secretion of Th2 cytokines and Th2-attracting chemokines [116]. TSL is considered a "master switch" in allergic inflammation [117] and in airway inflammation [118, 119]. IL-33 also increased mast cell response (TSL), a recently described potent mast cell activator [120].Adrenomedullin (AM) is a peptide that has been found to be involved in carcinogenesis [121], in the regulation of macrophage [122] and mast cell activation [123], as well as in complement fixation [124]. AM induced histamine [123] or beta-hexosaminidase [65] release from rat and human mast cell through a receptor-independent pathway. In a recent study, mast cells in the vicinity of tumors were shown to produce AM [125]. In the same study, AM was found to be chemotactic for human mast cell and stimulated mRNA expression of VEGF, MCP-1, and basic fibroblast growth factor (FGF) in this cell type; differentiated, but not undifferentiated human mast cell, responded to hypoxia with elevated AM mRNA/protein expression.

OxLDL has been implicated in the pathogenesis of atherosclerosis and has been shown to induce microvascular dysfunction through degranulation of mast cells [126]. OxLDL activates mast cells by increasing mRNA and protein levels of interleukin IL-8 [127].

Superallergens are proteins of various origins able to activate FcεRI+ cells (mast cells and basophils) through interaction with membrane-bound IgE. Several superallergens have been reported. Protein Fv, a sialoprotein produced in the human liver and released in biological fluids during viral hepatitis, is the most potent IgE-mediated stimulus for the activation of human basophils, as well as lung [128] and heart [129] mast cells. Other allergens include protein L, a bacterial cell-wall component that causes release of several mediators by human heart mast cells, as well as antigens of the HIV virus and Staphylococcus aureus [130].

Mast cells have been found to synthesize and secrete endothelins (ET) and also have ET receptors, therefore suggesting an autocrine path of action [131]. ET are cytokine-like agents that can be synthesized and bound by a large number of different cell types. Their role in the immune system and in the pathophysiology of different diseases is thus complicated [132]. There are 3 different ET peptides, ET1 ET2 and ET 3, as well as two different receptors ET-A and ET-B. ET-1 caused degranulation of fetal skin mast cell (FSMC), but not BMMC through ET(A)-mediated pathways; furthermore, ET-1 induced TNF-alpha and IL-6 production by FSMC, but not by BMMC, and significantly enhanced VEGF production and TGF-beta1 mRNA expression by FSMC. Finally, ET-1 was produced by FSMC, but not by BMMC in response to Toll-like receptor ligands [133]. A recent study [134] showed that mast cells may be implicated in preventing ET-1 toxicity through ET-1 degradation by chymase.

TLRs were shown to be important in recognition of ligands associated with bacterial or viral infections, and play a key role in the development of adaptive immune responses [135, 136] especially in asthma [137]. Ten human TLRs have been identified so far [136, 138, 139]. Rodent mast cells express bacterial Toll-like receptors (TLR) 2 and 4 [140, 141]. Human mast cells express viral TLR-9 [82], activation of which produced IL-6 [142], while TLR-3 activation produced IFN [143]. Lipopolysaccharide (LPS) induced TNF release of through TLR-4, while peptidoglycan induced histamine release through TLR-2 from rodent mast cells. Fetal rat skin-derived mast cells express TLR 3, 7 and 9 and activation by CPG oligodeoxynucleotide induces release of TNF and IL-6, as well as RANTES and MIP, but without degranulation [144, 145]. LPS could not induce release of GM-CSF, IL-1 or LTC$_4$ [81]. However, LPS did induce secretion of TH2 cytokines, IL-5, IL-10 and IL-13 and increased their production by FcεRI cross-linking [146]. Elsewhere, it was shown that TLR-2 activation produced IL-4, IL-6 and IL-13, but not IL-1 [147], while LPS produced TNF, IL-1, IL-6 and IL-13, but not IL-4 or IL-5, without degranulation [147].

CRH [148] and it structurally related peptide, urocortin (Ucn) [149] can activate skin mast cells and induce mast-cell dependent vascular permeability in rodents. CRH also increases vascular permeability in human skin [150], a process dependent on mast cells. CRH-2 receptor expression was shown to be upregulated in stress-induced alopecia in humans [151], while CRHR-1 expression was increased in chronic urticaria [152]. Acute restraint stress induces rat skin vascular permeability [153], an effect inhibited by a CRH receptor antagonist and absent in mast cell deficient mice [154]. Histamine is a major regulator of the hypothalamus [154] and can increase its CRH mRNA expression [155]. Moreover, human mast cells can synthesize and secrete large amounts of CRH [156], as well as IL-1 and IL-6 which are independent activators of the HPA axis [157].

Mast cells are frequently found in close proximity to mucosal nerves and vagal nerves have been reported to influence mast cells [158]. Very early studies have shown that vagal stimulation causes mast cells to degranulate [159, 160] in the gastrointestinal mucosa of rats and guinea pigs [161, 162]. Mediators released from mast cells such as histamine can then cause vagal stimulation [163, 164]. It has been, therefore, hypothesized that there is crosstalk between mast cells and nerves in vitro[165-166] and in the CNS [167]. A reversible increase of the surface of rat mesenteric mast cells was noted after vagal stimulation,feeding or even oldfactory stimulation of the animals [168]. Mast cell stabilizing agents reduced the bronchoconstriction caused by SP and neurokinin A and E [169]. In another study, histamine and serotonin released from the rat perfused heart by compound 48/80 or by allergen challenge increased noradrenaline or acetylcholine exocytotic release [170]. Vagal stimulation has also been found to exert a trophic effect on mast cells [171].

A number of drugs can also stimulate mast cells [Table 5], best known of which is morphine [172].

6. Mast Cell Mediators

Mast cells can secrete a multitude of biologically potent mediators (Table 6) that permit them to participate in innate or acquired immunity [64, 65, 173]. There are various vasodilatory and proinflammatory mediators, such as the preformed histamine, heparin, kinins, proteases, as well as the newly synthesized leukotrienes, prostaglandins, nitric oxide (NO) and cytokines [174-176].

A number of growth factors are also secreted such as Vascular Endothelial Growth Factor (VEGF) [65, 177, 178], which has been shown to be released selectively in response to PGE2 [179], adenosine [180] and CRH [181]. VEGF was specifically shown to induce dilation of microvessels [182].

Table 6. Mast Cell Mediators and their actions

Mediators	Main Pathophysiologic Effects
Prestored	
Biogenic Amines	
Histamine	Vasodilation, angiogenesis, mitogenesis,pain
5-Hydroxytryptamine (5-HT, serotonin)	Vasoconstriction, pain
Chemokines	
IL-8 (CXCL8), MCP-1 (CCL2),	
MCP-3 (CCL7), MCP-4 (CXCL13),	
RANTES (CCL5)	Chemoattraction and tissue infiltration of leukocytes
Enzymes	
Arylsulfatases	Lipid/proteoglycan hydrolysis
Carboxypeptidase A	Peptide processing
Chymase	Tissue damage, pain, angiotensin II synthesis
Kinogenases	Synthesis of vasodilatory kinins, pain
Mediators	*Main Pathophysiologic Effects*
Metalloproteinases	Tissue damage
Phospholipases	Arachidonic acid generation
Tryptase	Tissue damage, activation of PAR, inflammation,pain
Peptides/Proteins	
Corticotropin-releasing hormone (CRH)	Inflammation, vasodilation
Endorphins	Analgesia
Endothelin	Sepsis
Kinins (bradykinin)	Inflammation, pain, vasodilation
Neurotensin	Inflammation, pain
Renin(CTMC only)	Vascular contriction
Somatostatin (SRIF)	Anti-inflammatory (?)
Substance P (SP)	Inflammation, pain
Vasoactive intestinal peptide (VIP)	Vasodilation
Urocortin	Inflammation, vasodilation
Vascular endothelial growth factor (VGEF)	Neovascularization, vasodilation
Proteoglycans	
Chondroitin sulfate	Cartilage synthesis, anti-inflammatory
Heparin	Angiogenesis, NGF stabilization

Table 6. Mast Cell Mediators and their actions (Continued)

Mediators	*Main Pathophysiologic Effects*
Hyaluronic acid	Connective tissue
Angiogenic factors	
Adrenomedullin	
Angiogenin	
Angiopoietin	
EGF	
FGF α	
basic FGF	
IL-8	
Neuropillin	
PDGF	
TGF β	
VEGF	
De novo synthesized	
Cytokines	
Interleukins (IL)- 1,2,3,4,5,6,8,10,13,16,17,32	Inflammation, leukocyte migration, pain
IFN-γ; MIF; TNF-α,TGF-beta	Inflammation,leucocyte, proliferation, activation
Growth Factors	
SCF, GM-CSF, b-FGF, NGF, VEGF	Growth of a variety of cells
Phospholipid metabolites	
Leukotriene B_4 LTB_4	Leukocyte chemotaxis
Leukotriene C_4 (LTC_4)	Vasoconstriction, pain
Platelet activating factor (PAF)	Platelet activation, vasodilation
Prostaglandin D_2 (PGD_2)	Bronchonstriction, pain
Others	
Nitric oxide (NO)	Vasodilation
ROS	Inflammation

Proteases released from mast cells could act on plasma albumin to generate histamine releasing peptides [183, 184] that could further propagate mast cell activation and inflammation. Proteases could also stimulate protease activated receptors (PAR) inducing microleakage and widespread inflammation [185, 186]. Proteases can activate fibroblasts thereby promoting collagen deposition and fibrosis.

Reactive oxygen species (ROS) are produced in cells by a variety of enzymatic and non-enzymatic mechanisms. In a very early study, immunologic or nonimmunologic stimulation of rat peritoneal and human lung mast cells, as well as human leukemic basophils, induced parallel release of histamine and O(-) (2) within 2 min [187].

An increase in intracellular ROS production was observed in rat peritoneal mast cells (RPMCs) following stimulation with antigen [188-190], compound 48/80 [188-190] the calcium ionophore A23187 [190], SP [188], and NGF [188]. In contrast D-mannitol increased ROS production in stimulated mast cells without a marked effect on degranulation or histamine secretion [130].

In addition, chemicals such as mercuric chloride [191], silver [192], ionophore [193], phorbol myristate acetate (PMA) [144], vitamin K [195], silica [196], as well as bacteria [197] and fungal components [198] can produce ROS in mast cells. Recently it was reported that 5-Lipoxygenase (5-LO) was the primary enzyme involved in ROS production by human mast cells and mouse BMMC following FcεRI aggregation. Cyclooxygenase was also involved in ROS production, whereas NADPH oxidase was not [199].

Several studies implicate mast cells in the induction of intestinal ischemia reperfusion (IR) injury [200-202]. It has been shown that ROS play an essential role in the activation of mast cells in IR[203, 204]. Mast cell activation is also important in IR injury of the heart. In one study, use of the mast cell stabilizer cromolyn significantly reduced, while activation by compound 48/80 increased IR-dependent histamine levels [205].

In a model of myocardial ischemia and reperfusion injury in rat heart muscle cells in vivo, a superoxide dismutase mimetic significantly reduced myocardial damage, mast cell degranulation and the incidence of ventricular arrhythmias [206].

7. Selective Release of Mast Cell Mediator

Mast cell have been reported to secrete without degranulation but through ultrastructural alterations of the cell electron dense granular core indicative of secretion. This process has been termed "activation" [62, 207, 208], "intragranular activation" [89] or "piecemeal" degranulation [209]. During this process, mast cells can release many mediators differentially or selectively (Table 7) [210-212] as originally shown for serotonin [213] and eicosanoids [214-216]. IL-6 was shown to be released in response to IL-1 through small vesicles (40-80 nm in diameter), unrelated to the secretory granules (800-1000 nm) in diamerter [217]. VEGF could also be released selectively without degranulation by CRH [218]. PGE2 also induced VEGF release from human mast cells without degranulation [169], while adenosine induced selective release of the angiogenic factors IL-8 and VEGF [180].The only way to explain these observations would be through the ability of mast cells to undergo "differential" or "selective" release of mediators [213] without degranulation[219].

Exosomes are small, 30–100 nm membrane vesicles, which are released extracellularly after fusion of multivesicular endosomes with the cell membrane. They have emerged as a novel mechanism of genetic exchange since it has been shown that they are involved in transferring mRNAs and microRNAs between cells [220].

Exosomes containing MHC II antigens have been shown to be released by mast cells during degranulation[221]. In another study, it was demonstrated that mast cell associated exosomes induce immature dendritic cells (DCs) to up-regulate MHC class II, CD80, CD86, and CD40 molecules and to acquire potent Ag-presenting capacity to T cells [222].

Table 7. Mechanisms of mast cell secretion

Degranulation	Anaphylaxis
Selective release	Infection, Inflammation
Piecemeal degranulation	MS, scleroderma
Exosomes	Infection
Transgranulation	Brain

Exosomes have been implicated in the induction of tolerance in the gut epithelium towards food antigens [223], and in the maintenance of pregnancy [224] by several mechanisms.

8. Natural Mast Cell Secretion Inhibitors

There are no, so far, effective clinically available mast cell inhibitors (Table 8, Table 9). Disodium cromoglycate (cromolyn) is a potent inhibitor of rodent mast cell histamine secretion [225], but very weak inhibitor of human mast cells [66].

Table 8. Natural mast cell inhibitors

Chondroitin Sulfate
Flavonoids (luteolin,quercetin)
Heparin
Nitric Oxide
Somatostatin (mucosal must cells only)
Vitamin A (retinoic acid)
Vitamin E (tocopherol)

In the human mastocytoma cell line (HMC-1), vitamin E inhibits the PI3K/PKB signaling pathway with consequent inhibition of proliferation and reduced survival [226].

Vitamin E inhibits protein kinase C (PKC),which is involved in degranulation and cytokine production [227]. In many studies, vitamin E reduced mast cell degranulation by scavenging free radicals. However vitamin E also reduces the production of free radicals by NADPH-oxidase [228] or mitochondria [229], activates several drug-metabolizing enzymes (cytochrome P450 CYP3A and CYP4F2) 230], and modulates signal transduction and gene expression[171], suggesting that it may have additional modes of action.

Retinoic acid was also shown to inhibit proliferation of leukemic mast cells [232, 233].

Middleton and colleagues first showed that certain flavonoids could inhibit rodent mast cell secretion [234]. Flavonoids are polyphenolic compounds present in fruit, vegetables, nuts, seeds, wine, tea, and coffee with anti-oxidant and anti-inflammatory actions [234].

Table 9. Agents capable to stabilize mast cells

1. Simultaneous inhibition of H1 and H2
2. Lodoxamide
3. Sodium nedocromil (intal)
4. Sodium cromoglycate (lomuntal)
5. Ketotifen-H1-blocker (Zaditen)
6. Flavonoid quercetin (intacellular Ca)
7. Flavone luteolin inhibits T-cells, mast cells and mast cell-dependent T-cell activation
8. Relaxin (hormone from corpus luteus and prostate, generates NO)
9. IgG1 humanized monoclonal antibodies recognizing and masking corresponding IgEs in mast cell membrane)
10. NO inhibits IL-6 production through TNF-α inhibition
11. Peptides from C3α, C3α+, C3α9+, inhibit FcεRI-induced degranulation and TNF-α release
12. Zaprinast (phosphodiesterase inhibitor)
13. Stem cell factor (SCF) targeting drugs, since SCF is essential for mast cell development, proliferation, survival, adhesion, and homing

Kimata et al. [235] reported that luteolin, quercetin and baicalein inhibited the release of histamine, leukotrienes and prostaglandin D2, as well as the secretion of granulocyte macrophage-colony stimulating factor by human cultured mast cells in response to cross-linkage of FcεRI and subsequently showed that these compounds also inhibited IgE-mediated TNF-α and IL-6 production by bone marrow-derived cultured murine mast cells. It was also shown quercetin and other flavonoids could inhibit histamine, IL-6, IL-8, TNF-α and tryptase from IgE-stimulated human mast cells [236]. The same flavonoids could also inhibit leukemic mast cell proliferation [237].

Chondroitin sulphate, a major natural constituent of connective tissues, especially cartilage, and of mast cell secretory granules, had a dose-dependent inhibitory effect on rat peritoneal mast cell release of histamine induced by compound 48/80; this inhibition was stronger than that of the clinically available mast cell 'stabilizer' cromolyn. Moreover, inhibition by chondroitin sulphate increased with the length of preincubation and persisted after the drug was washed off, while the effect of cromolyn was limited by rapid tachyphylaxis [238].

Chondroitin sulphate's inhibitory actions have been recently tested with a traditional Korean formulation, OK205, which includes of water-soluble chitosan, glucosamine HCl, chondroitin sulfate used to treat rheumatoid arthritis. Choi et al [239] tested the inhibitory effects of OK205 on cytokine production in a human mast cell line (HMC-1 cells) and reported a decrease in production of TNF-α and IL-6. Heparin, the structure of which is quite similar to that of chondroitin sulphate and is also stored in mast cells, had been shown to inhibit in vivo release of histamine [240].

IL-10 inhibits the release of TNF-α and of IL-8, but not of IL-5, by activated CBMC. Interestingly, IL-10 also inhibits the release of histamine by activated CBMC, contrasting with data reported for rodent mast cell. These findings suggest that IL-10 might have anti-inflammatory effects on IgE/anti-IgE-challenged human mast cell by inhibiting their release of TNF-alpha, IL-8 and histamine [241]. However other studies have reported lack of an inhibitory action on human mast cell tryptase and IL-6 release [242], suggesting there may be species differences.

TGF-1b acts as a novel potent inhibitor and modulator of human intestinal mast cell effector functions [243]. It has also been found to downregulate FcERI expression [184] in mouse mast cells. This inhibition of mast cell function induced by TGF-1b might be of use in the control of mast cell associated disorders of the intestine such as allergic reactions, Crohn's disease, irritable bowel syndrome, and parasitic infection.

Somatostatin is an important regulator in the neuroendocrine-immune network. Several studies have shown that somatostatin inhibits mast cell activity and could prevent the intestinal responses to mast cell hyperplasia [245, 246]. In contrast, somatostatin was shown to stimulate connective tissue mast cells in vitro [214, 247].

Nitric oxide is a gas and free radical that has important physiological roles including defense against microorganisms, but also regulation of cellular activation[248] and gene expression [249]. It has been demonstrated that mast cells express NO synthases (NOS) and produce NO themselves[250]. Importantly, it has been shown that NO directly inhibits IgE depended mast cell degranulation [251, 252]. Endogenous and exogenous NO protects against IR injury in isolated guinea pig hearts; perfusion of the hearts with two inhibitors of the NOS pathway, (L-NMMA and L-NAME) significantly enhanced histamine and LDH release; these effects were attenuated by co-infusion with L-arginine. Perfusion of the heart with sodium nitroprusside (SNP), 3-morpholinosydnonimine (SIN-1), glyceryl trinitrate (GTN), reduced histamine release, effects that were amplified by concomitant perfusion with superoxide dismutase [253, 254]. Endogenous and exogenous NO inhibits mast cell degranulation and protease release [255], adherence to fibronectin [256], leukotriene [257], cytokine, and chemokine production [258, 259]. NOS-2 can be induced in response to pregnancy, IR injury, angiogenesis, antibody against CD8, and liver cirrhosis, as well as by several inflammatory stimuli such as IFN-γ, IL-1β and crosslinking of IgE on mast cell [258]. Recent data suggest that NO protects mast cells from activation-induced cell death [260]. Studies have also shown that the stabilizing effect of NO on mast cells may have a cardioprotective role [261].

9. Coronary Inflammation

The presence of mast cells has been established in human heart tissue [262, 263]. Their location and certain cytokines produced by mast cells, suggested they play an important role in cardiac diseases [264]. Mast cells are particularly prominent in coronary arteries during spasm [265] and accumulate in the shoulder region of human coronary plaque rupture [261-263].

Many mediators released from cardiac mast cells, such as TNF, basic fibroblast growth factor (bFGF or FGF-2), and transforming growth factor-β (TGF-β) could influence cardiovascular pathophysiology (Table 5). Cardiac mast cells can participate in the development of atherosclerosis, coronary inflammation and cardiac ischemia [262, 266-268]. Chymase can also induce the removal of cholesterol from HDL particles and increase uptake by macrophages that become "foam" cells, major components of coronary atheromas [269-272]. They do this, by impairing the ability of HDL to act as a high affinity cholesterol receptor [273] and destabilizing the LDL bound to the heparin proteoglycan component of the exocytosed granules of mast cells and by this way promoting LDL retention in the arterial intima [273]. Cardiac mast cell-derived histamine [274] can constrict the coronaries [275] and can sensitize nerve endings [164].

In a systematic study of the population density of mast cell in human coronary atherosclerosis, fewer mast cells were found in normal coronary intima, than in fatty streaks [266]. Chymase may also play a role in plaque destabilizaton by inhibiting collagen synthesis. Chymase inhibitors tested in animal models of myocardial infection, cardiomyopathy and heart failure have provided us with promising results [276].

Another important action of chymase is the ACE-independent coversion of angiotensin-I (ANG I) to angiotensin-II (ANG II), after vascular injury. It has recently been reported that mast cells are a novel and previously undescribed source of renin in human and rodent myocardium [277], and immediate- type allergic reaction elicits renin release from mast cells, which activates the local renin-angiotensin system, thereby promoting norepinephrine release [278]. As renin is stored in human mast cells, allergic reactins could initiate renin release, leading to local angiotensin formation and hyperadrenergic dysfunction. ANG I and ANG II concentrations in the interstitial fluid of the canine heart have been found to be 100-fold higher than plasma levels and are not modified by intravenous ANG I infusions [279]. This result indicates that ANG I found in the heart is synthesized in situ, and most of cardiac ANG II derives from the conversion of locally produced, rather than blood-derived, ANG I. In myocardial IR, mast cells degranulate and release renin to form ANG I; this is followed by the generation of ANG II via local ACE. ANG II then activates angiotensin type 1 (AT_1) receptors located on the membrane of sympathetic nerve terminals, promoting release of norepinephrine (NE) (277). NE and ANG II are known to contribute to reperfusion arrhythmias that are prevented by pharmacological mast cell stabilization, renin inhibition, or AT_1-receptor blockade [280].

Increasing evidence implicates acute psychological stress and cardiac mast cells in coronary heart disease (CHD), especially when occurring without angina, that appears to involve a sizable portion of myocardial infarction (MI) [281-284]. Acute stress induces rat cardiac mast cells activation, an effect blocked by cromolyn [285]. Both histamine [286] and IL-6 [287] are significant independent factors of CHD morbidity and mortality. Acute stress induced histamine release from mouse heart [288], as well as increase serum histamine and IL-6 [288, 289]. These effects are dependent on mast cells and are greater in apolipoprotein E (ApoE) knockout mice that develop atherosclerosis [288, 289]. Serum IL-6 elevations in patients with acute CHD were documented to derive primarily from the coronary sinus [290]. There are also reports of anaphylactic CHD that has been termed the "Kounis" syndrome [291-293].

Adrenomedullin (AM) also is a potent vasodilatory hypotensive peptide and is expressed in the heart, where it is known to play a protective role [244]. Cardiac mast cells are able to synthesize and store AM, and upon stimulation to release it near coronary arterioles and venules [295].

Adenosine and its receptors have also been shown to play an important role in cardiovascular disease. Adenosine acts on mast cells via A2a, A2b [296] receptors causing degranulation [297] and the release of IL-8 [298], as well as VEGF [299] that could participate in IR injury. Activation of A3 receptors has also been shown to cause more mast cells to degranulate [300, 301] and A3R knockout mice were tolerant to IR injury [301].

10. Common Pathway between Allergic and Non-Allergic Coronary Syndromes

Today, it is almost certain that the majority of cases of unstable angina and acute myocardial infarction are the result of combined coronary artery spasm and plaque erosion or rupture followed by thrombus formation. The following mediators, released during acute allergic episodes, have been found to be increased in blood or urine of patients suffering from acute coronary syndromes on non-allergic etiology.

Patients with acute coronary syndromes of non-allergic etiology have been found to have more than twice tile blood concentration of histamine than normal subjects [286]. Arachidonic acid metabolites such as thromboxane and leukotrienes have been found significantly higher in the systemic arterial circulation in the acute stage of non-allergic myocardial infarction than in circulation of normal controls [302]. Interleukin-6 levels, derived from inflamed coronary plaques and areas of myocardial necrosis, have been found elevated in patients with non-allergic acute coronary syndromes [303, 304]. In a recent study [305], tryptase levels were elevated in patients with non-allergic acute coronary syndromes with higher concentration in the ST segment depression group of patients and it was postulated that tryptase may be a potential new marker characterizing the unstable plaque. Tryptase levels were found all elevated in non-allergic patients with significant coronary artery disease as a result of chronic low-grade inflammatory activity present in the atherosclerotic plaques [66]. It is proposed that tryptase measurements may emerge as a novel way of identifying asymptomatic patients with coronary artery disease and represent a new biomarker of therapeutic efficacy in these patients [306].

Therefore, the same substances from the same cells are present in both acute allergic episodes and acute coronary syndromes.

11. Mast Cell Activation Precede Acute Coronary Events

The important question which arises in acute coronary events is whether inflammatory cells including mast cells and their contents are the cause or the result of the event.

There is now evidence that mast cells not only enter the culprit lesion before plaque erosion or rupture but also release their contents before an actual coronary event. Kaartinen et al. [307] showed that mast cells infiltrate not only the sites of coronary arteries at which plaque rupture or erosion has occurred but also sites of coronary plaques susceptible to erosion or rupture which means they invade before an actual initial event. The same applies also for other inflammatory cells such as macrophages and T lymphocytes. Therefore, there is much evidence to suggest that inflammatory cells infiltrate the lesions before erosion or rupture and they are not part of inflammatory response to rupture initiated by other processes. In another report, concerning patients who had died within 2 days after the acute coronary event [308], infiltrates of activated mast cells at the site of coronary atheromatous erosion or rupture were found in a ratio of 200 to 1 compared with normal endothelial segments. It is known mat circulating blood contains only mast cell precursors and these precursors take several days to weeks to differentiate into morphologically identifiable mast cells filled with cytoplasmic secretory granules [309, 310]. Therefore, the mast cells must already have been present at the erosion or rupture sites before the episode in the above patients. In fact, the number of mast cells was highest in one of the above patients who had the shortest interval between the onset of symptoms and death.

Histamine concentration was found to be elevated in the great cardiac vein in 8 of 11 patients suffering from attacks of variant angina [311] and in none of 8 control patients. In the same patients, the authors did not observe any histamine elevation during or after acetylocholine-induced coronary artery spasm. In contrast, elevation of plasma histamine levels was antecedent to angina attacks in 3 patients. In addition high levels of histamine were observed even in the absence of ST segment elevation in the same group of patients.

Tryptase levels were found elevated during spontaneous ischemic episodes in 8 patients suffering from unstable angina [312], but not after ergonovine-provoked ischemia in patients suffering from variant angina, suggesting that a primary yet unknown stimulus activates mast cells in patients suffering from episodes of unstable angina. In a recent report [313] it was found that arachidonic acid products such as leukotrienes and thromboxane were significantly higher in non-allergic patients with unstable angina than in patients with stable angina and in patients with nonischemic chest pain. In the same report it was shown that myocardial ischemia elicited by stress test in the stable angina patients was not accompanied by any change in leukotriene and thromboxane up to 6 days after positive exercise test. The authors of this study concluded that this can rule out a role of ischemia per se in the induction of increased eicosanoid products.

12. Ischemic Myocardial Damage seems to be the Primary Event during Allergic Episodes

It is generally believed, that during an allergic episode, systemic vasodilation, reduced venous return, leakage of plasma and volume loss due to increased vascular permeability and the ensuing depression of cardiac output contribute to coronary hypoperfusion with subsequent myocardial damage. Indeed, during severe acute allergic episodes circulating blood volume may decrease by as much as 35% within 10 min due to transfer of intravascular fluid to extravascular space and severe vasodilation resistant to epinephrine and responding only to other potent vasoconstrictors has been reported [314-316]. This effective shift of fluid volume is countered by compensatory vasopressor mechanisms involving the release of epinephrine and norepinephrine [317] as well as the activation of angiotensin system [318,

319]. The ensuing increase in catecholamines mighty produce varied effects. Some patients during acute allergic episodes experience maximum peripheral vaso-constriction [320] whereas others have decrease systemic vascular resistance [317]. These variable effects of internal compensatory mechanisms might explain why epinephrine injections sometimes fail to help acute and severe allergy. Furthermore, the endogenous catecholamine/release which can be enhanced by therapeutic administration can have an adverse effect in myocardium, including ischemic chest pain and electrocardiographic changes in the absence of diseased coronary arteries [321, 322].

However, experimental and clinical evidence indicates that the human heart can be the site and the primary target of anaphylaxis. In experimental anaphylaxis with ovalvumin sensitized guinea pigs [323] it was shown that within 3 min after the antigen administration the cardiac output decreased by 90%, the arterial blood pressure rose significantly by 35% as did the left ventricular end diastolic pressure indicating pump failure. In the same time range, electrocardiographic recordings uniformly showed signs of acute myocardial ischemia.

The blood pressure started declining steadily after 4 min. The authors of this paper concluded that "the idea that the registered anaphylactic damage might be due to peripheral vasodilation can be definitely excluded. In addition, the rapid increase in left ventricular end diastolic pressure suggests that decreased venous return and volume loss due to an increase of vascular permeability are unlikely to be the primary causes of the documented depression of cardiac output and blood pressure". In this study, it must be pointed out that, coronary vascular resistance and vasoconstriction of epicardial coronary arteries were not assessed.

However, in another study [324] with isolated guinea pig hearts undergoing anaphylaxis following intra-aortic injection of antigen, an abrupt heart rate increase reaching the peak within 2 min, a transient increase in ventricular contractile force followed by prolonged decrease, and a prompt and prolonged decrease in coronary blood flow were observed. Actually, the above reports were not the only ones, but they corroborated the findings of previous report [325] according to which the anaphylactic cardiac damage can be dissociated temporarily into two sets of events: an initial primary cardiac reaction caused by intracardiac release of histamine and a subsequent cardiovascular reaction secondary to systemic release of mediators.

In a group of patients with spontaneous angina [326], after infusion of histamine, with pre-treatment with cimetidine to antagonize H2 receptors, 40% of the patients developed angina with ST elevation, decrease coronary blood flow, increase coronary vascular resistance but with no significant changes in the mean arterial blood pressure.

Today, it is known that histamine acts via four different histamine receptors all of which contribute to the severity of the allergic myocardial damage. H1-histamine receptors mediate coronary vasoconstriction and increase vascular perneabilty. H2-histamine receptors mediate a minor degree of relaxation of the coronary arteries and increase atrial rate and atrial and ventricular contractility. The interaction of H1- and H2-receptor stimulation mediate decreased diastolic pressure and increased pulse pressure [327]. Histamine binding to H1-receptors during anaphylaxis stimulates endothelial cells to convert the amino acid L-arginine into nitric oxide (NO), a potent autocoid vasodilator [328, 329]. Enhanced NO production decreases venous return, thus contributing to the vasodilation that occurs during anaphylaxis [330]. H3-histamine receptors have been identified [331] on presynaptic terminals of the sympathetic effector nerves that innervate the heart ant the systemic vasculature. These receptors have been found to inhibit endogenous norepinephrine release which would be expected to enhance the degree of shock during anaphylactic events. The recently identified H4-histamine receptors control chemotaxis of murine mast cells [332] and human eosinophils [333, 334] and the release of interleukin -16 from human lymphocytes [335]. The recruitment of these specific inflammatory cells at the sites of me allergic response correlate with the severity of the allergic reaction [336, 337].

13. Frequency of Kounis Syndrome and Clinical Relevance

Acute coronary syndromes associated with acute allergic reactions are increasingly encountered in clinical practice, but it has been difficult to determine their true frequency because adequate reporting mechanisms do not exist. Indeed, unlike many disorders, mere is no requirement to report such reactions to any national registry [338]. For similar reasons, determining the incidence and prevalence of Kounis syndrome has been challenging. However, in a recent study [339] by pushing a single ant against the ventral forearm of 21 healthy volunteers, allowing it to sting for 60s, two of the subjects (9.5%) developed chest pain with electrocardiographic changes suggesting acute myocardial ischemia. In another survey concerning anaphylaxis during anesthesia, it was shown that cardiovascular symptoms were the most common (73.6%) clinical features [340]. In the canton Bern, Switzerland, during a 3-year period 226 individuals were diagnosed as having presented generalized anaphylaxis with circulatory problems [341].

There are several causes that have been reported as capable of inducing Kounis syndrome. These include a number of conditions, several drugs and a variety of environmental exposures (Table 9). Although many cases of Kounis syndrome might go unreported, searching the world literature shows that the reports concerning Kounis syndrome are increasing. Between them, there are reports of hymenoptera sting-induced Kounis syndrome and cases of drug-induced Kounis syndrome. A detailed list of drugs capable of inducing Kounis syndrome (Table 10) has been published recently [12]. The first report of acute myocardial infarction during a prolonged allergic reaction to penicillin was published in the American Heart journal in 1950 [342]. In the majority of cases of Kounis syndrome hypotension and increased oxygen demand were the consequence of the allergic coronary artery spasm and/or acute myocardial infarction. Adrenaline administration which can induce acute myocardial infarction [343] and venom hemorrhagins or endothelins [344] which can also induce coronary artery spasm have been definitely excluded. However, in patients with overt or quiescent pre-existing coronary artery disease or endothelial dysfunction, acute allergic episodes can induce plaque damage or artery spasm manifesting as type II or type I variant of Kounis syndrome, respectively.

Table 9. Causes capable of inducing Kounis syndrome

Conditions	Drugs	Environmental exposures
Angio-edema	Antibiotics	Ant stings
Bronchial asthma	Analgesics	Bee stings
Exercise induced anaphylaxis	Antineoplastics	Wasp stings
Food allergy	Contrast Media	Jellyfish sting
Idiopathic anaphylaxis	Corticosteroids	Grass cutting
Mastocytosis	Intravenous anaesthetics	Poison ivy
Serum sickness	Non steroidal	Latex contact
Urticaria	Anti-inflammatory	Limpet ingestion (the kiss of death)
Churg-Strauss syndrome	Drugs (NSAIDs)	Millet allergy
	Skin disinfectants	Shellfish eating
	Thrombolytics	Viper venom poisoning
	Anticoagulants	
	Others	

Table 10. Drugs that have been reported to induce Kounis syndrome

Antibiotics

Ampicillin
Ambicillin/sulfactam
Amoxicillin
Amikacin
Cafazolin
Cefoxitin
Cerufoxime
Cephradine
Cinoxacin
Lincomycin
Penicillin
Sulbactam/cefoperazone
Sulperazon
Trimethropin/sulfamethoxazol
Vancomycin

Contrast Media

Iohexone
Loxagate
Meglumine diatrizoate
Sodium indigotindisulfonate
Analgesics
Dipyrone

Antineoplasics

5-fluoroucacil
Capecitabine
Carboplatin
Denileukin
Interferons
Paclitaxel
Vinca alkaloids

Intravenous Anaesthetics

Etomidate
Rocuronium bromide
Suxamethonium
Trimethaphan

NSAIDs

Diclofenac
Naproxen

Thrombolytics and Anticoagulants

Heparin
Lepirudin
Streptokinase
Urokinase

Skin Disinfectants

Chlorhexidine
Povidone-iodine

Others

Allopurinol
Enalapril
Esmolol
Dextran 40
Fructose
Insulin
Iodine
Lanzoprasol
Protamine
Tetanus antitoxin
Glaphenine

It seems likely that atopic individuals are at higher risk of acute coronary syndromes than normal people. In a population based study [345] men with increased levels of IgE had significantly increased incidence of myocardial infarction, stroke and peripheral arterial disease. In the same study women had both significantly lower IgE levels and lower rates of cardiovascular disease. The authors of this study concluded that a causal role of IgE in the development of cardiovascular disease should not be excluded. It has been shown that in platelets isolated from atopic patients, the immunological stimulation with anti-lgE antibodies produced platelet aggregation and release of histamine [346]. The exposure of platelets from healthy donors to increasing concentrations of thrombin produced a progressive aggregation of platelets which was parallel to the release of histamine. Both effects were significantly enhanced in platelets isolated from atopic donors [347].

Table 11. Clinical and Electrocardiographic Features of Kounis Syndrome

Clinical Symptoms

- Chest discomfort
- Acute chest pain
- Dyspnea
- Faintness
- Nausea
- Vomiting
- Syncope
- Pruritus
- Urticaria
- Hypotention
- Diaphoresis
- Pallor
- Palpitations
- Bradycardia
- Tachycardia

Electrocardiographic Symptoms

- T-wave flattering
- T-wave inversion
- ST segment depression
- ST segment elevation
- QRS complex prolongation
- QT segment prolongation
- Sinus tachycardia
- Sinus bradycardia
- Nodal rhythm
- Atrial fibrillation
- Ventricular ectopics
- Bigeminal rhythm

Several reports have shown that type I variant of Kounis syndrome has better prognosis than type II variant [348]. However, in both types the prognosis depends on the magnitude of the initial allergic response, the patient's sensitivity, the patient's comorbidity, the site of antibody-antigen reaction, the allergen concentration and the route of allergen entrance. Patients who present with any grading [349] of systemic allergic reactions associated with clinical, laboratory and electrocardiographic findings of acute myocardial ischemia should be diagnosed as having Kounis syndrome (Table 11). Chest pain, during an allergic insult, with electrocardiographic ischemic changes but with normal cardiac enzymes, negative toponins, normal sestamibi scan, normal coronary angiogram and positive ergonovine or histamine test [350] are in favour of type I variant of the syndrome. Acute allergic reactions associated with acute myocardial infarction with angiographic evidence of coronary artery disease constitute type II variant of Kounis syndrome.

Since life threatening allergic reactions with circulatory compromise can occur at an annual rate of 7.9 - 9.1 per 100.000 populations with 10% of these due to food, 18% due to drugs, and 59% due to venoms [341] knowledge of individual hypersensitivity is crucial. Ischemic heart disease patients with history indicative of hypersensitivity must undergo a reliable diagnostic procedure including skin testing and antibody testing. Cases of Kounis syndrome are more often encountered in clinical practice than anticipated and we believe that many more causative factors will be incriminated in the future. Careful patient interrogation may reveal a mechanism involving mast cell activation to preceed acute coronary events. In patients with any grading of systemic allergic reactions routine evaluation of myocardial injury markers such as cardiac enzymes and troponins together with histamine and tryptase levels should be undertaken. Although allergic episodes are common in everyday practice only few patients develop chest pain with/or electrocardiographic changes during these episodes. We believe that there is a threshold level of mast cell content (histamine, tryptase, chymase, leukotriene, thromboxane, PAF and chemokines) above which it can provoke coronary artery spasm and/or plaque erosion or rupture.

14. An Emerging Clinical Problem: Kounis Syndrome and Coronary Stent Thrombosis

Stent thrombosis is an emerging serious clinical problem in patients treated with Drug Eluting Stents [351]. Recent data [352] have shown that a small but increasing number of patients develop stent thrombosis after insertion of drug eluting stents (DES). Stent thrombosis may lead to catastrophic consequences [353] including myocardial infarction with estimated 30-day mortality ranging from 20 to 48%. Several meta-analyses of large trials, have shown that the overall mortality from DES was increased by 2, 3, and 4 years in comparison with the bare metal stents [354]. Another study[355] showed that the rate of cardiac death and non fatal myocardial infarction between 7-18 months after DES insertion was 4.9% and additional up to 3 years data[356] showed that the rate of mortality and myocardial infarction after sirolimus eluting stent insertion raised to 6.3%. These studies have prompted a statement from Food and Drug Administration (FDA) warning about the small but significant increase in the rate of death and myocardial infarction from possible stent thrombosis followed 18 months to 3 years after stent implantation [357]. However, these rates have been challenged and three recent reports [358-360], showed no significant differences in the rates of death, myocardial infarction and stent thrombosis between DES and bare metal stents. It has been suggested that large randomized trials are necessary[361,362] in order to ascertain the long-term safety of DES.

Stent thrombosis has been classified as acute, occurring within 48 hours, subacute, occurring between the 2nd and the 30th day, late, occurring after the first 30 days to one year and very late occurring after one year of the implantation. This was followed by the "Academic Research Consortium " definitions which defines stent thrombosis as definite stent thrombosis which means acute coronary syndrome with angiographic or autopsy evidence of thrombus or occlusion, probable stent thrombosis which means either unexplained death within 30 days following stent insertion or acute myocardial infarction involving the target-vessel territory without angiographic confirmation and possible stent thrombosis which means unexplained death occurring at least 30 days following stent insertion[363].

Potential causes of stent thrombosis (Table 12) include delayed endothelialization, stent length, complex lesions, suboptimal stent insertion, flow disturbances and changes in shear stress, withdrawal of clopidogrel and/or aspirin, brachytherapy for in-stent restenosis, patient characteristics and hypersensitivity to stent components [364]. The concurrence of acute coronary syndromes with hypersensitivity reactions has been long ago established [1} and the question which arises is whether hypersensitivity to DES components could be associated with acute coronary events [365,366].

Table 12. procedural, clinical and angiographic variables of stent thrombosis

1. Supoptimal stent insertion
2. Stent length
3. Vessel calcification
4. Multivessel disease
5. Totally occluded lesion at baseline
6. Post-procedural TIMI flow <3
7. Insulin dependent diabetes
8. Advanced age
9. Low ejection fraction
10. Flow disturbances
11. Changes in shear stress
12. Withdrawal of clopidogrel and/or aspirin
13. Clopidogrel resistance
14. Brachytherapy
15. Delayed endothelialization
16. Hypersensitivity to stent components

Since it is not known if stent thrombosis is a time limited event, this might become a major clinical concern in patients who have been already treated with DES. Therefore, the search for causation and application of prophylactic and therapeutic measures for stent-associated coronary events must be of paramount importance for both patients and physicians.

15. Kounis Syndrome: Hypersensitivity to DES Components

Data deriving from FDA's Manufacturer and User Device Experience Center (MAUDE)[367] and the Research on Adverse Drug/Device events And Reports (RADAR)[368] project have shown that 262 cases of Drug-Eluding Stent implantation were associated with hypersensitivity reactions. RADAR project reviews in detail adverse event reports gathered from different sources and evaluates causal associations between drugs and potentially fatal adverse events. Although only 17 cases were classified as probably or certainly caused by the stent insertion, 4 of them developed fatal in-stent thrombosis and died at 4, 5, 18, and 18 months after implantation respectively[369]. These reactions included rash, itching, hives, dyspnea, fever, atypical chest pain, high or low blood pressure, joint pain, joint swelling, and anaphylaxis. The cutaneous rash was associated with hives, desquamation or blisters and covered the entire body in the 21% of the cases. Based on MAUDE seriousness codes, 95% of these reactions were classified as serious requiring hospitalizations, emergency interventions, intravenous steroids, cardiac catheterizations, or resulted in permanent disability and even death. Laboratory findings associated with the above reactions included eosinophilia and elevated IgE titers. Clinical or laboratory findings did not abate with discontinuation of the concurrent antiplatelet medications. MAUDE and RADAR project data may be biased because there are underreported events, lack of information for causality attribution and inclusion of reports deriving from concomitant medications. However, allergy to DES is regarded real clinical entity today[370] and there is obvious risk for serious complications. It has been proposed that health professionals should be vigilant and should submit detailed adverse event reports to the manufacturer of DES or to the FDA[369]. The proportion of 262 cases with allergic reactions in over six million DES implantation seems to be well below the 4% expected for allergy from drugs alone. However, new cases on serum sickness-like reactions after placement of sirolimus-eluting stents have been recently reported [371]. Apart from the risk of thrombosis, physicians should be aware also of the reports of life threatening paradoxical coronary vasoconstriction associated with DES implantation [372-375]. A series of 13 patients who developed severe life threatening coronary artery spasm after DES implantation has been recently published [376]. Two patients did not respond to vasodilators and died. The post mortem examination in one patient showed scattered mast cells infiltrating the adventitia of the left anterior coronary artery suggesting a hypersensitivity reaction to the stent [377]. Simultaneous multivessel acute drug-eluting stent thrombosis has been recently reported suggesting hypersensitivity reaction involving multiple vessels as a possible cause [378].

Coronary events associated with hypersensitivity reactions are not common and are dependent on allergen concentration, number of insulting allergens, route and rate of allergen entrance in the circulation, magnitude of the initial allergic response, area and localization of antibody-antigen reaction, patient's sensitivity and patient's comorbidity[379] . A threshold level of inflammatory cell content, closely associated with the above conditions, has been suggested, above which this can provoke smooth muscle contraction and plaque erosion or rupture [380].

16. Stent Components: Potential Allergens

DES components include the metal stent itself, the polymer coating and the impregmated drugs which for today are: the antimicrotubule antineoplastic agent paclitaxel for TAXUS brand and the anti-inflammatory, immunosuppressive and antiproliferative agent rapamycin for CYPHER brand. Other investigative agents such as zotarolimus, everolimus, biolimus, tacrolimus, pimecrolimus etc. are currently undergoing safety and efficacy trials either impregnated in metal stents or used in transplant recipients in order to prevent rejection. All DES components either separately or synergistically seem to be able to induce hypersensitivity reactions and hypersensitivity coronary events (Table 13). Allergic inflammation is initiated by allergens cross-bridging their corresponding, receptor-bound, immunoglobin IgE antibodies on the mast cell or basophil cell surface. These cells degranulate and release their mediators when the critical number of bridged IgE antibodies reaches the order of 2000 out of maximal number of some 500 000-1000 000 IgE antibodies on the cell surface [381]. However, recent findings indicate that mast cells can be activated by non allergic triggers often without degranulation, but with selective release of potent and vasoactive compounds [382, 383]. Clinical studies indicate that allergic patients simultaneously exposed to several allergens have more symptoms than mono-sensitized individuals [384]. A recent study showed that IgE antibodies with different specificities can have an additive effects and even small amounts of corresponding allergens can trigger mediator release when the patient is simultaneously exposed to them [385]. This data suggest that a possible sensitization to DES should not be clinically evaluated as a consequence of exposure to a single component but rather viewed in the context of potential sensitization to multiple DES compounds. In addition, recent in vitro studies [386] have shown that paclitaxel enhances tissue factor expression and activity in endothelial cells in concentrations comparable with those achieved locally after paclitaxel stent insertion [387]. Rapamycin also increases thrombin and tumor necrosis factor-α-induced endothelial tissue factor expression and activity at concentrations that are encountered in vivo [388]. Furthermore, histamine, the main amine released during hypersensitivity reactions, can also induce tissue factor expression and activity in human vascular smooth muscle cell and aortic endothelial cell [389]. Therefore, paclitaxel, rapamycin and the released histamine may contribute to a prothrombotic environment after insertion of DES.

Table 13. Hypersensitivity reactions to DES components

1. Sirolimus

- acrocyanosis
- angioedema
- flushing
- pruritus
- interstitial pneumonitis
- Schonlein-Henoch purpura
- localized eczematiform eruption
- palpable purpura due to leucocytoplastic vasculitis
- paradoxic coronary vasoconstriction

2. Paclitaxel

- angioedema
- atrioventricular block
- bronchospasm
- cutaneous flushing
- diaphoresis
- Kounis syndrome
- left bundle branch block
- ventricular tachycardia
- urticaria

3. Polymers and Latex

- allergic conjunctivitis
- allergic rhinitis
- allergic allergic stomatitis
- facial angioedema
- generalized anaphylactic reaction
- generalized urticaria
- interstitial asthma
- neurodermatitis
- stomatitis venenada

4. Nickel

- allergic contact dermatitis
- baboon syndrome
- bronchial asthma
- dependent edema
- diffuse exanthema
- fever
- flexural dermatitis
- itching erythema
- pericarditis
- pompholyx formation
- rosacea
- sarcoid granuloma (delayed hypersensitivity)

17. Paclitaxel and Sirolimus Induced Allergic Reations and Kounis Syndrome

Paclitaxel together with docetaxel belong to a dinstict type of antineoplastic drugs which in micromolar concentrations, easily achieved in patients, inhibit microtubule assembly (M-phase of the cell cycle) resulting in dissolution of the mitotic spindle structure, thereby inhibiting proliferation of cells[390]. They also promote microtubule resistance to depolymerization which results in the production of nonfunctional microtubules [391]. Morphological features and a DNA fragmentation pattern such as of programmed cell death indicate that paclitaxel may trigger cell apoptosis [392].

Most cytostatic drugs have reported to induce allergic reactions [393]. There are several reported instances of hypersensitivity reactions, mainly of anaphylactic type (type I) but also types II, III, and IV [394] . Severe and leathal reactions have also occurred [395,396]. Antineoplastics capable to induce acute coronary syndromes include [397] the antimicrotubule paclitaxel (Taxol), the antimetabolite 5-fluoruracil (Adrucil), its prodrug capecitabine (Xeloda), the alkaloids cisplatin (Platinol), the interleukin-2 agent denileukin diftitox (Ontak), the vinca alkaloids and interferons.

Apart from, neutropenia, thrombocytopenia, paralytic ileus, alopecia, gastrointestinal upset and peripheral neuropathy, hypersensitivity reactions are quite common with the use of paclitaxel with 90% of these occurring after the first or second dose [398].

According to a recent report [399] up to 42% of patients, receiving systemic paclitaxel for treatment of various types of cancer, experience some kind of hypersensitivity reactions and up to 2% of the patients developed serious allergic reactions. So far, there are several reports associating type I and type II variants of Kounis syndrome with paclitaxel systemic administration [400-411]. In another report [412], a patient experienced anaphylactic reaction during a Taxus stent implantation. This patient developed erythematous rash and hypotension immediately after the stent insertion. The case complicated with coronary spasm and thrombus formation. This reaction was successfully treated with steroids, antihistamines, epinephrine, dopamine and intraaortic balloon counterpulsation. Delayed severe multivessel coronary artery spasm and aborted sudden death has also been observed after systemic Taxus stent implantation [372]. Paclitaxel-induced hypersensitivity reactions can be decreased considerabley if a test dose of paclitaxel is implemented before the initiation of therapy [413]. In another study [414], involving 23 patients with recurred ovarian cancer, combination chemotherapy with carboplatin and paclitaxel induced hypersensitivity reactions in 5 patients. One of these patients exhibited severe allergic reaction compatible with Kounis syndrome. The rest of the patients developed eruptions, hypotension and tachycardia. It must be pointed out that all hypersensitivity reactions occurred immediately after carboplatin administration and not during paclitaxel administration. Perhaps, in this occasion, paclitaxel has acted as hapten. Low molecular weight antineoplastics have been proposed that have haptenic properties [13].

Sirolimus (rapamycin, Rapamune[R]) is a macrolide antibiotic derived from actinomycete streptomyces hygroscopius which for many years has been used as an immunosuppressive and antiproliferative agent in the treatment of organ rejection in transplant recipients. Unlike cyclosporine and tacrolimus, sirolimus does not inhibit the calcineurin pathway, but inhibits the mammalian target of rapamycin (mTOR), a multifunctional serine-threonine kinase that acts on IL-2-mediated signal transduction pathways, which is central regulator of cell growth proliferation and apoptosis [415]. Sirolimus prevents DNA and protein synthesis by regulation of p70S6 kinase phosphatase which leads in arrest of cell cycle [416]. These properties have been utilized also in coronary stents in order to reduce neointimal formation and restenosis.

Apart from the well known adverse effects associated with sirolimus use such as hyperlipidemia, hypercholesterolemia and thrombocytopenia some serious hypersensitivity reactions have been observed with its use.

Generalized, pruritic, ulcerating maculopapular rash necessitating cessation of sirolimus have been observed in a liver transplant patient [417]. A variety of cutaneous effects have been also reported in renal transplantation patients [418]. Sirolimus can induce allergic angioedema with diffuse swelling of eyelids, epiglottid edema, edema of floor of the mouth, tongue and soft Palate [419]. Despite vigorous therapy of these patients with angioedema complete resolution of this effect may occur only after withdrawal of sirolimus.

Furthermore, sirolimus-induced pulmonary hypersensitivity have been reported [420,421]. Acneiform eruption [422], leucocytoclastic vasculitis [423,424], even cardiac tamponade [425] are some additional but rare side effects.

In an experimental study [426] the side effects of rapamycin on treated rats were evaluated by histopathological examination of heart, kidney and eyes. Rapamycin administration at doses of 1.5 and 1.0 mg/kg/day resulted in focal myocardial infarction in 60% and 9% of rats respectively. In one animal a small area of focal retina ischemic necrosis was evident at the higher dose while no rat nephrotoxicity found in any rapamycin dose. In addition, animal experiments indicate a propensity for thombus formation in a rat model with synthetic vascular grafts treated by systemic or local administration of rapamycin [427]. Although no evidence of hypersensitivity was noted in this experiment, thrombus formation was largest in animals that received high dose of rapamycin either orally or intraperitoneally, when compared with the control group [428].

In humans, paradoxical coronary vasoconstriction[373] and life threatening coronary spasm[374] followed sirolimus eluting stent deployment has been also reported and was attributed to severe endothelial dysfunction[375] as in type I variant of Kounis syndrome. For example, localized hypersensitivity and late coronary thrombosis secondary to a sirolimus eluting stent has been reported in a 58-year old man who died 18 months later after stent implantation [429,430]. The inflammatory cells found at autopsy to infiltrate the intima, the media and the adventitia were the same namely macrophages, eosinophils, lymphocytes, and plasma cells with those participating in the process of Kounis syndrome.

18. Investigative Agents: Everolimus, Zotarolimus, Biolimus Induced Allergic Reactions

Several efficacy and safety trials are currently under way in order to evaluate the ability of some new sirolimus analogues for better inhibition of neointimal proliferation, even more reduction of the stenotic area, further increase of the lumen area and to avoid local

rapidly growing end of actin filaments. Actin filaments are components of cytoskeleton. They are required for intracellular signaling, cell migration, replication and protein synthesis [466].

21. Hypersensitivity to Polymers and Latex

Synthetic biodegradable polymers are commonly used in drug eluting stents as a vehicle for local drug delivery and as a solution to improve their quality. The impregnated drugs are released by diffusion through and/or breakdown of the base polymer. Cypher stents are coated with a thin layer of poly-n-butyl methacrylate and polyethylene-vinyl acetate copolymer. In sirolimus eluting stens, about 80% of the rapamycin is eluted by 30 days, leaving a polymer-coated metal stent with small drug amounts. In Taxus stents, about 10% of paclitaxel is eluted by 10 days and the rest remains in the polymer for long period [467].

Hypersensitivity reactions have been reported with the use of polymers (Table 4) like those in latex and vinyl gloves as well as with polyurethane and methyl-methacrylate in dentistry[468,469[. The latter has induced labial edema and allergic stomatitis confirmed by patch tests in orthodontic patients [470,471]. Chronic urticaria [472], stomatitis venenata [473] and allergic erythema of the hard palate [474] have been also reported to auto-polymerized acrylic resin. These allergic reactions are usually type IV reactions caused by compounds of low molecular weight that are acting as haptens. They can initiate an allergic reaction when they carried by a protein. For acrylic resins these would be formaldehyde, benzyl peroxide, methyl-methacrylate, and plasticizers such as dibutyl phthalate [475].

Nonbioerodable polymers such as polyurethane polydimethyl siloxane (silicone) and polyethylene terephthalate (Dacron) can promote inflammation when implanted in swine coronary arteries [476-478]. Macrophages, giant cells, tissue damage and fibrosis are seen during subcutaneous implantation of poly-n-butylmethacrylate which is a component of bone cement and the polymer coating of cypher stents [479]. Furthermore, the polyethylene-vinyl acetate compound of the cypher copolymer induces inflammatory reaction in 25% of rabbits when used as an antigen delivery matrix [480]. Cases of immediate and delayed allergic reactions to anionic cellulose polymers carboxymethylcellulose and methyl hydroxyethylcellulose have been reported recently [481].

It should be emphasized that the allergic reactions to latex components can be exacerbated when a variety of foods are ingested. Latex can cross react with the hevemine in fruits and cause an immediate hypersensitivity reaction [482]. The inflammatory and allergic properties of polymers have made their use problematic in gene delivery[483], although polymer-coated gene-delivery stents have been shown in animal studies to be effective for both reporter[484] and therapeutic[485] vector delivery. However, encouraging results have been achieved recently through gene vector delivery from the direct metal alloy surfaces of stents which had been pretreated with polyallylamine bisphosphonate [486].

22. Hypersensitivity to Metals

The majority of intracoronary stents are made from 316L stainless steel which contains nickel, chromium, and molybdenum. Ions from the above metals are eluted through the action of blood, saline, proteins, and mechanical stress.

It has been already known that allergy and inflammatory reactions have occurred in patients with prosthetic valves and other endovascular prostheses [487]. Allergic reactions to metallic implants have been incriminated for postoperative complications such as loosening or formation of new tissue around the metals [488,489]. In a patient with aseptic loosening of an orthopaedic chromium/cobalt alloy and positive patch tests to potassium dichromate, peri-inplantar tissue examination showed oligoclonal T-cell infiltration and Th1-type cytokine expression [490].

Hypersensitivity reactions to nickel occur in up to 17.2% of the population and are the most frequent cause of allergic contact dermatitis [491]. In patients undergoing percutaneous atrial septal defect and patent foramen ovale closure, nickel allergy can be the cause of systemic effects such as chest discomfort, palpitation, and migraine headache with or without aura [492]. It is postulated that local allergic reaction to the implanted device could result in formation of platelet adhesions which could embolize in heart and brain causing chest discomfort and headache [492]. Local nickel allergy from intracardiac devices and subsequent systemic allergic reactions confirmed by patch tests as an allergy to nitinol (nickel-titanium alloy) have necessitated the removal of these devices[493-495].

Reports concerning hypersensitivity reactions to various metals used in orthodontics have been also published [496]. Nickel is the metal which can provoke the most severe responses [497]. Delayed hypersensitivity reactions to nickel and molybdenum might be part of inflammatory process and one of the triggering factors for development of in-stent restenosis [498]. The rate of nickel allergy following initial stent implantation has been estimated [499] to be 9.2%.

Skin clips containing nickel, chromium, molybdenum, cobalt, and titanium can induce allergic reactions and may be the cause of delayed wound healing [500]. Hypersensitivity to molybdenum has been incriminated to induce a syndrome resembling systemic lupus erythematosus [501].

Contact allergy to gold has been associated with increase incidence of restenosis when patients are stented with gold-plated stents and these stents have been abandoned [502]. On the other hand, the titan stent which is a stainless steel stent coated with titanium-nitride oxide (TINOX) can prevent discharge of nickel, chromium and molybdenum and it seems promising in eliminating local allergy and inflammation[503].

23. Delayed Hypersensitivity to DES and Late Coronary Events

Release kinetics of drugs from DES polymers is a complex phenomenon depending on multiple factors. The release varies with the type of polymer, layering, drug to polymer formulation ratio, overcoat, dose density and total amount loaded [504]. Important determinants for tissue drug accumulation include drug physicochemical properties, distribution of drug in the arterial wall, rate and duration of release, endothelial function and arterial wall condition [505]. Drug release from stents is characterized by an initial fast release followed by sustained slow release [506]. Lipophilic drugs are released slowly allowing. Hydrophilic drugs tend to elute faster into the blood and need higher amounts and shorter duration of delivery in order to achieve optimum local levels [507]. However, in human atherosclerotic intimas, drug release kinetics seems to differ considerably and might be prolonged.

The time of appearance of hypersensitivity events depend on these kinetics and can include immediate reactions (type I), antibody mediated cytotoxic reactions (type II), immune complex mediated reactions (type III), and delayed hypersensitivity reactions (type IV). When hypersensitivity is considered as the cause of DES thrombosis, the time of appearance of hypersensitivity events depends on allergen release kinetics, number and level of the insulting allergens and existence of drug-reactive lymphocytes [508]. Atopic patients with increased propensity to hypersensitivity reactions possess long lasting reactivity due to high frequency of drug-specific lymphocytes, thus potentially making them prone to react again even years after drug avoidance [509].

24. Future Directions Concerning DES

At the present, as it was stated by the FDA, coronary DES remain safe and effective when used in patients according to approved by the agency indications. However, it seems likely that, with these sophisticated devices, cases of mild hypersensitivity reactions to DES might go unreported; thus it is anticipated that many more cases will be encountered in the coming years.

Therefore, in atopic patients, in patients with food allergy and who have already experienced a first Kounis syndrome and are going to have DES implantation, and until further studies characterizing the incidence, the course, the risk of occurrence in a given patient, the circumstances and the definite cause of coronary stent thrombosis will be undertaken, one can make a good case for:

- detailed history taking regarding allergies and drug hypersensitivity reactions, patch-testing,
- antibody testing, macrophage and T-cell activation studies, and desensitization strategies when and where applicable, monitoring the levels of inflammatory mediators after implantation, and considering the use of corticosteroids and mast cell stabilizers since the latter have abrogated late thrombotic events experimentally[510].

Thousands of patients worldwide every year are benefited with DES treatment because it reduces significantly the need of second procedures to treat restenosis. New DES development targeting to prevention of stent thrombosis are under evaluation. Eptifibatite-eluting stents are currently being evaluated in vitro as antiproliferative and antithrombotic devices [511]. The proposed dimethyl sulfoxide eluting stent which suppresses tissue factor expression and activity, as well as thrombus formation seems to be a novel strategy [512]. Accelerated endothelialization could be achieved with stents loaded with an integrin-binding cyclic Arg-Gly-Asp peptide attracting endothelial progenitor cells [513]. Again, stents coated with CD34 antibodies can attract endothelial progenitor cells and accelerate endothelialization5 [514]. An interesting new approach for DES is the use of peroxisome proliferator-activated receptor-γ agonists which diminish inflammation and enhance endothelialization [515]. Hypersensitivity to DES components and the Kounis syndrome should be always considered as a possibility. New DES combining drugs with anti-inflammatory, antiallergic, and/or antithrombotic agents might be the solution of the problem.

25. Management of Kounis Syndrome

Treatment of Kounis syndrome is directed firstly towards the alleviation of the acute allergic insult and secondly the therapy of the acute coronary event. The first is achieved by administration of H1 and H2 blockers together with the administration of corticosteroids. This treatment alone can be successful in cases of type I Kounis syndrome without any additional effort. Administration of corticosteroids is mandatory because these drugs:

- Suppress the release of arachidonic acid from cell membrane and inhibit eicosanoid biosynthesis (via phospholipase A2 inhibition)
- Induce cell apoptosis and reduce inflammation via up-regulation of death receptor CD95 and its ligand CD95L
- Induce synthesis of proteins called   annexins (lipocortins) which modulate inflammatory cell activation, adhesion molecule expression and transmigratory and phagocytic functions.

In the cases where type I Kounis syndrome progresses to acute myocardial infarction with increased cardiac enzymes and troponins and in the cases where the acute allergic episode induces type II Kounis syndrome with plaque erosion or rupture manifesting as an acute myocardial infarction then, antiallergic treatment is combined with classical treatment of acute myocardial infarction.

26. Conclusion

So far, attempts have been made to counteract the actions of inflammatory mediators by using, experimentally, mediator antagonists, inhibitors of mediator biosynthesis and mediator receptor blockers [516]. However, in the medical armamentarium drugs such as sodium nedocromil, sodium cromoglycate, ketotifen, lodoxamide and others which are currently used experimentally that are interfering with mast cell stabilization (Table 8, Table 9) might be useful tools in the future. There is also considerable evidence today that the polyphenolic plant compounds such as flavonoids that block basophils and mast cells and inhibit mediator release [517] may be used. In a recent study [518], anti-IgE therapy with humanized IgG1 nonoclonal antibodies was recognized and masked the region of mast cell surface responsible for IgE binding thus offering protection against mast cell degranulation. Following this study, it has been suggested [519] that in atopic patients, who produce large amounts of interleukin-4 and interleukin-13, treatment with anti-IL-4Rα antibodies might inhibit acute and severe allergic episodes. All these agents and natural molecules capable to stabilize and protect mast cell membrane could prevent also acute thrombotic events, at least in some instances. It has been stated [307] that "a new possibility emerges for the prevention of the progression of coronary plaques to unstable lesions, and that is; inhibition of mast cell degranulation". This has already been achieved experimentally by Nemmar et al. [510]. These investigators managed to abrogate late thrombotic events by stabilizing mast cell membrane with sodium cromoglycate and reducing inflammation with dexamethasone. Clinical reports have also showed that corticosteroids can reduce the risk of myocardial infarction. For example, in patients with no indication of severe asthma , the risk of myocardial infarction was 22% lower with the use of inhaled corticosteroids and in patients with severe asthma the risk of myocardial infarction was 81% lower with the use of inhaled corticosteroids [520]. Corticosteroids may be considered as a treatment of choise for patients with refractory vasospastic angina, particularly when the patient has an allergic tendency, such as bronchial asthma [521].

Does, therefore, Kounis syndrome represent a magnificent natural paradigm and nature's own experiment in a final trigger pathway implicated in cases of coronary artery spasm and plaque rupture?

Whether this question will be answered in future clinical trials is unknown. If so, case selective mast cell surface membrane protection and stabilization should be considered a potential therapeutic strategy for patients prone to food-induced allergy, for allergic patients to stent components, for atopic patients in general and for patients who have already experienced a first Kounis syndrome.

References

[1]   Kounis, N.G. and Zavras, G.M. Histamine-induced coronary artery spasm: the concept of allergic angina. *Br J Clin Pract*. 1991; 45:121-8.

[2]   Zosin, P., Miclea, F. and Munteanu, M. Allergic myocardial infarction. *Rom Med Review*, 1965; 19:26-8.

[3]   Kounis, N.G. and Zavras, G.M. Allergic angina and allergic myocardial infarction. *Circulation*, 1996; 94:1789.

[4]   Kounis, N.G., Grapsas, G.M. and Goudevenos, J.A. Unstable angina, allergic angina and allergic myocardial infarction. *Circulation*, 1999; 100: el 56.

[5]   Constantinides, P. Infiltrates of activated mast cells at the site of coronary atheromalous erosion or rupture in myocardial infarction. *Circulatory*, 1995; 92:1083.

[6]   Brawnvald, E. Unstable angina. An etiologic approach to management. *Circulation*, 1998; 98:2219-22.

[7]   Zavras, G.M., Papadaki, P.J., Kokkinis, S.E., et al. Kounis syndrome secondary to allergic reaction following shellfish ingestion. *Int J Clin Pract.* 2003; 57:622-4.

[8]   Koutsojannis, C.M. and Kounis, N.G. Lepirudin anaphylaxis and Kounis syndrome. *Circulation,* 2004; 109:e315.

[9]   Koutsojannis, C.M., Mallioris, C.N. and Kounis, N.G. Corticosteroids, Kounis syndrome and the treatment of refractory vasospastic angina. *Circulation J.* 2004; 68:806-7.

[10]   Mallioris, C.N, and Kounis, N.G. Glucocorticoids, Kounis syndrome and the prevention of atrial fibrillation. *Eur Heart J.* 2004; 25:2175-6.

[11]   Kounis, N.G., Kouni, S.N. and Koutsojannis, C.M. Myocardial infarction after aspirin, and Kounis syndrome. J R Soc Med. 2005; 98:296.

[12]   Mazarakis, A., Koutsojannis, C.M., Kounis, N.G., and Alexopoulos, D. Cefuroxime-induced coronary artery spasm manifesting as Kounis syndrome. *Acta Cardiol.* 2005; 60:341-5.

[13]   Soufras, G.D., Ginopoulos, P.V., Papadaki, P.J., et al Penicillin allergy in cancer patients manifesting as Kounis syndrome. *Heart Vessels,* 2005; 20:159-63.

[14]   Waller, B.F. Non atherosclerotic coronary heart disease, In: Fuster V, Wane Alexander A, O'Rourke RA, editors. Hurst's The Heart, 11th edn. New York: McGraw-Hill; 2004. p. 1183.

[15]   Nikolaidis, L.A., Kounis, N.G. and Grandman, A.H. Allergic angina and allergic myocardial infarction: a new twist on an old syndrome. *Can J Cardiol.* 2002; 18:508-11.

[16]   Galli, S.J., Nakae, S. and Tsai, M. Mast cells in the development of adaptive immune responses. Nat Immunol 2005; 6:135-42.

[17]   Galli, S.J., Kalesnikoff, J., Grimbaldeston, M.A., et al Mast cells as "tunable" effector and immunoregulatory cells: recent advances. *Annu Rev Immunol.* 2005; 3:749-86.

[18]   Ishizaka, T. and Ishizaka, K. Activation of mast cells for mediator release through IgE receptors. *Prog Allergy,* 1984; 34:188-235.

[19]   Liu, M.C., Proud, D., Lichtenstein, L.M., et al Human lung macrophage-derived histamine-releasing activity is due to IgE-depended factors. *J Immunol.* 1986; 136:2588-95.

[20]   Sedgwick, J.D., Holt, P.G. and Tunner, K.J. Production of a histamine-releasing lymphokine by antigen - or mitogen-stimulated human peripheral T cells. *Clin Exp Immunol.* 1981; 45:409-18.

[21]   Metcalfe, D.D., Kaliner, M. and Donlon, M.A. The mast cell. *Crit Rev Immunol.* 1981; 3:23-74.

[22]   McCurdy, J.D., Olynych, T.J., Maher, L.H., and Marshall, J.S. Cutting edge: distinct Toll-like receptor 2 activators selectively induce different classes of mediator production from human mast cells. *J Immunol.* 2003; 170:1625-9.

[23]   Barke, K.E. and Hough, L.B. Opiates, mast cells and histamine release. *Life Scil.* 993; 53:1391-9.

[24]   Di Lorenzo, G., Pacor, M.L., Vignola, A.M., et al Urinary metabolites of histamine and leukotrienes before and after placebo-controlled challenge with ASA and food additives in chronic urticaria patients. *Allergy,* 2002; 57: 1 180-6.

[25]   Murray, D.B., Gardner, J.D., Brower, G.L., and Janicki, J.S. Endothelin-1 mediates cardiac mast cell degranulation, matrix metalloproteinase activation, and myocardial remodeling in rats. *Am J Physiol Heart Circ Physiol.* 2004; 287:H2295-9.

[26]   Lindstedt, K.A. and Kovanen, P.T. Mast cells in vulnerable coronary plaques: potential mechanisms linking mast cell activation to plaque erosion and rupture. *Curr Opin Lipidol.* 2004; 15:567-73.

[27]   Dvorak, A.M. Basophils and mast cells: piecemeal degranulation in situ and ex vivo: a possible mechanism for cytokine-induced function in disease. *Immunol Ser.* 1992; 57:169-271.

[28]   van Haaster, C.M.C.J., Engels, W., Lemmens, P.J.M.R., Hornstra, G., van der Vusse, G.J., and Heemskerk, J.W.M. Differential release of histamine and prostaglandin D2 in rat peritonal mast cells; roles of cytosolic calcium and protein tyrosine kinases. *Biochim Biophys Acta*, 1995; 1265:79-88.

[29]   Gagari, E., Tsai, M., Lantz, C.S., Fox, L.G., and Galli, S.J. Differential release of mast cell interleukin-6 via c-kit. *Blood*, 1997; 89:2654-63.

[30]   Kandere-Grzybowska, K., Letourneau, R., Donelan, J., Kempuraj, D., and Theoharides, T.C. Interleukin-1-induced secretion of interleukin-6 without degranulation from human mast cells. *J Immunol.* 2003; 171:4830-6.

[31]   Silver, R.B., Reid, A.C., Mackins, C.J., et al. Mast cells: a unique source of rennin. Proc Natl Acad Sci USA 2004; 101:13607-12.

[32]   Hara, M., Ono, K., Wada, H., Sasayama, S., and Matsumori, A. Preformed angiotensin II is present in human mast cells. *Cardiovasc Drugs Ther.* 2004; 18:415-20.

[33]   Genovese, A. and Spadaro, G. Highlights in cardiovascular effects of histamine and H1-receptor antagonists. *Allergy*, 1997; 52 (suppl 34): 67-78.

[34]   Christian, E.P., Undem, B.J. and Weinreich, D. Endogenous histamine excites neurones in guinea-pig superior cervical ganglion in vitro. *J Physiol.* 1989; 409:297-312.

[35]   Laine, P., Naukkarinen, A., Heikkila, L., and Kovanen, P.T. Adventitial mast cells connect with sensory nerve fibers in atherosclerotic coronary arteries. *Circulation*, 2000; 101:1665-9.

[36]   Masini, E., Di Bello, M.G., Raspanti, S., et al. The role of histamine in platelet aggregation by physiological and immunological stimuli. *Inflamm Res.* 1998;47:211-20.

[37]   Saxena, S.P., Brandes, L.J., Becker, A.B., Simons, K.J., La Bella, F.S., and Gerrard, J.M. Histamine is an intracellular mediating platelet aggregation. *Science,* 1989; 43:1596-9.

[38]   Shah, B.H., Lashari, I., Rana, S., Saeed, O., Rasheed, H., and Arshad Saeed, S. Synergistic interaction of adrenaline and histamine in human platelet aggregation is mediated through activation of phospholipase, nap kinase and cyclo-oxygenase pathways. *Pharmacol Res.* 2000; 42:479-83.

[39]   Benbarek, H., Mouithys-Michkalad, A., Deby-Dupont, G., et al. High concentrations of histamine stimulates equine polymorphonuclear neutronphils to produce reactive oxygen species, *Inflamm Res.* 1999; 48:594-601.

[40] Elenkov, L.J., Webster, E., Papanikolaou, D.A., Fleisher, T.A., Chrousos, G.P., and Wilder, R.L. Histamine potently suppresses human 1L-12 and stimulates IL-10 production via H2 receptors. *J Immunol.* 1998; 161: 2586-93.

[41] Clark, R.A., Sandier, J.A., Gallin, J.L., and Kaplan, A.P. Histamine modulation of eosinophil migration. *J Immunol.* 1977; 118:137-45.

[42] Li, Y., Chi, L., Stechschuh, O.J., and Dileepan, K.N. Histamine induced production of interleukin-6 and interieukin-8 by human coronary artery endothelial cells is enhanced by endotoxin and tumor necrosis factor-alpha. *Microvasc Res.* 2001; 61:253-62.

[43] Asako, H., Kurose, I., Wolf, R., et al. Rote of HI receptors and P-selectin in histamine-induced leucocyte rolling and adhesion in post capillary venules. *J Clin Inest.* 1994, 93:1508-15.

[44] Eppihimer, M.J., Wolitzky, B., Anderson, D.C., Labow, M.A., and Granger, D.N. Heterogenicity of expression of E- and P-selectins in vivo. *Circ Res.* 1996; 79:560-9.

[45] Miyazawa, N., Watanabe, S., Matsuda, A., et al. Role of histamine H1 and H2 receptor antagonists in the prevention of intimal thichening. *Eur J Pharmacol.* 1998; 362:53-9.

[46] Huang, M., Pang, X., Letourneau, R., Boucher, W., and Theoharides, T.C. Acute stress induces cardiac mast cell activation and histamine release, effects that are increased in Apolipoprotein E knockout mice. *Cardiovasc Res.* 2002; 5:150-60.

[47] Pang, X., Alexacos, N., Letourneau, R., et al. A neurotensin receptor antagonist inhibits acute immobilization stress-induced cardiac mast cell degranulation, a corticotropin-releasing hormone-dependent process. *J Pharmacol Exp Ther.* 1988; 287:307-14.

[48] Theoharides, T.C., Donelan, J.M., Papadopoulou, N., Cao, J., Kempuraj, D., and Conti, P. Mast cells as targets of corticotropin-releasing factor and related peptides. *Trends Pharmacol Sci.* 2004; 5:563-8.

[49] Cao, J., Papadopoulou, N., Kempuraj, D., et al. Human mast cells express corticotropin-releasing hormone (CRH) receptors and CRH leads to selective secretion of vascular endothelial growth factor. *J Immunol.* 2005; 174:7665-75.

[50] Steffel, J., Akhmedov, A., Greutert, H., Luscher, T.F., and Tanner, F.C. Histamine induces tissue factor expression. Implications for acute coronary syndromes. *Circulation,* 2005; 1 12:341-9.

[51] Moons, A.H., Levi, M. and Peters, R.J. Tissue factor and coronary artery disease. *Cardiovasc Res.* 2002; 53:313-25.

[52] Johnson, J.C., Jackson, C.L., Angelini, G.D., and George, S. Activation of matrix-degrating metalloproteinases by mast cell proteases in atherosclerotic plaques. *Arterioscler Thromb Vase Biol.* 1998; 18: 707-1715.

[53] Laine, P., Kaartinen, M., Pentila, A., Panula, P., Paavonen, T., and Kovanen, P.T. Association between myocardial infarction and mast cells in the adventitia of the infarct-related coronary artery. *Circulation,* 1999; 99:361-9.

[54] Tselepis, A.D., Goudevenos, J.A., Tambaki, A.P., et al. Platelet aggrega-tory response to platelet activating factor (PAF), ex vive, and PAF-acetylhydrolase activity in patients with unstable angina: effect of c7E3 (abciximab) therapy. *Cardiovasc Res.* 1999; 43:183-91.

[55] Carry, M., Korley, W., Wfllerson, J.T., Weigelt, L., Ford-Hutchinson, A.W., and Taga-
      ri, P. Increased urinary leucotriene excretion in patients with cardiac ischemia: in vivo
      evidence for 5-lipoxygenase activation. *Circulation,* 1992; 85:230-6.

[56] Ellis, E.F., Oelz, O., Roberts, L.J., 2nd, et al. Coronary arterial smooth muscle
      contraction by a substance released from platelets: evidence that is TXA2. *Science,*
      1976; 193:1135-7.

[57] Montrucchio, G., Alloatti, G. and Camussi, G. Role of platelet activating factor in
      cardiovascular pathophysiology. *Physiol Rev.* 2000; 80:1669-99.

[58] Feuerstein, G., Rabinovici, R., Leor, J., Winkler, J.D., and Vonhof, S. Platelet-
      activating factor and cardiac diseases: therapeutic potential for PAF inhibitors. *J Lipid
      Cell Signalling,* 1997; 15:255-84.

[59] Abete, P., Ferrara, N., Leosco, D., et al. Age-related effects of platelet activating factor
      (PAF) in the isolated perfused rat heart. *J Mol Cell Cardiol.* 1992; 24:1399-407.

[60] Tarmiere, M. and Rochette, L. Direct effects of platelet-activating factor (PAF) on
      cardiac function in isolated guinea pig heart. *Drug Rev Res.* 1987; ll: 177-86.

[61] Metcalfe, D. D., Kaliner, M. and Donlon, M. A. . The mast cell. CRC Crit Rev
      Immunol 1981; 3: 23-74.

[62] Wedemeyer, J., Tsai, M. and Galli, S. J. . Roles of mast cells and basophils in innate
      and acquired immunity. *Curr Opin Immunol.* 2000; 12: 624-31.

[63] Puxeddu, I., Piliponsky, A. M., Bachelet, I. and Levi-Schaffer, F. Mast cells in allergy
      and beyond. *Int J Biochem Cell Biol.* 2003;35: 1601-1607.

[64] Galli, S. J., Kalesnikoff, J., Grimbaldeston, M. A., Piliponsky, A. M., Williams, C. M.
      and Tsai, M. (2005). Mast cells as "tunable" effector and immunoregulatory cells:
      recent advances. *Annu Rev Immunol.* 2005;23:749-86.

[65] Theoharides, T. C. and Kalogeromitros, D. The critical role of mast cell in allergy and
      inflammation. *Ann NY Acad Sci* 2006;1088: 78-99.

[66] Theoharides, T. C. and Cochrane, D. E. Critical role of mast cells in inflammatory
      diseases and the effect of acute stress. *J Neuroimmunol* 2004; 146: 1-12.

[67] Kirshenbaum, A. S., Goff, J. P., Semere, T., Foster, B., Scott, L. M. and Metcalfe, D.
      D. Demonstration that human mast cells arise from a progenitor cell population that is
      CD34(+), c-kit(+), and expresses aminopeptidase N (CD13). *Blood* 1999; 94: 2333-
      2342.

[68] Czarnetzki, B. M., Figdor, C. G., Kolde, G., Vroom, T., Aalberse, R. and de Vries, J. E.
      Development of human connective tissue mast cells from purified blood monocytes.
      Immunology 1984; 51: 549-554.

[69] Valent, P., Spanblöchl, E., Sperr, W. R., Sillaber, C., Zsebo, K. M., Agis, H. et al.
      Induction of differentiation of human mast cells from bone marrow and peripheral
      blood mononuclear cells by recombinant human stem cell factor/kit-ligand in long-term
      culture. *Blood* 1992; 80: 2237-2245.

[70] Aloe, L. and Levi-Montalcini, R. Mast cells increase in tissues of neonatal rats injected
      with the nerve growth factor. *Brain Res* 1977; 133: 358-366.

[71] Conti, P., Pang, X., Boucher, W., Letourneau, R., Reale, M., Barbacane, R. C. et al.
      Impact of Rantes and MCP-1 chemokines on in vivo basophilic mast cell recruitment in

rat skin injection model and their role in modifying the protein and mRNA levels for histidine decarboxylase. *Blood* 1977; 89: 4120-4127.

[72]   Conti, P., Reale, M., Barbacane, R. C., Letourneau, R. and Theoharides, T. C. Intramuscular injection of hrRANTES causes mast cell recruitment and increased transcription of histidine decarboxylase: lack of effects in genetically mast cell-deficient W/W^v mice. *FASEB J* 1998; 12: 1693-1700.

[73]   Tsuji, K., Nakahata, T., Takagi, M., Kobayashi, T., Ishiguro, A., Kikuchi, T. et al. Effects of interleukin-3 and interleukin-4 on the development of "connective tissue-type" mast cells: interleukin-3 supports their survival and interleukin-4 triggers and supports their proliferation synergistically with interleukin-3. *Blood* 1990; 75: 421-427.

[74]   Bischoff, S.C., Sellge, G., Lorentz, A., Sebald, W., Raab, R. and Manns, M. P. IL-4 enhances proliferation and mediator release in mature human mast cells. *Proc Natl Acad Sci USA* 1999; 96: 8080-8085.

[75]   Toru, H., Eguchi, M., Matsumoto, R., Yanagida, M., Yata, J. and Nakahata, T. (1998). Interleukin-4 promotes the development of tryptase and chymase double-positive human mast cells accompanied by cell maturation. *Blood* 91: 187-195.

[76]   van der Kleij, H. P., Ma, D., Redegeld, F. A., Kraneveld, A. D., Nijkamp, F. P. and Bienenstock, J. (2003). Functional expression of neurokinin 1 receptors on mast cells induced by IL-4 and stem cell factor. *J Immunol* 171: 2074-2079.

[77]   Tainsh, K. R. and Pearce, F. L. (1992). Mast cell heterogeneity: evidence that mast cells isolated from various connective tissue locations in the rat display markedly graded phenotypes. *Int Arch Allergy Immunol* 98: 26-34.

[78]   Bradding, P., Okayama, Y., Howarth, P. H., Church, M. K. and Holgate, S. T. (1995). Heterogeneity of human mast cells based on cytokine content. *J Immunol* 155: 297-307.

[79]   Levi-Schaffer, F., Austen, K. F., Gravallese, P. M. and Stevens, R. L. (1986). Co-culture of interleukin 3-dependent mouse mast cells with fibroblasts results in a phenotypic change of the mast cells. *Proc Natl Acad Sci USA* 83: 6485-6488.

[80]   Shanas, U., Bhasin, R., Sutherland, A. K., Silverman, A.-J. and Silver, R. (1998). Brain mast cells lack the c-kit receptor: immunocytochemical evidence. *J Neuroimmunol* 90: 207-211.

[81]   Dimitriadou, V., Lambracht-Hall, M., Reichler, J. and Theoharides, T. C. (1990). Histochemical and ultrastructural characteristics of rat brain perivascular mast cells stimulated with compound 48/80 and carbachol. *Neuroscience* 39: 209-224.

[82]   Robinson-White, A. and Beaven, M. A. (1982). Presence of histamine and histamine-metabolizing enzyme in rat and guinea-pig microvascular endothelial cells. *J Pharmacol Exp Ther* 223: 440-445.

[83]   Bienenstock, J., Tomioka, M., Matsuda, H., Stead, R. H., Quinonez, G., Simon, G. T. et al. (1987). The role of mast cells in inflammatory processes: evidence for nerve mast cell interactions. *Int Arch Allergy Appl Immunol* 82: 238-243.

[84]   Pang, X., Marchand, J., Sant, G. R., Kream, R. M. and Theoharides, T. C. (1995). Increased number of substance P positive nerve fibers in interstitial cystitis. *Br J Urol* 75: 744-750.

[85] Newson, B., Dahlström, A., Enerbäck, L. and Ahlman, H. (1983). Suggestive evidence for a direct innervation of mucosal mast cells. *Neuroscience* 10: 565-570.

[86] Stead, R. H., Tomioka, M., Quinonez, G., Simon, G. T., Felten, S. Y. and Bienenstock, J. (1987). Intestinal mucosal mast cells in normal and nematode-infected rat intestines are in intimate contact with peptidergic nerves. *Proc Natl Acad Sci USA 84*: 2975-2979.

[87] Dvorak, A. M., McLeod, R. S., Onderdonk, A.B., Monahan-Earley, R. A., Cullen, J. B., Antonioli, D. A. et al. (1992). Human gut mucosal mast cells: ultrastructural observations and anatomic variation in mast cell-nerve associations in vivo. *Int Arch Allergy Immunol* 98: 158-168.

[88] Letourneau, R., Pang, X., Sant, G. R. and Theoharides, T. C. (1996). Intragranular activation of bladder mast cells and their association with nerve processes in interstitial cystitis. *Br J Urol* 77: 41-54.

[89] Theoharides, T. C. (1996). Mast cell: a neuroimmunoendocrine master player. *Int J Tissue React* 18: 1-21.

[90] Theoharides, T. C., Spanos, C. P., Pang, X., Alferes, L., Ligris, K., Letourneau, R. et al. (1995). Stress-induced intracranial mast cell degranulation. A corticotropin releasing hormone-mediated effect. *Endocrinology* 136: 5745-5750.

[91] Blank, U. and Rivera, J. (2004). The ins and outs of IgE-dependent mast-cell exocytosis. *Trends Immunol* 25: 266-273.

[92] Kraft, S., Rana, S., Jouvin, M. H. and Kinet, J. P. (2004). The role of the FcepsilonRI beta-chain in allergic diseases. *Int Arch Allergy Immunol* 135: 62-72.

[93] Redegeld, F. A. and Nijkamp, F. P. (2005). Immunoglobulin free light chains and mast cells: pivotal role in T-cell-mediated immune reactions? *Trends Immuno.l* 24: 181-185.

[94] Kraneveld, A. D., Kool, M., van Houwelingen, A. H., Roholl, P., Solomon, A., Postma, D. S. et al. (2005). Elicitation of allergic asthma by immunoglobulin free light chains. *Proc Natl Acad Sci USA* 102: 1578-1583.

[95] Redegeld, F. A., van der Heijden, M. W., Kool, M., Heijdra, B. M., Garssen, J., Kraneveld, A. D. et al. (2002). Immunoglobulin-free light chains elicit immediate hypersensitivity-like responses. *Nat Med* 8: 694-701.

[96] Church, M. K., Lowman, M. A., Rees, P. H. and Benyon, R. C. (1989). Mast cells, neuropeptides and inflammation. *Agents Actions* 27: 8-16.

[97] Goetzl, E. J., Cheng, P. P. J., Hassner, A., Adelman, D. C., Frick, O. L. and Speedharan, S. P. (1990). Neuropeptides, mast cells and allergy: novel mechanisms and therapeutic possibilities. *Clin Exp Allergy* 20: 3-7.

[98] Foreman, J.C. (1987). Peptides and neurogenic inflammation. *Brain Res Bull.* 43: 386-398.

[99] Swieter, M., Hamawy, M. M., Siraganian, R. P. and Mergenhagen, S. E. (1993). Mast cells and their microenvironment: the influence of fibronectin and fibroblasts on the functional repertoire of rat basophilic leukemia cells. *J Periodontol* 64: 492-496.

[100] Janiszewski, J., Bienenstock, J. and Blennerhassett, M.G. (1994). Picomolar doses of substance P trigger electrical responses in mast cells without degranulation. *Am J Physiol.* 267: C138-C145.

[101] Mousli, M., Hugli, T. E., Landry, Y. and Bronner, C. (1994). Peptidergic pathway in human skin and rat peritoneal mast cell activation. *Immunopharmacol* 27: 1-11.

[102] Ali, H., Leung, K. B. P., Pearce, F. L., Hayes, N. A. and Foreman, J. C. (1986). Comparison of the histamine-releasing action of substance P on mast cells and basophils from different species and tissues. *Int Arch Allergy Appl Immunol* 79: 413-418.

[103] Matsuda, H., Kawakita, K., Kiso, Y., Nakano, T. and Kitamura, Y. (1989). Substance P induces granulocyte infiltration through degranulation of mast cells. *J Immunol* 142: 927-931.

[104] Theoharides, T. C. (1987). Substance P-induced release of brain mast cell nociceptive mediators. *Pain* 40, 262. Ref Type: Abstract.

[105] Carraway, R., Cochrane, D. E., Lansman, J. B., Leeman, S. E., Paterson, B. M. and Welch, H. J. (1982). Neurotensin stimulates exocytotic histamine secretion from rat mast cells and elevates plasma histamine levels. *J Physiol* 323: 403-414.

[106] Tal, M. and Liberman, R. (1997). Local injection of nerve growth factor (NGF) triggers degranulation of mast cells in rat paw. *Neurosci Lett* 221: 129-132.

[107] De Simone, R., Alleva, E., Tirassa, P. and Aloe, L. (1990). Nerve growth factor released into the bloodstream following intraspecific fighting induces mast cell degranulation in adult male mice. *Brain Behav Immun* 4: 74-81.

[108] Camarda, V., Rizzi, A., Galo, G., Guerrini, R., Salvadori, S. and Regoli, D. (2002). Pharmacological profile of hemokinin 1: a novel member of the tachykinin family. *Life Sci* 71: 363-370.

[109] Seebeck, J., Kruse, M. L., Schmidt-Choudhury, A. and Schmidt, W. E. (1998). Pituitary adenylate cyclase activating polypeptide induces degranulation of rat peritoneal mast cells via high-affinity PACAP receptor-independent activation of G proteins. *Ann NY Acad Sci* 865: 141-146.

[110] Odum, L., Petersen, L. J., Skov, P. S. and Ebskov, L. B. (1998). Pituitary adenylate cyclase activating polypeptide (PACAP) is localized in human dermal neurons and causes histamine release from skin mast cells. *Inflamm Res* 47: 488-492.

[111] Iikura, M., Suto, H., Kajiwara, N., Oboki, K., Ohno, T., Okayama, Y. et al. (2007). IL-33 can promote survival, adhesion and cytokine production in human mast cells. *Lab Invest* 87: 971-978.

[112] Moulin, D., Donze, O., Talabot-Ayer, D., Mezin, F., Palmer, G. and Gabay, C. (2007). Interleukin (IL)-33 induces the release of pro-inflammatory mediators by mast cells. *Cytokine 40*: 216-225.

[113] Ho, L. H., Ohno, T., Oboki, K., Kajiwara, N., Suto, H., Iikura, M. et al. (2007). IL-33 induces IL-13 production by mouse mast cells independently of IgE-FcepsilonRI signals. *J Leukocyte Biol 82*: 1481-1490.

[114] Ho, L. H., Ohno, T., Oboki, K., Kajiwara, N., Suto, H., Iikura, M. et al. (2007). IL-33 induces IL-13 production by mouse mast cells independently of IgE-Fc{epsilon}RI signals. *J Leukoc Biol 82*: 1481-1490.

[115] Allakhverdi, Z., Smith, D. E., Comeau, M. R. and Delespesse, G. (2007). Cutting edge: The ST2 ligand IL-33 potently activates and drives maturation of human mast cells. *J Immunol* 179: 2051-2054.

[116] Liu, Y. (2006). Thymic stromal lymphopoietin: master switch for allergic inflammation. *The Journal of Experimental Medicine* 203: 269-273.

[117] Al-Shami, A., Spolski, R., Kelly, J., Keane-Myers, A. and Leonard, W. J. (2005). A role for TSLP in the development of inflammation in an asthma model. *The Journal of Experimental Medicine* 202: 829-839.

[118] Zhou, C.-Y., Comeau, M. R., Smedt, T. D., Light, A. E., Dahl, M. E., Lewis, D. B. et al. (2005). Thymic stromal lymphopoietin as a key initiator of allergic airway inflammation in mice. *Nat Immunol* 6: 1047.

[119] Allakhverdi, Z., Comeau, M. R., Jessup, H. K., yoon, B. P., Breuer, A., Chartier, S. et al. (2007). Thymic stromal lymphopoietin is released by human epithelial cell in response to microbes, trauma, or inflammation and potently activates mast cells. *J Exp Med.* 19: 253-258.

[120] Cuttitta, F., Pio, R., Garayoa, M., Zudaire, E., Julian, M., Elsasser, T. H. et al. (2002). Adrenomedullin functions as an important tumor survival factor in human carcinogenesis. *Microsc Res Tech* 57: 110-119.

[121] Wong, L. Y., Cheung, B. M., Li, Y. Y. and Tang, F. (2005). Adrenomedullin is both proinflammatory and antiinflammatory: its effects on gene expression and secretion of cytokines and macrophage migration inhibitory factor in NR8383 macrophage cell line. *Endocrinology* 146: 1321-1327.

[122] Yoshida, M., Yoshida, H., Kitaichi, K., Hiramatsu, K., Kimura, T., Ito, Y. et al. (2001). Adrenomedullin and proadrenomedullin N-terminal 20 peptide induce histamine release from rat peritoneal mast cells. *Regul Pept* 101: 163-168.

[123] Pio, R., Martinez, A., Unsworth, E. J., Kowalak, J. A., Bengoechea, J. A., Zipfel, P. F. et al. (2001). Complement factor H is a serum-binding protein for adrenomedullin, and the resulting complex modulates the bioactivities of both partners. *J Biol Chem* 276: 12292-12300.

[124] Zudaire, E., Martinez, A., Garayoa, M., Pio, R., Kaur, G., Woolhiser, M. R. et al. (2006). Adrenomedullin is a cross-talk molecule that regulates tumor and mast cell function during human carcinogenesis. *Am J Pathol* 168: 280-291.

[125] Liao, L. X. and Granger, D. N. (1996). Role of mast cells in oxidized low-density lipoprotein-induced microvascular dysfunction. *Am J Physiol Heart Circ Physiol* 271: H1795-H1800.

[126] Kelley, J., Hemontolor, G., Younis, W., Li, C., Krishnaswamy, G. and Chi, D. S. (2006). Mast cell activation by lipoproteins. *Methods Mol Biol* 315: 341-348.

[127] Patella, V., Bouvet, J. P. and Marone, G. (1993). Protein Fv produced during vital hepatitis is a novel activator of human basophils and mast cells. *J Immunol* 151: 5685-5698.

[128] Genovese, A., Borgia, G., Bouvet, J. P., Detoraki, A., de Paulis, A., Piazza, M. et al. (2003). Protein Fv produced during viral hepatitis is an endogenous immunoglobulin superantigen activating human heart mast cells. *Int Arch Allergy Immunol* 132: 336-345.

[129] Marone, G., Rossi, F. W., Detoraki, A., Granata, F., Marone, G., Genovese, A. et al. (2007). Role of superallergens in allergic disorders. *Chem Immunol Allergy* 93: 195-213.

[130] Ehrenreich, H., Burd, P. R., Rottem, M., Hultner, L., Hylton, J. B., Garfield, M. et al. (1992). Endothelins belong to the assortment of mast cell-derived and mast cell-bound cytokines. *New Biol* 4: 147-156.

[131] Kedzierski, R. M. and Yanagisawa, M. (2001). Endothelin system: the double-edged sword in health and disease. *Annu Rev Pharmacol Toxicol* 41: 851-876.

[132] Matsushima, H., Yamada, N., Matsue, H. and Shimada, S. (2004). The effects of endothelin-1 on degranulation, cytokine, and growth factor production by skin-derived mast cells. *Eur J Immunol* 34: 1910-1019.

[133] Maurer, M., Wedemeyer, J., Metz, M., Piliponsky, A. M., Weller, K., Chatterjea, D. et al. (2004). Mast cells promote homeostasis by limiting endothelin-1-induced toxicity. *Nature* 432: 512-516.

[134] Rock, F. L., Hardiman, G., Timans, J. C., Kastelein, R. A. and Bazan, J. F. (1998). A family of human receptors structurally related to Drosophila Toll. *Proc Natl Acad Sci USA* 95: 588-593.

[135] Aderem, A. and Ulevitch, R. J. (2000). Toll-like receptors in the induction of the innate immune response. Nature 406: 782-787.

[136] Cristofaro, P. and Opal, S. M. (2006). Role of toll-like receptors in infection and immunity: clinical implications. *Drugs* 66: 15-29.

[137] Akira, S., Takeda, K. and Kaisho, T. (2001). Toll-like receptors: critical proteins linking innate and acquired immunity. *Nat Immunol* 2: 675-680.

[138] Heine, H. and Lien, E. (2003). Toll-like receptors and their function in innate and adaptive immunity. *Int Arch Allergy Immunol* 130: 180-192.

[139] Varadaradjalou, S., Feger, F., Thieblemont, N., Hamouda, N. B., Pleau, J. M., Dy, M. et al. (2003). Toll-like receptor 2 (TLR2) and TLR4 differentially activate human mast cells. *Eur J Immunol* 33: 899-906.

[140] McCurdy, J. D., Olynych, T. J., Maher, L. H. and Marshall, J. S. (2003). Cutting edge: distinct Toll-like receptor 2 activators selectively induce different classes of mediator production from human mast cells. *J Immunol* 170: 1625-1629.

[141] Ikeda, R. K., Miller, M., Nayar, J., Walker, L., Cho, J. Y., McElwain, K. et al. (2003). Accumulation of peribronchial mast cells in a mouse model of ovalbumin allergen induced chronic airway inflammation: modulation by immunostimulatory DNA sequences. *J Immunol* 171: 4860-4867.

[142] Kulka, M., Alexopoulou, L., Flavell, R. A. and Metcalfe, D. D. (2004). Activation of mast cells by double-stranded RNA: evidence for activation through Toll-like receptor 3. *J Allergy Clin Immunol* 114: 174-182.

[143] Anthony, M. and Lance, J. W. (1971). Whole blood histamine and plasma serotonin in cluster headache. *Proc Aust assoc Neurol* 8: 43-46.

[144] Cairns, J. A. and Walls, A. F. (1996). Mast cell tryptase is a mitogen for epithelial cells. Stimulation of IL-8 production and intercellular adhesion molecule-1 expression. *J Immunol* 156: 275-283.

[145] Masuda, A., Yoshikai, Y., Aiba, K. and Matsuguchi, T. (2002). Th2 cytokine production from mast cells is directly induced by lipopolysaccharide and distinctly regulated by c-Jun N-terminal kinase and p38 pathways. *J Immunol* 169: 3801-3810.

[146] Supajatura, V., Ushio, H., Nakao, A., Akira, S., Okumura, K., Ra, C. et al. (2002). Differential responses of mast cell Toll-like receptors 2 and 4 in allergy and innate immunity. *J Clin Invest* 109: 1351-1359.

[147] Theoharides, T. C., Singh, L. K., Boucher, W., Pang, X., Letourneau, R., Webster, E. et al. (1998). Corticotropin-releasing hormone induces skin mast cell degranulation and increased vascular permeability, a possible explanation for its pro-inflammatory effects. *Endocrinology* 139: 403-413.

[148] Singh, L. K., Boucher, W., Pang, X., Letourneau, R., Seretakis, D., Green, M. et al. (1999). Potent mast cell degranulation and vascular permeability triggered by urocortin through activation of CRH receptors. *J Pharmacol Exp Ther.* 288: 1349-1356.

[149] Clifton, V. L., Crompton, R., Smith, R. and Wright, I. M. (2002). Microvascular effects of CRH in human skin vary in relation to gender. J Clin Endocrinol Metab 87: 267-270.

[150] Katsarou-Katsari, A., Singh, L. K. and Theoharides, T. C. (2001). Alopecia areata and affected skin CRH receptor upregulation induced by acute emotional stress. *Dermatology* 203: 157-161.

[151] Papadopoulou, N., Kalogeromitros, D., Staurianeas, N. G., Tiblalexi, D. and Theoharides, T. C. (2005). Corticotroopin-releasing hormone receptor-1 and histidine decarboxylase expression in chronic urticaria. *J Invest Dermatol* 125: 952-955.

[152] Singh, L. K., Pang, X., Alexacos, N., Letourneau, R. and Theoharides, T. C. (1999). Acute immobilization stress triggers skin mast cell degranulation via corticotropin-releasing hormone, neurotensin and substance P: A link to neurogenic skin disorders. *Brain Behav Immunity* 13: 225-239.

[153] Roberts, F. and Calcutt, C. R. (1983). Histamine and the hypothalamus. *Neuroscience* 9: 721-739.

[154] Kjaer, A., Larsen, P. J., Knigge, U., Jorgensen, H. and Warberg, J. (1998). Neuronal histamine and expression of corticotropin-releasing hormone, vasopressin and oxytocin in the hypothalamus: relative importance of H_1 and H_2 receptors. *Eur J Endocrinol* 139: 238-243.

[155] Lytinas, M., Kempuraj, D., Kandere, K., Huang, M., Madhappan, B., Christodoulou, S. et al. (2003). Human mast cells synthesize and secrete corticotropin-releasing hormone (CRH) which triggers them to secrete IL-6. *Endocrinology*. Ref Type: In Press

[156] Bethin, K. E., Vogt, S. K. and Muglia, L. J. (2000). Interleukin-6 is an essential, corticotropin-releasing hormone-independent stimulator of the adrenal axis during immune system activation. *Proc Natl Acad Sci USA* 97: 9317-9322.

[157] Stead, R. H., Colley, E. C., Wang, B., Partosoedarso, E., Lin, J., Stanisz, A. et al. (2006). Vagal influences over mast cells. *Auton Neurosci* 125: 53-61.

[158] Blandina, P., Fantozzi, R., Mannaioni, P. F. and Masini, E. (1980). Characteristics of histamine release evoked by acetylcholine in isolated rat mast cells. *J Physiol* 301: 281-293.

[159] Fantozzi, R., Masini, E., Blandina, P., Mannaioni, P. F. and Bani-Sacchi, T. (1978). Release of histamine from rat mast cells by acetylcholine. *Nature* 273: 473-474.

[160] Cho, C. H. and Ogle, C. W. (1977). The effects of zinc sulphate on vagal-induced mast cell changes and ulcers in the rat stomach. *Eur J Pharmacol* 43: 315-322.

[161] Bani-Sacchi, T., Barattini, M., Bianchi, S., Blandina, P., Branelleschi, S., Fantozzi, R. et al. (1986). The release of histamine by parasympathetic stimulation in guinea pig auricle and rat ileum. *J Physiol* 371: 29-43.

[162] Casale, T. B. and Marom, Z. (1983). Mast cells and asthma. The role of mast cell mediators in the pathogenesis of allergic asthma. *Ann Allergy* 51: 2-6.

[163] Christian, E. P., Undem, B. J. and Weinreich, D. (1989). Endogenous histamine excites neurones in the guinea-pig superior cervical ganglion in vitro. *J Physiol* 409: 297-312.

[164] Blennerhassett, M. G., Tomioka, M. and Bienenstock, J. (1991). Formation of contacts between mast cells and sympathetic neurons in vitro. *Cell Tissue Res* 265: 121-128.

[165] Suzuki, R., Furuno, T., McKay, D. M., Wolvers, D., Teshima, R., Nakanishi, M. et al. (1999). Direct neurite-mast cell communication in vitro occurs via the neuropeptide substance P. *J Immunol* 163: 2410-2415.

[166] Rozniecki, J. J., Dimitriadou, V., Lambracht-Hall, M., Pang, X. and Theoharides, T. C. (1999). Morphological and functional demonstration of rat dura mast cell-neuron interactions in vitro and in vivo. *Brain Res* 849: 1-15.

[167] Rothschild, A. M., Gomes, E. L. and Rossi, M. A. (1991). Reversible rat mesenteric mast cell swelling caused by vagal stimulation or sham-feeding. *Agents Actions* 34: 295-301.

[168] Joos, G. F., Pauwels, R. A. and van der Straeten, M. E. (1988). The mechanism of tachykinin-induced bronchoconstriction in the rat. *Am Rev Respir Dis* 137: 1038-1044.

[169] Fuder, H., Ries, P. and Schwarz, P. (1994). Histamine and serotonin released from the rat perfused heart by compound 48/80 or by allergen challenge influence noradrenaline or acetylcholine exocytotic release. *Fundam Clin Pharmacol* 8: 477-490.

[170] Gottwald, T., Lhotak, S. and Stead, R. H. (1997). Effect of truncal vagotomy and capsaicin on mast cells and IgA-positive plasma cells in rat jejunal mucosa. *Neurogastroenterol Motil* 9: 25-32.

[171] Barke, K. E. and Hough, L. B. (1993). Opiates, mast cells and histamine release. *Life Sci* 53: 1391-1399.

[172] Rottem, M. and Mekori, Y. A. (2005). Mast cells and autoimmunity. *Autoimmun Rev* 4: 21-27.

[173] Lagunoff, D., Martin, T. W. and Read, G. (1983). Agents that release histamine from mast cells. *Annu Rev Pharmacol Toxicol* 23: 331-351.

[174] Dvorak, A. M. (1997). New aspects of mast cell biology. *Int Arch Allergy Immunol* 114: 1-9.

[175] Hogan, A. D. and Schwartz, L. B. (1997). Markers of mast cell degranulation. *Methods Enzymol* 13: 43-52.

[176] Grutzkau, A., Kruger-Krasagakes, S., Baumeister, H., Schwarz, C., Kogel, H., Welker, P. et al. (1998). Synthesis, storage and release of vascular endothelial growth factor/vascular permeability factor (VEGF/VPF) by human mast cells: Implications for the biological significance of VEGF$_{206}$. *Mol Biol Cell* 9: 875-884.

[177] Boesiger, J., Tsai, M., Maurer, M., Yamaguchi, M., Brown, L. F., Claffey, K. P. et al. (1998). Mast cells can secrete vascular permeability factor/vascular endothelial cell growth factor and exhibit enhanced release after immunoglobulin E-dependent upregulation of Fce receptor I expression. *J Exp Med* 188: 1135-1145.

[178] Abdel-Majid, R. M. and Marshall, J. S. (2004). Prostaglandin E2 induces degranulation-independent production of vascular endothelial growth factor by human mast cells. J Immunol 172: 1227-1236.

[179] Feoktistov, I., Ryzhov, S., Goldstein, A. E. and Biaggioni, I. (2003). Mast cell-mediated stimulation of angiogenesis: cooperative interaction between A2B and A3 adenosine receptors. *Circ Res* 92: 485-492.

[180] Kempuraj, D., Papadopoulou, N. G., Lytinas, M., Huang, M., Kandere-Grzybowska, K., Madhappan, B. et al. (2004). Corticotropin-releasing hormone and its structurally related urocortin are synthesized and secreted by human mast cells. *Endocrinology* 145: 43-48.

[181] Laham, R. J., Li, J., Tofukuji, M., Post, M., Simons, M. and Sellke, F. W. (2003). Spatial heterogeneity in VEGF-induced vasodilation: VEGF dilates microvessels but not epicardial and systemic arteries and veins. *Ann Vasc Surg* 17: 245-252.

[182] Carraway, R. E., Cochrane, D. E., Boucher, W. and Mitra, S. P. (1989). Structures of histamine-releasing peptides formed by the action of acid proteases on mammalian albumin(s). *J Immunol* 143: 1680-1684.

[183] Cochrane, D. E., Carraway, R. E., Feldberg, R. S., Boucher, W. and Gelfand, J. M. (1993). Stimulated rat mast cells generate histamine-releasing peptide from albumin. *Peptides* 14: 117-123.

[184] Schmidlin, F. and Bunnett, N. W. (2001). Protease-activated receptors: how proteases signal to cells. *Curr Opin Pharmacol 1*: 575-582.

[185] Molino, M., Barnathan, E. S., Numerof, R., Clark, J., Dreyer, M., Cumashi, A. et al. (1997). Interactions of mast cell tryptase with thrombin receptors and PAR-2. *J Biol Chem* 272: 4043-4049.

[186] Henderson, W. R. and Kaliner, M. (1978). Immunologic and nonimmunologic generation of superoxide from mast cells and basophils. *J Clin Invest* 61: 187-196.

[187] Brooks, A. C., Whelan, C. J. and Purcell, W. M. (1999). Reactive oxygen species generation and histamine release by activated mast cells:modulation by nitric oxide synthase inhibition. *Br J Pharmacol* 128: 585-590.

[188] Swindle, E. J., Metcalfe, D. D. and Coleman, J. W. (2004). Rodent and human mast cells produce functionally significant intracellular reactive oxygen species but not nitric oxide. *J Biol Chem* 279: 48751-48759.

[189] Tsinkalovsky, O. R. and Laerum, O. D. (1994). Flow cytometric measurement of the production of reactive oxygen intermediate in activated rat mast cells. *APMIS 102*: 474-480.

[190] Wolfreys, K. and Oliveira, D. B. (1997). Alterations in intracellular reactive oxygen species generation and redox potential modulate mast cell function. *Eur J Immunol* 27: 297-306.

[191] Yoshimaru, T., Suzuki, Y., Inoue, T., Niide, O. and Ra, C. (2006). Silver activates mast cells through reactive oxygen species production and a thiol-sensitive store-independent Ca2+ influx. *Free Radic Biol Med 40*: 1949-1959.

[192] Cho, S. H., Woo, C. H., Yoon, S. B. and Kim, J. H. (2004). Protein kinase Cdelta functions downstream of Ca2+ mobilization in FcepsilonRI signaling to degranulation in mast cells. *J Allergy Clin Immunol 114*: 1085-1092.

[193] Kim, J. Y. and Ro, J. Y. (2005). Signal pathway of cytokines produced by reactive oxygen species generated from phorbol myristate acetate-stimulated HMC-1 cells. *Scand J Immunol* 62: 25-35.

[194] Kawamura, F., Hirashima, N., Furuno, T. and Nakanishi, M. (2006). Effects of 2-methyl-1,4-naphtoquinone (menadione) on cellular signaling in RBL-2H3 cells. *Biol Pharm Bull* 29: 605-607.

[195] Brown, J. M., Swindle, E. J., kushnir-Sukhov, N. M., Holian, A. and Metcalfe, D. D. (2007). Silica-directed mast cell activation is enhanced by scavenger receptors. *Am J Respir Cell Mol Biol* 36: 43-52.

[196] Malaviya, R., Ross, E. A., MacGregor, J. I., Ikeda, T., Little, J. R., Jakschik, B. A. et al. (1994). Mast cell phagocytosis of FimH-expressing enterobacteria. *J Immunol*. 152: 1907-1914.

[197] Niide, O., Suzuki, Y., Yoshimaru, T., Inoue, T., Takayama, T. and Ra, C. (2006). Fungal metabolite gliotoxin blocks mast cell activation by a calcium- and superoxide-dependent mechanism: implications for immunosuppressive activities. *Clin Immunol* 118: 108-116.

[198] Swindle, E. J., Coleman, J. W., DeLeo, F. R. and Metcalfe, D. D. (2007). FcepsilonRI- and Fcgamma receptor-mediated production of reactive oxygen species by mast cells is lipoxygenase- and cyclooxygenase-dependent and NADPH oxidase-independent. *J Immunol* 179: 7059-7071.

[199] Kanwar, S. and Kubes, P. (1994). Mast cells contribute to ischemia-reperfusion-induced granulocyte infiltration and intestinal dysfunction. *Am J Physiol* 267: G316-G321.

[200] Boros, M., Takaichi, S., Masuda, J., Newlands, G. F. J. and Hatanaka, K. (1995). Response of mucosal mast cells to intestinal ischemia-reperfusion injury in the rat. *Shock* 3: 125-131.

[201] Kimura, T., Fujiyama, Y., Sasaki, M., Andoh, A., Fukuda, M., Nakajima, S. et al. (1998). The role of mucosal mast cell degranulation and free-radical generation in intestinal ischaemia-reperfusion injury in rats. *Eur J Gastroenterol Hepatol* 10: 659-666.

[202] Boros, M., Kaszaki, J., Bako, L. and Nagy, S. (1992). Studies on the relationship between xanthine oxidase and histamine release during intestinal ischemia-reperfusion. *Circ Shock* 38: 108-114.

[203] Kurose, I., Argenbright, L. W., Wolf, R., Lianxi, L. and Granger, D. N. (1997). Ischemia/reperfusion-induced microvascular dysfunction: role of oxidants and lipid mediators. *Am J Physiol* 272: H2976-H2982.

[204] Davani, S., Muret, P., Royer, B., Kantelip, B., Frances, C., Millart, H. et al. (2002). Ischaemic preconditioning and mast cell histamine release: microdialysis of isolated rat hearts. *Pharmacol Res* 45: 383-390.

[205] Masini, E., Cuzzocrea, S., Mazzon, E., Marzocca, C., Mannaioni, P. F. and Salvemini, D. (2002). Protective effects of M40403, a selective superoxide dismutase mimetic, in myocardial ischaemia and reperfusion injury in vivo. *Br J Pharmacol* 136: 905-917.

[206] Dimitriadou, V., Buzzi, M. G., Moskowitz, M. A. and Theoharides, T. C. (1991). Trigeminal sensory fiber stimulation induces morphologic changes reflecting secretion in rat dura mast cells. *Neuroscience* 44: 97-112.

[207] Theoharides, T. C., Sant, G. R., El-Mansoury, M., Letourneau, R. J., Ucci, A. A., Jr. and Meares, E. M., Jr. (1995). Activation of bladder mast cells in interstitial cystitis: a light and electron microscopic study. *J Urol* 153: 629-636.

[208] Dvorak, A. M., McLeod, R. S., Onderdonk, A., Monahan-Earley, R. A., Cullen, J. B., Antonioli, D. A. et al. (1992). Ultrastructural evidence for piecemeal and anaphylactic degranulation of human gut mucosal mast cells in vivo. *Int Arch Allergy Immunol* 99: 74-83.

[209] Kops, S. K., Van Loveren, H., Rosenstein, R. W., Ptak, W. and Askenase, P. W. (1984). Mast cell activation and vascular alterations in immediate hypersensitivity-like reactions induced by a T cell derived antigen-binding factor. *Lab Invest* 50: 421-434.

[210] Van Loveren, H., Kops, S. K. and Askenase, P. W. (1984). Different mechanisms of release of vasoactive amines by mast cells occur in T cell-dependent compared to IgE-dependent cutaneous hypersensitivity responses. *Eur J Immunol* 14: 40-47.

[211] Kops, S. K., Theoharides, T. C., Cronin, C. T., Kashgarian, M. G. and Askenase, P. W. (1990). Ultrastructural characteristics of rat peritoneal mast cells undergoing differential release of serotonin without histamine and without degranulation. *Cell Tissue Res* 262: 415-424.

[212] Theoharides, T. C., Bondy, P. K., Tsakalos, N. D. and Askenase, P. W. (1982). Differential release of serotonin and histamine from mast cells. *Nature* 297: 229-231.

[213] Benyon, R., Robinson, C. and Church, M. K. (1989). Differential release of histamine and eicosanoids from human skin mast cells activated by IgE-dependent and non-immunological stimuli. *Br J Pharmacol* 97: 898-904.

[214] Levi-Schaffer, F. and Shalit, M. (1989). Differential release of histamine and prostaglandin D_2 in rat peritoneal mast cells activated with peptides. *Int Arch Allergy Appl Immunol* 90: 352-357.

[215] van Haaster, C. M., Engels, W., Lemmens, P. J. M. R., Hornstra, G., van der Vusse, G. J. and Heemskerk, J. W. M. (1995). Differential release of histamine and prostaglandin D_2 in rat peritoneal mast cells; roles of cytosolic calcium and protein tyrosine kinases. *Biochim Biophys Acta* 1265: 79-88.

[216] Kandere-Grzybowska, K., Letourneau, R., Kempuraj, D., Donelan, J., Poplawski, S., Boucher, W. et al. (2003). IL-1 induces vesicular secretion of IL-6 without degranulation from human mast cells. *J Immunol* 171: 4830-4836.

[217] Cao, J., Curtis, C. L. and Theoharides, T. C. (2006). Corticotropin-releasing hormone induces vascular endothelial growth factor release from human mast cells via the cAMP/protein kinase A/p38 mitogen-activated protein kinase pathway. *Mol Pharmacol.* 69: 998-1006.

[218] Theoharides, T. C., Kempuraj, D., Tagen, M., Conti, P. and Kalogeromitros, D. (2007). Differential release of mast cell mediators and the pathogenesis of inflammation. *Immunol Rev* 217: 65-78.

[219] Valadi, H., Ekstrom, K., Bossios, A., Sjostrand, M., Lee, J. J. and Lotvall, J. O. (2007). Exosome-mediated transfer of mRNAs and microRNAs is a novel mechanism of genetic exchange between cells. *Nat Cell Biol* 9: 654-659.

[220] Raposo, G., Tenza, D., Mecheri, S., Peronet, R., Bonnerot, C. and Desaymard, C. (1997). Accumulation of major histocompatibility complex class II molecules in mast cell secretory granules and their release upon degranulation. *Mol Biol Cell* 8: 2631-2645.

[221] Skokos, D., Botros, H. G., Demeure, C., Morin, J., Peronet, R., Birkenmeier, G. et al. (2003). Mast cell-derived exosomes induce phenotypic and functional maturation of dendritic cells and elicit specific immune responses in vivo. *J Immunol* 170: 3037-3045.

[222] Karlsson, M., Lundin, S., Dahlgren, U., Kahu, H., Pettersson, I. and Telemo, E. (2001). "Tolerosomes" are produced by intestinal epithelial cells. *Eur J Immunol* 31: 2892-2900.

[223] Taylor, D. D., Akyol, S. and Gercel-Taylor, C. (2006). Pregnancy-associated exosomes and their modulation of T cell signaling. *J Immunol* 176: 1534-1542.

[224] Theoharides, T. C., Sieghart, W., Greengard, P. and Douglas, W. W. (1980). Antiallergic drug cromolyn may inhibit histamine secretion by regulating phosphorylation of a mast cell protein. *Science* 207: 80-82.

[225] Kempna, P., Reiter, E., Arock, M., Azzi, A. and Zingg, J. M. (2004). Inhibition of HMC-1 mast cell proliferation by vitamin E: involvement of the protein kinase B pathway. *J Biol Chem* 279: 50700-50709.

[226] Ricciarelli, R., Tasinato, A., Clement, S., Ozer, N. K., Boscoboinik, D. and Azzi, A. (1998). alpha-Tocopherol specifically inactivates cellular protein kinase C alpha by changing its phosphorylation state. *Biochem J* 334 (Pt 1): 243-249.

[227] Cachia, O., Benna, J. E., Pedruzzi, E., Descomps, B., Gougerot-Pocidalo, M. A. and Leger, C. L. (1998). alpha-tocopherol inhibits the respiratory burst in human monocytes. Attenuation of p47(phox) membrane translocation and phosphorylation. *J Biol Chem* 273: 32801-32805.

[228] Chow, C. K. (2001). Vitamin E regulation of mitochondrial superoxide generation. *Biol Signals Recept* 10: 112-124.

[229] Brigelius-Flohe, R. (2005). Induction of drug metabolizing enzymes by vitamin E. *J Plant Physiol* 162: 797-802.

[230] Azzi, A., Gysin, R., Kempna, P., Munteanu, A., Negis, Y., Villacorta, L. et al. (2004). Vitamin E mediates cell signaling and regulation of gene expression. *Ann N Y Acad Sci* 1031: 86-95.

[231] Arici, A., Tazuke, S. I., Attar, E., Kliman, H. J. and Olive, D. L. (1996). Interleukin-8 concentration in peritoneal fluid of patients with endometriosis and modulation of interleukin-8 expression in human mesothelial cells. *Mol Hum Reprod* 2: 40-45.

[232] Ishida, S., Kinoshita, T., Sugawara, N., Yamashita, T. and Koike, K. (2003). Serum inhibitors for human mast cell growth: possible role of retinol. *Allergy* 58: 1044-1052.

[233] Middleton, E., Jr., Kandaswami, C. and Theoharides, T. C. (2000). The effects of plant flavonoids on mammalian cells: implications for inflammation, heart disease and cancer. *Pharmacol Rev* 52: 673-751.

[234] Kimata, M., Shichijo, M., Miura, T., Serizawa, I., Inagaki, N. and Nagai, H. (2000). Effects of luteolin, quercetin and baicalein on immunoglobulin E-mediated mediator release from human cultured mast cells. *Clin Exp Allergy* 30: 501-508.

[235] Kempuraj, D., Madhappan, B., Christodoulou, S., Boucher, W., Cao, J., Papadopoulou, N. et al. (2005). Flavonols inhibit proinflammatory mediator release, intracellular calcium ion levels and protein kinase C theta phosphorylation in human mast cells. *Br J Pharmacol* 145: 934-944.

[236] Alexandrakis, M. G., Letourneau, R., Kempuraj, D., Kandere, K., Huang, M., Christodoulou, S. et al. (2003). Flavones inhibit proliferation and increase mediator content in human leukemic mast cells (HMC-1). *Eur J Haematol* 71: 448-454.

[237] Theoharides, T. C., Patra, P., Boucher, W., Letourneau, R., Kempuraj, D., Chiang, G. et al. (2000). Chondroitin sulfate inhibits connective tissue mast cells. *Br J Pharmacol* 131: 1039-1049.

[238] Choi, I. Y., Jung, H. S., Kim, H. R., Lee, E. J., Lee, E. H., Shin, T. Y. et al. (2004). OK205 regulates production of inflammatory cytokines in HMC-1 cells. *Biol Pharm Bull* 27: 1871-1874.

[239] Inase, N., Schreck, R. E. and Lazarus, S. C. (1993). Heparin inhibits histamine release from canine mast cells. *Am J Physiol* 264: L387-L390.

[240] Phillips, G. D., Pickering, E. C. and Wilkinson, K. (1975). Renal responses of the cow to alteration of the dietary intake of nitrogen and sodium chloride. *J Physiol* 245: 95P-96P.

[241] Conti, P., Kempuraj, D., Kandere, K., Gioacchino, M. D., Barbacane, R. C., Castellani, M. L. et al. (2003). IL-10, an inflammatory/inhibitory cytokine, but not always. *Immunol Lett* 86: 123-129.

[242] Gebhardt, T., Lorentz, A., Detmer, F., Trautwein, C., Bektas, H., Manns, M. P. et al. (2005). Growth, phenotype, and function of human intestinal mast cells are tightly regulated by transforming growth factor beta1. *Gut* 54: 928-934.

[243] Gomez, G., Ramirez, C. D., Rivera, J., Patel, M., Norozian, F., Wright, H. V. et al. (2005). TGF-beta1 inhibits mast cell FceRI expression. *J Immunol* 174: 5987-5993.

[244] Saavedra, Y. and Vergara, P. (2003). Somatostatin inhibits intestinal mucosal mast cell degranulation in normal conditions and during mast cell hyperplasia. *Regul Pept* 111: 67-75.

[245] Tang, C., Lan, C., Wang, C. and Liu, R. (2005). Amelioration of the development of multiple organ dysfunction syndrome by somatostatin via suppression of intestinal mucosal mast cells. *Shock* 23: 470-475.

[246] Kassessinoff, T. A. and Pearce, F. L. (1988). Histamine secretion from mast cells stimulated with somatostatin. *Agents Actions* 23: 211-213.

[247] Grisham, M. B., Jourd'Heuil, D. and Wink, D. A. (1999). Nitric oxide. I. Physiological chemistry of nitric oxide and its metabolites:implications in inflammation. *Am J Physiol.* 276: G315-G321.

[248] Ray, A., Chakraborti, A. and Gulati, K. (2007). Current trends in nitric oxide research. *Cell Mol Biol* (Noisy -le-grand) 53: 3-14.

[249] Bidri, M., Feger, F., Varadaradjalou, S., Ben, H. N., Guillosson, J. J. and Arock, M. (2001). Mast cells as a source and target for nitric oxide. *Int Immunopharmacol* 1: 1543-1558.

[250] Eastmond, N. C., Banks, E. M. and Coleman, J. W. (1997). Nitric oxide inhibits IgE-mediated degranulation of mast cells and is the principal intermediate in IFN-gamma-induced suppression of exocytosis. *J Immunol* 159: 1444-1450.

[251] Deschoolmeester, M. L., Eastmond, N. C., Dearman, R. J., Kimber, I., Basketter, D. A. and Coleman, J. W. (1999). Reciprocal effects of interleukin-4 and interferon-gamma on immunoglobulin E-mediated mast cell degranulation: a role for nitric oxide but not peroxynitrite or cyclic guanosine monophosphate. *Immunology* 96: 138-144.

[252] Masini, E., Salvemini, D., Ndisang, J. F., Gai, P., Berni, L., Moncini, M. et al. (1999). Cardioprotective activity of endogenous and exogenous nitric oxide on ischaemia reperfusion injury in isolated guinea pig hearts. *Inflamm Res* 48: 561-568.

[253] Masini, E., Gambassi, F., Bianchi, S., Mugnai, L., Lupini, M., Pistelli, A. et al. (1991). Effect of nitric oxide generators on ischemia-reperfusion injury and histamine release in isolated perfused guinea pig heart. *Int Arch Allergy Appl Immunol* 94: 257-258.

[254] Jorens, P. G., van Overveld, F. J., Bult, H., Vermeire, P. A. and Herman, A. G. (1993). Muramyldipeptide and granulocyte-macrophage colony-stimulating factor enhance interferon-gamma-induced nitric oxide production by rat alveolar macrophages. *Agents Actions* 38: 100-105.

[255] Wills, F. L., Gilchrist, M. and Befus, A. D. (1999). Interferon-gamma regulates the interaction of RBL-2H3 cells with fibronectin through production of nitric oxide. *Immunology* 97: 481-489.

[256] Gilchrist, M., McCauley, S. D. and Befus, A. D. (2004). Expression, localization, and regulation of NOS in human mast cell lines: effects on leukotriene production. *Blood* 104: 462-469.

[257] Sekar, Y., Moon, T. C., Munoz, S. and Befus, A. D. (2005). Role of nitric oxide in mast cells: controversies, current knowledge, and future applications. *Immunol Res* 33: 223-239.

[258] Coleman, J. W. (2002). Nitric oxide: a regulator of mast cell activation and mast cell-mediated inflammation. *Clin Exp Immunol* 129: 4-10.

[259] Inoue, T., Suzuki, Y., Yoshimaru, T. and Ra, C. (2008). Nitric oxide protects mast cells from activation-induced cell death: the role of the phosphatidylinositol-3 kinase-Akt-endothelial nitric oxide synthase pathway. *J Leukoc Biol*.

[260] Parikh, V. and Singh, M. (2001). Possible role of nitric oxide and mast cells in endotoxin-induced cardioprotection. *Pharmacol Res* 43: 39-45.

[261] Patella, V., de Crescenzo, G., Ciccarelli, A., Marino, I., Adt, M. and Marone, G. (1995). Human heart mast cells: a definitive case of mast cell heterogeneity. *Int Arch Allergy Immunol* 106: 386-393.

[262] Kovanen, P. T. (2007). Mast cells: multipotent local effector cells in atherothrombosis. *Immunol Rev* 217: 105-122.

[263] Frangogiannis, N. G. (2007). Chemokines in ischemia and reperfusion. *Thromb Haemost* 97: 738-747.

[264] Forman, M. B., Oates, J. A., Robertson, D., Robertson, R. M., Roberts, L. J., II and Virmani, R. (1985). Increased adventitial mast cells in a patient with coronary spasm. *N Engl J Med* 313: 1138-1141.

[265] Kaartinen, M., Penttilä, A. and Kovanen, P. T. Accumulation of activated mast cells in the shoulder region of human coronary atheroma, the predilection site of atheromatous rupture. *Circulation* 1994; 90: 1669-1678.

[266] Constantinides, P. Infiltrates of activated mast cells at the site of coronary atheromatous erosion or rupture in myocardial infarction. *Circulation* 1995; 92: 1083-1088.

[267] Laine, P., Kaartinen, M., Penttilä, A., Panula, P., Paavonen, T. and Kovanen, P. T. Association between myocardial infarction and the mast cells in the adventitia of the infarct-related coronary artery. *Circulation* 1999; 99: 361-369.

[268] Lee, M., Kovanen, P. T., Tedeschi, G., Oungre, E., Franceschini, G. and Calabresi, L. Apolipoprotein composition and particle size affect HDL degradation by chymase: effect on cellular cholesterol efflux. *J Lipid Res2003*; 44: 539-546.

[269] Lee, M., Calabresi, L., Chiesa, G., Franceschini, G. and Kovanen, P. T. Mast cell chymase degrades apoE and apoA-II in apoA-I-knockout mouse plasma and reduces its ability to promote cellular cholesterol efflux. *Arterioscler Thromb Vasc Biol* 2002; 22: 1475-1481.

[270] Kovanen, P. T. Mast cells in human fatty streaks and atheromas: Implications for intimal lipid accumulation. *Curr Opin Lipidol* 1`996; 7: 281-286.

[271] Lindstedt, L., Lee, M., Castro, G. R., Fruchart, J. C. and Kovanen, P. T. Chymase in exocytosed rat mast cell granules effectively proteolyzes apolipoprotein AI-containing lipoproteins, so reducing the cholesterol efflux-inducing ability of serum and aortic intimal fluid. *J Clin Invest* 1996; 97: 2174-2182.

[272] von Eckardstein, A., Nofer, J. R. and Assmann, G. High density lipoproteins and arteriosclerosis. Role of cholesterol efflux and reverse cholesterol transport. *Arterioscler Thromb Vasc Biol* 2001; 21: 13-27.

[273] Gristwood, R. W., Lincoln, J. C., Owen, D. A. and Smith, I. R. Histamine release from human right atrium. *Br J Pharmacol* 1981; 74: 7-9.

[274] Genovese, A. and Spadaro, G. Highlights in cardiovascular effects of histamine and H1-receptor antagonists. *Allergy* 1997; 52: 67-78.

[275] Doggrell, S. A. and Wanstall, J. C. Cardiac chymase: pathophysiological role and therapeutic potential of chymase inhibitors. *Can J Physiol Pharmacol* 2005; 83: 123-130.

[276] Doggrell, S. A. and Wanstall, J. C. Vascular chymase: pathophysiological role and therapeutic potential of inhibition. *Cardiovasc Res* 2004; 61: 653-662.

[277] Silver, R. B., Reid, A. C., Mackins, C. J., Askwith, T., Schaefer, U., Herzlinger, D. et al. Mast cells: A unique source of renin. *Proc Natl Acad Sci USA* 2004; 101: 13607-13612.

[278] Kano, S., Tyler, E., SAlazar-Rodriguez, M., Estephan, R., Mackins, C.J., Veerappan, A., et al. Immediate hypersensitivity elicits renin release from cardiac mast cells. *Int Arch Immunol.* 2008; 146: 71-75

[279] Dell'Italia, L. J., Meng, Q. C., Balcells, E., Wei, C. C., Palmer, R., Hageman, G. R. et al. Compartmentalization of angiotensin II generation in the dog heart. Evidence for

independent mechanisms in intravascular and interstitial spaces. *J Clin Invest* 1997; 100: 253-258.

[280] Mackins, C. J., Kano, S., Seyedi, N., Schafer, U., Reid, A. C., Machida, J. et al. Cardiac mast cell-derived renin promotes local angiotensin formation, norepinephrine release, and arrhythmias in ischemia-reperfusion. *J Clin Invest* 2006; 116: 1063-1070.

[281] Deedwania, P. C. Mental stress, pain perception and risk of silent ischemia. *JACC* 1995; m 25: 1504-1506.

[282] Freeman, L. J., Nixon, P. G. F., Sallabank, P. and Reaveley, D. Psychological stress and silent myocardial ischemia. *Am Heart J* 1987; 114: 477-482.

[283] Deanfield, J. E., Shea, M., Kensett, M., Horlock, P., Wilson, R. A., deLandsheere, C. M. et al. Silent myocardial ischaemia due to mental stress. *Lancet* 1984; 2: 1001-1005.

[284] Rozanski, A., Bairey, C. N., Krantz, D. S., Friedman, J., Resser, K. J., Morell, M. et al. Mental stress and the induction of silent myocardial ischemia in patients with coronary artery disease. *N Engl J Med* 1988; 318: 1005-1012.

[285] Pang, X., Alexacos, N., Letourneau, R., Seretakis, D., Gao, W., Cochrane, D. E. et al. A neurotensin receptor antagonist inhibits acute immobilization stress-induced cardiac mast cell degranulation, a corticotropin-releasing hormone-dependent process. *J Pharm and Exp Therap* 1998; 287: 307-314.

[286] Clejan, S., Japa, S., Clemetson, C., Hasabnis, S. S., David, O. and Talano, J. V. Blood histamine is associated with coronary artery disease, cardiac events and severity of inflammation and atherosclerosis. *J Cell Mol Med* 2002; 6: 583-592.

[287] Suzuki, M., Inaba, S., Nagai, T., Tatsuno, H. and Kazatani, Y. Relation of C-reactive protein and interleukin-6 to culprit coronary artery plaque size in patients with acute myocardial infarction. *Am J Cardiol* 2003; 91: 331-333.

[288] Huang, M., Pang, X., Letourneau, L., Boucher, W. and Theoharides, T. C. Acute stress induces cardiac mast cell activation and histamine release, effects that are increased in apolipoprotein E knockout mice. *Cardiovasc Res* 2002; 55: 150-160.

[289] Huang, M., Pang, X., Karalis, K. and Theoharides, T. C. Stress-induced interleukin-6 release in mice is mast cell-dependent and more pronounced in Apolipoprotein E knockout mice. *Cardiovasc Res* 2003; 59: 241-249.

[290] Deliargyris, E. N., Raymond, R. J., Theoharides, T. C., Boucher, W. S., Tate, D. A. and Dehmer, G. J. Sites of interleukin-6 release in patients with acute coronary syndromes and in patients with congestive heart failure. *Am J Cardiol* 2000; 86: 913-918.

[291] Kounis, N. G. and Zavras, G. M. Allergic angina and allergic myocardial infarction. *Circulation* 1996; 94: 1789.

[292] Kounis, N. G., Grapsas, N. D. and Goudevenos, J. A. Unstable angina, allergic angina, and allergic myocardial infarction. *Circulation* 1999; 100: e156.

[293] Kounis, N. G., Hahalis, G. and Theoharides, T. C. Coronary stents, hypersensitivity reactions and the Kounis syndrome. *J Interv Cardiol* 2007; 20: 314-323.

[294] Beltowski, J. and Jamroz, A. Adrenomedullin--what do we know 10 years since its discovery? *Pol J Pharmacol* 2004; 56: 5-27.

[295] Belloni, A. S., Petrelli, L., Guidolin, D., De, T. R., Bova, S., Spinazzi, R. et al. Identification and localization of adrenomedullin-storing cardiac mast cells. *Int J Mol Med* 2006; 17: 709-713.

[296] Schmidt, H. D. and Brunner, H. Ascending choledochal papillomatosis (author's transl). *MMW Munch Med Wochenschr* 1976; 118: 163-166.

[297] Marquardt, D. L., Parker, C. W. and Sullivan, T. J. Potentiation of mast cell mediator release by adenosine. *J Immunol* 1978; 120: 871-878.

[298] Feoktistov, I. and Biaggioni, I. Adenosine A_{2b} receptors evoke interleukin-8 secretion in human mast cells - An enprofylline-sensitive mechanism with implications for asthma. *J Clin Invest* 1995; 96: 1979-1986.

[299] Feoktistov, I., Ryzhov, S., Goldstein, A. E. and Biaggioni, I. Mast cell-mediated stimulation of angiogenesis: cooperative interaction between A2B and A3 adenosine receptors. *Circ Res* 2003; 92: 485-492.

[300] Fozard, J. R., Pfannkuche, H. J. and Schuurman, H. J. Mast cell degranulation following adenosine A3 receptor activation in rats. *Eur J Pharmacol* 1996; 298: 293-297.

[301] Cerniway, R. J., Yang, Z., Jacobson, M. A., Linden, J. and Matherne, G. P. Targeted deletion of A(3) adenosine receptors improves tolerance to ischemia-reperfusion injury in mouse myocardium. *Am J Physiol Heart Circ Physiol* 2001; 281: H1751-H1758.

[302] Takase, B., Maruyama, T., Kurita, A., et al Arachidonic acid metabolites in acute myocardial infarction. *Angiology,* 1996; 47:649-61.

[303] Deliargyris, E.N., Raymond, R.J., Theoharides, T.C., Boucher, W.S., Tate, D.A., and Dehmer, G.J. Sites of interleukin-6 release in patients with acute coronary syndromes and in patients with congestive heart failure. *Am J Cardiol.* 2000; 86:913-8.

[304] Huang, M., Pang, X., Karalis, K., and Theoharides, T.C. Stress-induced interleukin-6 release in mice is mast cell-dependent and more pronounced in Apolipoprotein E knockout mice. *Cardiovasc Res.* 2003; 59:241-9.

[305] Filipiak, K.J., Tarchsalska-Krynska, B., Opolski, G., et al. Tryptase levels in patients with acute coronary syndromes: the potential new marker in unstable plaque? *Clin Cardiol.* 2003; 26:366-72.

[306] Deliargyris, E.N., Upadhya, B., Sane, D.C., et al. Mast cell tryptase: a new biomarker in patients with stable coronary artery disease. *Atherosclerosis,* 2005; 178:381-6.

[307] Kaartinen, M., Penttila, A. and Kovanen, P.T. Accumulation of activated mast cells in the shoulder region of human coronary atheroma, the prediction site of atheromatous rupture. *Circulation,* 1994; 90: 1669-78.

[308] Kovanen, P.T., Kaartinen, M. and Paavonen, T. Infiltrates of activated mast cells at the site of coronary atheromatous erosion or rupture in myocardial infarction. *Circulation,* 1995; 92:1083-8.

[309] Irani, A.A., Nilsson, G., Miettinen, U., et al. Recombinant human stem cell factor stimulates differentiation of mast cells from dispersed human fetal liver cells. *Blood,* 1992; 80:3009-21.

[310] Vatent, P., Spanbloshe, E., Sperr, W.R., et al. Induction of differentiation of human mast cells from bone marrow and peripheral blood mononuclear cells by recombinant human stem cell factor (CSF)/kit ligand (KL) in long-term culture. *Blood,* 1992; 80: 2337-2245.

[311] Sakata, V., Komamura, K., Hirayama, A., et al. Elevation of plasma histamine concentration in the coronary circulation in patients with variant angina. *Am J Cardiol.* 1996; 77:1121-6.

[312] Cuculo, A., Summaria, F., Schiavino, D., et al. Tryptase levels are elevated during spontaneous ischemic episodes in unstable angina but not after ergonovine test in variant angina. *Cardiologia,* 1998; 43:189-93.

[313] Cipollone, F., Ganci, A.A., Greco, M., et al. Modulation of aspirin-insensitive eicosanoid biosynthesis by 6-methylprednisolone in unstable angina. *Circulation,* 2003; 107:55-61.

[314] Fisher, M.M. Clinical observations on the pathophysiology and treatment of anaphylactic cardiovascular collapse. *Anaesth Intensive Care,* 1986; 14:17-21.

[315] Schummer, W., Schummer, C., Wippennan, J., and Fuchs, J. Anaphylactic shock: is vasopressin the drug of choice? *Anesthesiology,* 2004; 101: 1025-7.

[316] Heytman, M. and Rainbird, A. Use of alpha-agonists for management of anaphylaxis occurring under anaesthesia: case studies and review. *Anaesthesia,* 2004; 9:1210-5.

[317] Fahmy, N.R. Hemodynamics, plasma histamine and catecholamine concentrations during an anaphylactoid reaction to morphine. *Anesthesiology,* 1981; 55:329-31.

[318] van der Linden, P.W., Struyvenberg, A., Kraaijenhagen, R.J., Hack, C.E., and van der Zwang, J.K. Anaphylactic shock after insect-sting challenge in 138 persons with a previous insect-sting reaction. *Ann Intern Med.* 1993; 118:161-8.

[319] Hermann, K., Rittweger, R. and Ring, J. Urinary excretion of angiotensin I, II, arginine vasopressin and oxytocin in patients with anaphylactoid reactions. *Clin Exper Allergy,* 1992; 22:845-53.

[320] Hanashiro, R.K. and Weil, M.H. Anaphylactic shock in man: report of two cases with detailed hemodynamics and metabolic studies. *Arch Intern Med.* 1967; 119:129-40.

[321] Brown, S.G.A. Cardiovascular aspects of anaphylaxis: implications for treatment and diagnosis. *Curr Opin Allergy Immunol.* 2005; 5: 359-64.

[322] Wittstein, I.S., Thiermann, D.R., Lima, J.A, et al. Neurohumoral features of myocardial stunning due to sudden emotional stress. *N Engl J Med.* 2005; 352:539-538.

[323] Felix, S.B., Baumann, G. and Berdel, W.E. Systemic anaphylaxis separation of cardiac reactions from respiratory and peripheral vascular events. *Res Exp Med.* 1990; 190:239-52.

[324] Levi, R. Cardiac anaphylaxis: models, mediators, mechanisms, and clinical considerations. In: Marone G, Lichtenstein LM, Condorelli M, Fauci AS, editors. Human Inflammatory Disease Clinical Immunology, vol 1. Toronto: Decker; 1988. p. 93-105.

[325] Zavecz, J.H. and Levi, R. Separation of primary and secondary cardiovascular events in systemic anaphylaxis. *Circ Res.* 1977; 40:15-9.

[326] Vigorito, C., Poto, S., Picotti, G.B., Triggiani, M., and Marone, G. Effect of activetion of HI receptor on coronary hemodynamics in man. *Circulation,* 1986; 73:1175-82.

[327] Bristow, M.R., Ginsburg, R. and Harisson, D.C. Histamine and the human heart: the other receptor system. *Am J Cardiol.* 1982; 49:249-51.

[328] Mitsuhata, H., Shimizu, R. and Yokoyama, M.M. Role of nitric oxide in anaphylactic shock. *J Clin Immunol.* 1995; 15:277-83.

[329] Palmer, R.M.J., Ferrige, A.G., and Moncada, S. Nitric oxide release accounts for the biological activity of endothelium derived relaxing factor. *Nature,* 1987; 27:524-6.

[330] Kemp, S.F. and Lockey, R.F. Anaphylaxis: a review of causes and mechanisms. *J Allergy Clin Immunol.* 2002; 110:341 -8.

[331] Mink, S., Becker, A., Sharma, S., Unruh, H., Duke, K., and Kepron, W. Role of autacoids in cardiovascular collapse in anaphylactic shock in anesthetized dogs. *Cardiovasc Res.* 1999; 43:173-82.

[332] Hofstra, C.L., Desai, P.I., Thurmond, R.L., and Fung-Leung, W.P. Histamine H4 receptor mediates chemotaxis and calcium mobilization of mast cells. *J Pharmacol Exp Ther.* 2003; 305:1212-21.

[333] O'Reilly, M., Alpert, R., Jenkinson, S., et al. Identification of a histamine H4 receptor on human eosinophil-role in eosinophil chemotaxis. *J Recept Signal Transduct Res.* 2002; 22:431 -48.

[334] Ling, P., Ngo, K., Nguyen, S., et al Histamine H4 receptor mediates eosinophil chemotaxis with cell shape change and adhesion molecule upregulation. *Brit J Pharmacol.* 2004; 142:161-71.

[335] Gantner, F., Sakai, K., Tusche, M.W., Cruikabank, W.W., Center, D.M., and Bacon, K.B. Histamine h(4) and h(2) receptors control histamine-induced interleukin-16 release from human CD8(+) t cells. *J Pharmacol Exp Ther.* 2002; 303:300-7.

[336] Bousquet, J., Chanez, P., Lacoste, J.Y., et al. Eosinophilic inflammation in asthma. *N Engl J Med.* 1990; 23:1033-9.

[337] Macfarlane, A.J., Kon, O.M., Smith, S.J., et al Basophils, eosinophils and mast cells in atopic and nonatopic asthma and in late-phase allergic reactions in the lung and skin. *J Allergy Clin Immunol.* 2000; 10S:99-107.

[338] Burks, W., Bannon, G.A., Sicheter, S., and Sampson, H.A. Peanut-induced anaphylactic reactions. *Int Arch Allergy Immunol.* 1999; 119:165-72.

[339] Brown, S.G.A., Blackman, K.E., Stenlake V, and Heddle, R.J. Insect sting anaphylaxis; prospective evaluation of treatment with intravenous adrenaline and volume resuscitation. *Emerg Med J.* 2004; 21:149 -54.

[340] Laxenaire, M.C. and Metres, P.M. Anaphylaxis during anaesthesia: results of a two-year survey in France. Br J Anaesth 2001; 87:549-58.

[341] Helbling, A., Humi, T., Mueller, U.R. and Pichler, W.J. Incidence of anaphylaxis with circulatory symptoms: a study over a 3-year period comprising 940.000 inhabitants of the Swiss Canton Bern. *Clin Exp Allergy,* 2004; 4:285-90.

[342] Pfister, C.W. and Plice, S.G. Acute myocardial infarction during a prolonged allergic reaction to penicillin. *Am Heart J.* 1950; 40:945-7.

[343] Johnston, S.L., Unsworth, J. and Gompels, M.M. Adrenaline given outside the context of life threatening allergic reactions. *BMJ,* 2003; 326: 589-90.

[344] Saadeh, A.M. Case report: acute myocardial infarction complicating a viper bite. *Am J Trop Med Hyg.* 2001; 64:280-2.

[345] Criqui, M.H., Lee, E.R., Hamburger, R.N., Klauber, M.R., and Coughli, S.S. IgE and cardiovascular disease. Results from a population-based study. *Am J Med.* 1987; 82:964-8.

[346] Masini, E., Di Bello, M.G., Raspanti, S., Bani Sacchi, T., Maggi, E., and Mannaioni, P.F. Platelet aggregation and histamine release by immunological stimuli, hnmunopharmacology 1994;28:19-29.

[347] Masini, E., Di Bello, M.G., Cappugi, P., Bemi, L., Mirabella, C., and Mannaioni, P.F. Platelet aggregation and platelet histamine release by immunological stimulation in atopic patients: modulation by nitric oxide. *Infamm Res.* 1997; 46 (Suppl 1):S81-2.

[348] Mori, E., Iceda, H., Ueno, T., et al Vasospastic angina induced by nonsteroidal anti-inflammatory drugs. *Clin Cardiol.* 1997; 20:656-8.

[349] Brown, S.G.A. Clinical features and severity grading of anaphylaxis. *J Allergy Clin Immunol.* 2004;114:371 -6.

[350] Ginsburg, R., Bristow, M.R., Kantrowitz, N., Bain, D.S., and Harrison, D.C. Histamine provocation of clinical coronary artery spasm: implications concerning pathogenesis of variant angina pectoris. *Am Heart J.* 1981; 102:819-22.

[351] Iakovou, I., Schmidt, T., Bonizzoni, E., Ge, L., Sangiorgi, G.M., Stankovic, G., Airoldi, F., Chieffo, A., Montorfano, M., Carlino, M., Michev, I., Corvaja, N., Briguori, C., Gerckens, U., Grube, E., and Colombo, A. Incidence, predictors, and outcome of thrombosis after successful implantation of drug-eluting stents. *JAMA*, 2005; 293: 2126-213.

[352] Joner, M., Finn, A.V., Farb, A., Mont, E.K., Kolodgie, F.D., Ladich, E., Kutys, R., Skorija, K., Gold, H.K., and Virmani, R. Pathology to drug-eluting stents in humans. Delayed healing and late thrombotic risk. *J Am Coll Cardiol.* 2006; 48: 193-202.

[353] Cutlip, D.E., Baim, D.S., Ho, K.K., Popma, J.J., Lansky, A.J., Cohen, D.J., Carrozza, J.P., Jr., Chauhan, M.S., Rodriguez, O., and Kuntz, R.E. Stent thrombosis in the modern era: A pooled analysis of multicenter coronary stent trials. *Circulation,* 2001; 103: 1967-1971.

[354] Nordmann, A.J., Briel, M. and Bucher, H.C. Mortality in randomized controlled trials comparing drug-eluting vs. metal stents in coronary artery disease: a meta-analysis. *Eur Heart J.* 2006; 27: 2784-2814.

[355] Pfisterer, M.E., Brunner-La Rocca, H.P., Buser, P.T., Rickenbacher, P., Hunziker, P., Mueller, C., Jeger, R., Bader, F., Osswald, S., and Kaiser, C. BASKET-LATE Investigators. Late clinical events after clopidogrel discontinuation may limit the benefit of drug-eluting stents. An observational study of drug-eluting versus bare-metal stents. *J Am Coll Cardiol.* 2006; 48: 2584-2591.

[356] Camenzind, E., Steng, P.G. and Wijns, W. A meta-analysis of first generation drug eluting stent programs. Presented at Hotline Session I, World Congress of Cardiology 2006, Barcelona, September 2-5, 2006. abstract

[357] FDA statement on coronary drug-eluting stents.http://www.fda.gov/cdrh/news/010407.html.

[358] Spaulding, C., Daemen, J., Boersma, E., Cutlip, D.E., and Serruys, P.W. A pooled analysis of data comparing sirolimus-eluting stents with bare-metal stents. *N Engl J Med.* 2007; 356: 989-997.

[359] Stone, G.W., Moses, J.W., Ellis, S.G., Schofe, J., Dawkins, K.D., Morice, M.C., Colombo, A., Schampaert, E., Grude, E., Kirtane, A.J., Cutlip, D.E., Fahy, M., Pocock,

S.J., Mehran, R., and Leon, M.B. Safety and efficacy of sirolimus-and paclitaxel-eluting stents. *N Engl J Med.* 2007; 356: 998-1008.

[360] Kastrati, A., Mehilli, J., Pache, J., Kaiser, C., Valgimigli, M., Kelbaek, H., Menichelli, M., Sabate, M., Suttorp, M.J., Baumgart, D., Seyfarth, M., Pfisterer, M.E., and Schomig, A. Analysis of 14 trials comparing sirolimus-eluting stents with bare-metal stents. *N Engl J Med.* 2007; 356: 1030-1039.

[361] Lagerqvist, B., James, S.K., Stenestrand, U., Lindback, J., Nilsson, T., and Wallentin, L. Long-term outcomes with drug-eluting stents versus bare-metal stents. *N Engl J Med.* 2007; 356: 1009-1019.

[362] Luscher, T.F., Steffel, J., Eberli, F.R., Joner, M., Nakazawa, G., Tanner, F.C., and Virmani, R. Drug-eluting stent and coronary thrombosis. Biological mechanisms and clinical implications. *Circulation,* 2007; 115: 1051-1058.

[363] Cutlip, D.E., Windecker, S., Mehran, R., et al. Clinical end points in coronary stent trials: a case for standardise definitions. *Circulation,* 2007; 115: 2344-2351.

[364] Farb, A., Burke, A.P., Kolodgie, F.D., and Virmani, R. Pathological mechanisms of fatal late coronary stent thrombosis in humans. *Circulation,* 2003; 108: 1701-1706.

[365] Kounis, N.G., Kounis, G.N. and Kouni, S.N. Coronary-artery stents, *N Engl J Med.* 2006; 354: 2076-2077.

[366] Kounis, N.G., Kounis, G.N., Kouni, S.N., Niarchos, C., and Mazarakis, A. Allergic reactions following implantation of drug-eluting stents: A manifestation of Kounis syndrome? *J Am Coll Cardiol.* 2006; 48: 592-593.

[367] Manufacturer and User Facility Device Experience Database. Rockville.MD: Food and Drug Administration, 2004.

[368] Bennett, C.L., Nebeker, J.R., Lyons, E.A., Samore, M.H., Feldman, M.D., McKoy, J.M., Casron, K.R., Belknap, S.M., Trifilio, S.M., Schumock, G.T., Yarnold, P.R., Davidson, C.J., Evens, A.M., Kuzel T.M., Parada, J.P., Cournoyer, D., West, D.P., Sartor, O., Tallman, M.S., and Raisch, D.W. The Research on Adverse Drug Events and Reports (RADAR) project. *JAMA,* 2005; 293: 2131-2140.

[369] Nebeker, J.R., Virmani, R., Bennet, C.L., Hoffman, J.M., Samore, M.H., Alvarez, J., Davidson, C.J., McKoy, J.M., Raisch, D.W., Whisenant, B.K., Yarnold, P.R., Belknap, S.M., West, D.P., Gage, J.E., Morse, R.E., Gligoric, G., Davidson, L., and Feldman, M.D. Hypersensitivity cases associated with drug-eluding stents. A review of available cases from the research on adverse drug events and reports (RADAR) project. *J Am Coll Cardiol.* 2006; 47: 175-181.

[370] Azarbal, B. and Currier, J.W. Allergic reactions after the implantation of drug-eluding stents. *J Am Coll Cardiol.* 2006; 47: 182-183.

[371] Rana, J.S. and Sheikh, J. Serum sickness-like reactions after placement of sirolimus – eluting stents. *Ann allergy Asthma Immunol.* 2007; 98: 201202.

[372] Kim, J.W., Park, C.G., Seo, H.S., Oh, D.J. Delayed severe multivessel spasm and aborted sudden death after Taxus stent implantation. *Heart.* 2005; 91: e15.

[373] Togni, M., Winddecker, S., Cocchia, R., Wenaweser, P., Cook, S.,Billinger, M., Meier, B., and Hess, O.M. Sirolimus-eluting stents associated with paradoxic coronary vasoconstriction. *J Am Coll Cardiol.* 2005;46: 231-236

[374] Wheatcroft, S.W., Byrne, J., Thomas, M., and MacCarthy, P. Life-threatening coronary artery spasm following sirolimus-eluting stent deployment. *J Am Coll Cardiol.* 2006; 47: 1911-1912.

[375] Maekawa, K., Kawamoto, K., Fuke, S., Yoshioka, R., Saito, H., Sato, T., and Hioka, T. Severe endothelial dysfunction after sirolimus-eluting stent implantation. *Circulation,* 2006;113: e850-e851.

[376] Brott, B.C., Anayiotos, A., Chapman, G., Anderson, P.G., and Hillegass, W.B. Severe, diffuse coronary artery spasm after drug-eluting stent placement. *J Invasive Cardiol.* 2006; 18: 584-592.

[377] Togni, M. and Eberli, F.R. Vasoconstriction and coronary artery spasm after drug-eluting stent placement. *J Invasive Cardiol.* 2006; 18: 593.

[378] Garcia, J.A., Hansgen, A. and Casserly, I.P. Simultaneously multivessel acute drug-eluting stent thrombosis. *Int J Cardiol.* 2006; 113: E11-E15

[379] Kounis, N.G. Kounis syndrome (allergic angina and allergic myocardial infarction): a natural paradigm? *Int J Cardiol.* 2006; 110: 7-14.

[380] Kounis, N.G. and Zavras, G.M. Allergic angina and allergic myocardial infarction. *Circulation,* 1996; 94: 1789.

[381] Wickman, M. When allergies complicate allergies. *Allergy,* 2005;60: 14-18.

[382] Galli, S.J., Nakae, S. and Tsai, M. Mast cells in the development of adaptive immune responses. *Nat Immunol.* 2005; 6: 135-142.

[383] Theoharides, T.C. and Kalogeromitros, D. The critical role of mast cells in allergy and inflammation. *Ann NY Acad Sci.* 2006; 1088: 78-99.

[384] MacGlashan, D.W., Jr., Brochner, B.S., Adelman, D.C., Jardieu, P.M., Togias, A., Mckenzie-White, J., Sterbinsky, S.A., Hamilton, R.G., and Lichtenstein, L.M. Down-regulation of FcεRI expression in human basophils during in vivo treatment of atopic patients with anti-IgE antibody. *J Immunol.* 1997; 158: 1438-1445.

[385] Nopp, A., Johansson, S.G.O., Lundberg, M., and Oman, H. Simultaneous exposure of several allergens has an additive effect on multisensitized basophils. *Allergy,* 2006; 61: 1366-1368.

[386] Stahli, B.E., Camici, G.G., Steffel, J., Akhmedov, A., Shojaati, K., Graber, M., Luscher, T.F., and Tanner, F.C. Paclitaxel enhances thrombin-induced endothelial tissue factor expression via c-jun terminal NH2 kinase activation. *Circ Res.* 2006; 99: 149-155.

[387] Finn, A.V., Kolodgie, F.D., Hamek, J., Guerrero, L.J., Acampado, E., Tefera, K., Skorija, K., Weber, D.K., Gold, H.K., and Virmani, R. Differential response of delayed healing and persistent inflammation at sites of overlapping sirolimus- or paclitaxel – eluting stents. *Circulation,* 2005; 112: 270-278.

[388] Steffel, J., Latini, R.A., Akhmedov, A., Zimmermann, D., Zimmerling, P., Luscher, T.F., and Tanner, F.C. Rapamycin, but not FK-506, increases endothelial tissue factor expression: implications for drug-eluting stent design. *Circulation,* 2005; 112: 2002-2011.

[389] Steffel, J., Akhmedov, A., Greutert, H., Luscher, T.F., and Tanner, F.C. Histamine induces tissue factor expression. Implications for acute coronary syndromes. *Circulation,* 2005; 112: 341-349.

[390] Blagosklonny, M.V., Darzyziewicz, Z., Halicka, H.D., Pozarowski, P., Demidenko, Z.N., Barry, J.J., Kamath, K.R., and Herrmann, R.A. Paclitaxel induces primary and postmitotic G1 arrest in human arterial muscle cells. *Cell Cycle*, 2004; 3: 1050-1056.

[391] Parker, W.B. and Cheng, Y.C. Metabolism and mechanism of action of 5-fluoruracil. *Pharmacol Ther.* 1990; 48: 381.

[392] Trent, J.M., Buick, R.N., Olson, S., Horns, R.C., Jr., and Schimke, R.T. Cytologic evidence for gene amplification in methotrexate-resistance cells obtained from a patient with ovarian adenocarcinoma. *J Clin Oncol.* 1984; 2: 8.

[393] Weidmann, B., Mulleneisen, N., Bojko, P., and Niederle, N. Hypersensitivity reactions to carboplatin. Report of two patients, review of ythe literature, and discussion of diagnostic procedures and management. *Cancer,* 1994; 73: 2218-2222.

[394] Gell, P.G.H. and Coombs, R.R.A. Clinical Aspects of Immunology. 2nd edition. Blackwell Scientific, Oxford and Edinburgh, 1968;580.

[395] O`Brien, M.E.R. and Souberbielle, B.E. Allergic reactions to cytotoxic drugs-an update. *Ann Oncol.* 1992; 3: 605-610.

[396] Weiss, R.B. Hypersensitivity reactions. *Semin Oncol.* 1992; 19: 458-477.

[397] Yeh, E.T.H., Tong, A.T., Lenihan, D.J., Yusuf, S.W., Swafford, J., Champion, C., Durand, J.B., Gibbs, H., Zafarmand, A.A., and Ewer, M.S. Cardiovascular complications of cancer therapy. Diagnosis, pathogenesis, and management. *Circulation,* 2004; 109: 3122-31.

[398] Grem, J.L., van Groeningen, C.J., Ismail, A.A., Johnston, P.G., Alexander, H.R., and Allegra, C.J. The3 role of interferon-alpha as a modulator of fluorouracil and leucovorin. *Eur J Cancer*, 1995; 31A: 1316- 1320.

[399] Zanotti, K.M. and Markman, M. Prevention and management of antineoplastic-induced hypersensitivity reactions. *Drug Saf.* 2001; 24: 767-77.

[400] Weiss, R.B., Donchover, R.C., Wiernik, P.H., Ohnuma, T., Gralla, R.G., Trump, D.L., Baker, G.R., Jr., Van Echo, D.A., Von Hoff, D.D., and Leyland-Jones, B. Hypersensitivity reactions from taxol. *J Clin Oncol.* 1990; 8: 1263-1268.

[401] Rowinsky, E.K., McGuire, W.P., Guarnieri, T., Fisherman, J.S., Christian, M.C., and Donehover, R.C. Cardiac disturbances during the administration of taxol. *J Clin Oncol.* 1991; 9: 1704-1712.

[402] Rowinsky, E.K., Eisenhauer, E.A., Chaudhry, V., Arbuck, S.G., and Donchover, R.C. Clinical toxicities encountered with paclitaxel (Taxol). *Sem Oncol.* 1993; 20 Suppl 3: S1-S15.

[403] Sevelda, P., Mayerhofer, K., Obermair, A., Stolzlechner, J., and Kurz, C. Thrombosis with paclitaxel. *Lancet,* 1994; 343: 727.

[404] Hekmat, E. Fatal myocardial infarction potentially induced by paclitaxel. *Ann Pharmacother.* 1996; 30: 1110-1112.

[405] Laher, S. and Karp, S.J. Acute myocardial infarction following paclitaxel administration for ovarian carcinoma. *Clin Oncol* (R Coll Radiol) 1997; 9: 124-126.

[406] Pai, V.B. and Nahata, M.C. Cardiotoxicity of chemotherapeutic agents: incidence, treatment and prevention. *Drug Saf.* 2000; 22: 263-302.

[407] Mersin, N., Boulbair, F., Davani, S., Hehn, M., and Kantelip, J.P. Myocardial infarction after paclitaxel use. *Therapie.* 2003; 58: 467-469.

[408] Nguyen-Ho, P., Keiman, N.S. and Verani, M.S. Acute myocardial infarction and cardiac arrest in a patient receiving paclitaxel. *Can J Cardiol.* 2003; 19: 300-302.

[409] Kloover, J.S., den Bakker, M.A., Gelderblon, and van Meerbeeck, J.P. Fatal outcome of a hypersensitivity reaction to paclitaxel: a critical review of premedication regimens. *Br J Cancer,* 2004; 90:304-305.

[410] Schrader, C., Keussen, C., Bewig, B., von Freier, A., and Lins, M. Symptoms and signs of acute myocardial ischemia caused by chemotherapy with paclitaxel (Taxol) in a patient with metastatic ovarian carcinoma. *Eur J Med Res.* 2005;10: 498-501.

[411] Ruiz-Casado, A., Calzas, J., Garcia, J., Soria, A., and Guerra, J. Life-threatening adverse drug reaction to paclitaxel. Postmarketing surveillance. *Clin Transl Oncol.* 2006; 8: 60-62.

[412] Turkoglu, S., Simsek, V. and Abasi, A. Possible anaphylactic reaction to Taxus stent: A case report. *Catheter Cardiovasc Interv.* 2005; 66: 554-556.

[413] Henry, A., Charpiat, B., Perol, M., Vial, T., de Saint Hilaire, P.J., and Descotes, J. Paclitaxel hypersensitivity reactions: assessment of the utility of a test-dose program. *Cancer J.* 2006; 12: 237-245.

[414] Watanabe, Y., Nakai, H., Ueda, H., Nozaki, K., and Hoshiai, H. Carboplatin hypertsensitivity induced by low-dose paclitaxel/carbop[latin in multiple platinum-treated patients with recurrent ovarianj cancer. *Int J Gynecol Cancer,* 2005; 15: 224-227.

[415] Vasquez, E.M. Sirolimus: a new agent for prevention of renal allograft rejection. *Am J Health Syst Pharm.* 2000; 57: 437-448.

[416] Marx, S.O., Jayaraman, T., Go, L.O., and Marks, A.R. Rapamycin-FKBP inhibits cell cycle regulators of proliferation in vascular smooth muscle cells. *Circ Res.* 1995; 76: 412-417.

[417] Tracey, C., Hawley, C., Griffin, A.D., Strutton, G., and Lynch, S. Generalized, pruritic, ulcerating maculopapular rash necessitating cessation of sirolimus in a liver transplantation patient. *Liver Transpl.* 2005; 11: 987-989.

[418] Warino, L. and Libecco, J. Cutaneous effects of sirolimus in renal transplant recipients. *J Drugs Dermatol.* 2006; 5: 273-274.

[419] Wadei, H., Gruber, S.A., El-Amm, J.M., Garnick, J.,West, M.S., Granger, D.K., Sillix, D.H., Migdal, S.D., and Haririan, A. Sirolimus-induced angioedema. *Am J Transplant,* 2004; 4: 1002-1005.

[420] Mingos, M.A. and Kane, G.C. Sirolimus-induced interstitial pneumonitis in a renal transplant patient. *Respir Care,* 2005; 50: 1659-1661.

[421] Howard, L., Gopalan, D., Griffiths, M., and Mahadeva, R. Sirolimus-induced pulmonary hypersensitivity with a CD4 T-cell infiltrate. *Chest,* 2006; 129: 1718-1721.

[422] Kunzle, N., Venetz, J.P., Pascual, M., Panizzon, R.G., and Laffitte, E. Sirolimus-induced acneiform eruption. *Dermatology,* 2005; 211: 305-306.

[423] Hardinger, K.L., Cornelius, L.A., Trulock, E.P., 3rd, and Brennan, D.C. Sirolimus-induced leukocytoclastic vasculitis. *Transplantation,* 2002; 74: 739-743.

[424] Pasqualotto, A.C., Bianco, P.D., Sukiennik, T.C., Furian, R., and Garcia, V.D. Sirolimus-induced leukocytoclastic vasculitis: the second case reported. *Am J Transplant,* 2004; 4: 1549-1551.

[425] Truong, U., Moon-Grady, A.J. and Butani, L. Cardiac tamponade in a pediatric renal transplant recipient on sirolimus therapy. *Pediatr Transplantation*, 2005; 9: 541-544.

[426] Chan, C.C., Martin, D.F., Xu, D., and Roberge, F.G. Side effects of rapamycin in the rat. *J Ocul Pharmacol Ther.* 1995; 11: 177-181.

[427] Walpoth, B.H. and Hess, O.M. Late coronary thrombosis secondary to a sirolimus-eluting stent. *Circulation,* 2004; 110: e309.

[428] Walpoth, B.H., Pavlicek, M., Celik, B., Nikolaus, B., Schaffner, T., Althaus, U., Hess, O.M., Carrel, T., and Morris, R.E. Prevention of neointimal proliferation by immunosuppression in synthetic vascular grafts. *Eur J Cardiothorac Surg.* 2001; 19: 487-492.

[429] Virmani, R., Guagliumi, G., Farb, A., Musumeci, G., Grieco, N., Motta, T., Mihalcsik, L., Tespili M., Valsecchi, O., and Kolodgie, F.D. Localized hypersensitivity and late coronary thrombosis secondary to a sirolimus stent. Should we be cautious? *Circulation,* 2004; 109: 701-705.

[430] Virmani, R., Farb, A., Kolodgie, F.D., Guagliumi, G., Musumeci, G., Grieco, N., Mihalcsik, L., Tespili, M., Valsecchi, O., and Motta, T. Late coronary thrombosis secondary to a sirolimus-eluting stent. *Circulation,* 2004; 110: e309.

[431] Hummel, M. Recommendations for use of Certican (everolimus) after heart transplantation: results from a German and Austian concensus conference. *J Heart Lung Transplant*, 2005; 24: S196-S200.

[432] Fuchs, U., Zittermann, A., Berthold, H.K., Tenderich, G., Deyerling, K., Minami, K., and Koerfer, R. Immunosuppressive therapy with everolimus can be associated with potentially life-threatening lingual angioedema. *Transplantation*, 2005; 79: 981-983.

[433] Grube, E., Sonoda, S., Ikeno, F., Honda, Y., Kar, S., Chan, C., Gerckens, U., Lansky, A.J., and Fitgerald, P.J. Six-and twelve-month results from first human experience using everolimus-eluting stents with bioabsorbable polymer. *Circulation,* 2004; 109: 2168-2171.

[434] Serruys, P.W., Ong, A.T.L. and Piek, J.J. A randomized comparison of a durable polymer Everolimus-eluting stent with a bare metal coronary stent: the SPIRIT first trial. *Eurointervention,* 2005; 1: 58-65.

[435] Serruys, P.W., Kutryk, M.J.B. and Ong, A.T.L. Coronary-artery stents. *N Engl J Med.* 2006; 354: 483-495.

[436] Costa, R.A., Lansky, A.J., Abizaid, A., Mueller, R., Tsuchiya, Y., Mori, K., Cristea, E., Leon, M.B., Sousa, J.E., Schmidt, T., Hauptmann, K.E., and Grube, E. Angiographic results of the first human experience with the biolimus A9 drug-eluting stent for De Novo coronary lesions. *Am J Cardiol.* 2006; 98: 443-446.

[437] Clingiroglu, M., Elliott, J., Patel, T., Tio, F., Matthews, H., McCasland, M., Trauthen, B., Elicker, J., and Bailey, S.R. Long-term effects of novel biolimus elutng DEVAX AXXESS plus nitinl self-expanding stent in porcine coronary model. *Catheter Cardiovasc Interv.* 2006; June: ahead of print.

[438] Garcia-Touchard, A., Burke, S.E., Toner, J.L., Cromack, K., and Schwartz, R.S. Zotarolimus-eluting stents reduce experimental coronary artery neointimal hyperplasia after 4 weeks. *Eur Heart J.* 2006; 27: 988-993.

[439] Fajadet, J., Wijns, W., Laarman, G.J., Kuck, K.H., Ormiston, J., Munzel, T., Popma, J.J., Fitzgerald, P.J., Bonon, R., and Kuntz, R.E. For the ENDEAVOR II Investigators. Randomized, double-blind, multicenter study of the endeavour zotarolimus-eluting phosphorylcholine-encapsulated stent for treatment of native coronary artery lesions. Clinical and angiographic results of the ENDEAVOR II trial. *Circulation*, 2006; 114: 798-806.

[440] Woodside, K.J., Hu, M., Liu, Y., Song, W., Hunter, G.C., and Daller, J.A. Apoptosis of allospecifically activated human helper T cells is blocked by calcineurin inhibition. *Transplant Immunol.* 2006; 15: 229-234.

[441] Lacaille, F., Laurent, J. and Bousquet, J. Life threatening food allergy in a child treated with FK506. *J Pediatr Gastroenterol Nutr.* 1997; 25: 228-229.

[442] Inui, A., Komatsu, H., Fujisawa, T., Matsumoto, H., and Miyagawa, Y. Food allergy and tacrolimus. *J Pediatr Gastroenterol Nutr.* 1999; 28: 355-356.

[443] Lacaille, F., Laurent, J. and Bousquet, J. Life threatening food allergy in a child treated with FK506. *J Pediatr Gastroenterol Nutr.* 1997; 25: 228-229.

[444] Nowak –Wegrzyn, A.H., Sicherer, S.H., Conover-Walker, M.K., and Wood, R.A. Food allergy after pediatric organ transplantation with tacrolimus immunosuppression. *J Allergy Clin Immunol.* 2001; 108: 146-147.

[445] Lykavieris, P., Fraauger E., Habes, D., Bernard, O., and Debray, D. Angioedema in pediatric liver transplant recipients under tacrolimus immunosuppression. *Transplantation*, 2003; 75: 152-165.

[446] Ozdemir, O., Mensah-Arrey, A. and Sorensen, R.U. Development of multiple food allergies in children taking tacrolimus after heart and liver transplantation. *Pediatr Transplantation*, 2006; 10: 380-383.

[447] Huang, Y., Salu, K., Wang, L., Liu, X., Li, S., Lorenz, G., Wnedt, S., Verbeken, E., Bosmans, J., Van de Werf, F., and De Scheerder, I. Use of tacrolimus-eluting stents inhibit neointimal hyperplasia in a porcine coronary model. *J Invasive Cardiol.* 2005; 17: 142-148.

[448] Bavandi, A., Fahrngruber, H., Aschauer, H., Hartmann, B., Meingassner, J.G., and Kalthoff, F.S. Pimecrolimus and tacrolimus differ in their inhibition of lymphocyte activation during the sensitization phasev of contact hypersensitivity. *J Dermatol Sci.* 2006; June: ahead of print.

[449] FDA Statement. New warnings for two eczema drugs. FDA Consum 2006; 40: 5

[450] Suissa, S., Assimes, T., Brassard, P., and Ernst, P. Inhaled corticosteroids in asthma and the prvention of myocardial infarction. *Am J med.* 2003; 115: 377-381.

[451] Takagi, S., Goto, Y., Hirose, E., Terashima, M., Sakuragi, S., Suzuki, S., et al. Successful treatment of refractory vasospastic angina with corticosteroids: Coronary arterial hyperactivity caused by local inflammation? *Circ J.* 2004; 68: 17-22.

[452] Gaspardone, A., Versaci, F., Tomai, F., Citone, C., Proietti, I., Gioffre, G., and Skossyreva, O. C-reactive protein, clinical outcome, and restenosis rates after implantation of different drug-eluting stents. *Am J Cardiol.* 2006; 97: 1311-1316.

[453] Wang, L., Salu, K., Verbeken, E., Bosmans, J., van de Werf, F., De Scheerder, I., De Scheerrder, I., and Huang, Y. Stent-mediated methylprednisolone delivery reduces

macrophage contents and in-stent neointimal formation. *Coron Artery Dis.* 2005; 16: 237-243.

[454] Huang, Y., Liu, X., Wang, L., Verbeken, E., Li, S., and De Scheerder, I. Local methylprednisolone delivery using a biodivYsio phosphorylcholine-coated drug-delivery stent reduces inflammation and neointimal hyperplasia in a porcine coronary stent model. *Int J Cardiovasc Intervent.* 2003; 5: 166-171.

[455] Patti, G., Chello, M., Pasceri, V., Colonna, D., Carminati, P., Covino, E., and Di Germano, S. Dexamethasone-eluting stents and plasma concentrations of adhesion molecules in patients with unstable cornary syndromes.: results of the historically SESAME study. *Clin Ther.* 2005; 27: 1411-1419.

[456] Patti, G., Pasceri, V., Carminati, P., D`Ambrozio, A., Carcagni, A., and Di Sciascio, G. Effect of dexamethasone-eluting stents on systemic inflammatory response in patients with unstable angina pectoris or recent myocardial infarction undergoing percutaneous coronary intervention. *Am J cardiol.* 2005; 95: 502-505.

[457] Hoffmann, R., Langenberg, R., Radke, P., Franke, A., Blindt, R.,Ortlepp, J., Popma, J.J., Weber, C., and Hanrath, P. Evaluation of a high-dose dexamethasone eluting stent. *Am J Cardiol.* 2004; 94: 193-195.

[458] Pires, N.M., Schepers, A., van der Hoeven, B.L., de Vries, M.R., Boesten, L.S., Jukema, J.W., and Quax, P.H. Histopathologic alterations following local delivery of dexamethasone to inhibit restenosis in murine arteries. *Cardiovasc Res.* 2005; 68: 415-424.

[459] Kounis, N.G. Bronchospasm induced by althesin and pancuronium bromide. *Br J Anaesth.* 1974; 46: 281.

[460] Kounis, N.G. Untoward reactions to corticosteroids: intolerance to hydrocortisone. *An Allergy,* 1976; 36: 203-206.

[461] Peng, Y.S., Shyur, S.D., Lin, H.Y., and Wang, C.Y. Steroid allergy: report of two cases. *J Microbiol Immunol Infect.* 2001; 34: 150-154.

[462] Nakamura, H., Matsuse, H., Obase, Y., et al. Clinical evaluation of anaphylactic reactions to intravenous corticosteroids in adult asthmatics. *Respiration,* 2002; 69: 309-313.

[463] Swanson, N., Hogrefe, K., Malik, N., and Gershlick, A.H. Vascular endothelial growth factor (VEGF)-eluting stents: in vivo effects on thrombosis, endothelialization and intimal hyperplasia. *J Invasive Cardiol.* 2003; 15: 688-692.

[464] Walter, D.H., Cejna, M., Diaz-Sandoval, L., Willis, S., Kirkwood, L., Stratford, P.W., Tietz, A.B., Kirchmair, R., Silver, M., Wecker, A., Yoon, Y.S., Heidenreich, R., Hanley, A., Kearney, M., Tio, F.O., Kuenzler, P., Isner, J.M., and Losordo, D.W. Local gene transfer of phVEGF-2 plasmid by gene-eluting stents: an alternative strategy for inhibition of restenosis. *Circulation,* 2004; 110: 36-45.

[465] Salu, K.J., Bosmans, J.M., Huang, Y., Hendriks, M., Verhoeven, M., Levels, A., Cooper, S., De Scheerrder, I.K., Vrints, C.J., and Bult, H. Effects of cytochalasin D-eluting stents on intimal hyperplasia in a porcine coronary artery model. *Cardiovasc Research* 2006: 69: 536-544.

[466] Carpenter, C.L. Actin cytoskeleton and cell signalling. *Crit Care Med.* 2000; 28: N94-N99.

[467] McFadden, E.P., Stabile, E., Regar, E., Cheneau, E., Ong, A.T.L., Kinnaird, T., Suddath, W.O., Weissman, N.J., Kent, K.M., Pichard, A.D., Satler, L.F., Waksman, R., and Serruys, P.W. Late thrombosis in drug-eluting coronary stents after discontinuation of antiplatelet therapy. *Lancet,* 2004; 364: 1519-1521.

[468] Leggat, P.A. and Ketjarune, U. Toxicity of methyl methacrylate in dentistry. *Int Dent J.* 2003; 53: 126-131.

[469] Ahmed, D.D., Sobczak, S.C. and Yunginger, J.W. Occupational allergies caused by latex. *Immunol Allergy Clin North Am.* 2003; 23: 205-219.

[470] Ruiz-Genao, D.P., Moreno, De Vega, M.J., Sanchez Perez, J., and Garcia-Diez, A. Labial edema due to an acrylic dental prosthesis. *Contact Dermatitis,* 2003; 48: 273-274.

[471] Giunta, J. and Zablotsky, N. Allergic stomatitis caused by self-polymerizing resin. *Oral Surg Med Oral Pathol.* 1976; 41: 631-637.

[472] Lunder, T. and Rogl-Butina, M. Chronic urticaria from an acrylic dental prosthesis. *Contact Dermatitis,* 2000; 43: 222-223.

[473] Nealey, E.T. and Del Rio, C.E. Stomatitis venenata: reaction of a patient to acrylic resin. *J Prosthet Dent.* 1969; 21: 480-484.

[474] Concalves, T.S., Morganti, M.A., Campos, L.C., Rizzatto, S.M.D., and Menezes, L.M. Allergy to auto-polymerized acrylic resin in an orthodontic patient. *Am J Orthod Dentof Orthoped.* 2006; 129: 431-435.

[475] Devlin, H. and Watts, D.C. Acrylic "allergy"? *Br Dent J.* 1984; 157: 272-275.

[476] van Beusekom, H.M., Schwartz, R.S. and van der Giessen, W.J. Synthetic polymers. *Semin Interv Cardiol.* 1998; 3: 145-148.

[477] van Der Giessen, W.J., Lincoff, A.M., Schwartz, R.S., van Beusekom, H.M., Holmes, D.R. Jr., Ellis, S.G., and Topol, E.J. Marked inflammatory sequelae to implantation of biodegradable and nonbiodegradable polymers in porcine coronary arteries. *Circulation,* 1996; 94: 1690-1697.

[478] van Beusekom, H.M., Serruys, P.W. and van der Giessen, W.J. Coronary stent coatings. *Coron Artery Dis.* 1994; 5: 590-596.

[479] Revell, P.A., Braden, M. and Freeman, M.A. Review of the biological response to a novel bone cement containing poly(ethyl methacrylate) and n-butyl methacrylate. *Biomaterials,* 1998; 19: 1579-1586.

[480] Niemi, S.M., Fox, J.G., Brown, L.R., and Langer, R. Evaluation of ethylene-vinyl acetate copolymer as a non-inflammatory alternative to Freund's complete adjuvant in rabbits. *Lab Anim Sci.* 1985; 35: 609-612.

[481] Moreau, L., Alomer, G., Dube, N., and Sasseville, D. Contact urticaria from carboxymethylcellulose in white chalk. *Dermatitis,* 2006; 17: 29-31.

[482] Ownby, D.R. Mechanisms in adverse reactions to food: the whole body. *Allergy,* 1995; 50(20 suppl): 26-30.

[483] Carter, A.J., Aggarwal, M., Kopia, G.A., Tio, F., Kolata, R., Lianos, G., Dooley, J., and Falotico, R. Long-term effects opf polymer-based, slow release, sirolimus-eluting stents in a porcine coronary model. *Cardiovasc Res.* 2004; 63: 617-624.

[484] Takahashi, A., Palmer-Opolski, M., Smith, R.C., and Walsh, K. Transgene delivery of plasmid DNA to smooth muscle cells and macrophages from a biostable polymer-coated stent. *Gene Ther.* 2003; 10: 1471-1478.

[485] Johnson, T.W., Wu, Y.X., Herdeg, C., Baumbach, A., Newby, A.C., Karsch, K.R., and Oberhoff, M. Stent-based delivery of tissue inhibitor of metalloproteinase-3 adenovirus inhibits neointimal formation in porcine coronary arteries. *Arterioscler Thromb Vasc Biol.* 2005; 25: 754-759.

[486] Fishbein, I., Alferiev, I.S., Nyanguile, O., Gaster, R., Vohs, J.M., Wong, G.S., Felderman, H., Chen, I.W., Choi, H., Wilensky, R.L., and Levy, R.J. Biphosphonate-mediated gene vector delivery from the metal surfaces of stents. *Proc National Acad Sci.* 2006; 103: 159-164.

[487] Lyell, A., Bain, W.H. and Thomson, R.M. Repeated failure of nickel-containing prosthetic valves in a patient allergic to nickel. *Lancet*, 1978; 2: 657-659.

[488] Kanerva, L., Sipilainen-Malm, T., Estlander, T., Zitting, A., Jolanki, R., and Tarvainen, K. Nickel rease from metals, and a case of allergic contact dermatitis from stainless steel. *Contact Dermat.* 1994; 31: 299-303.

[489] Hillen, U., Haude, M., Erbel, R., and Goos, M. Evaluation of metal allergies in patients with coronary stents. *Contact Dermat.* 2002; 47: 353-356.

[490] Thomas, P., Summer, B., Sander, C.A., Przybilla, B., Thomas, M., and Naumann, T. Intolerance of osteosynthesis material: evidence of dichromate contact allergy with concomitant oligoclonal T-cell infiltrate and TH1-type cytokine expression in the peri-inplantar tissue. *Allergy,* 2000; 55: 969-972.

[491] Oppei, T. and Schnuch, A. The most frequent allergens in allergic contact dermatitis. Dtsch Med Wochennschr 2006; 131: 1584-1589.

[492] Wertman, B., Azarbal, B., Riedl, M., and Tobis, J. Adverse events associated with nickel allergy in patients undergoing percutaneous atrial septal defect or patent foramen ovale closure. *J Am Coll Cardiol.* 2006; 47: 1226-1227.

[493] Fukahara, K., Minami, K., Reiss, N., Fassbender, D., and Koerfer, R. Systemic allergic reactions to the percutaneous patent foramen ovale closure. *J Thoracic Cardiovasc Surg.* 2003; 125: 213-214.

[494] Dasika, U.K., Kanter, K.R. and Vincent, R. Nickel allergy to percutaneouis patent foramen ovale occluder and subsequent systemic nickel allergy. *J Thoracic Cardiovasc Surg.* 2003; 125: 2112-2113.

[495] Sharifi, M. and Burks, J. Efficacy of clopidogrel in the treatment of post-ASD closure migraines. *Catheter Cardiovasc Inter.* 2004; 63: 255.

[496] Menezes, L.M., Campos, L.C., Quintao, C.C., and Bolognese, A.M. Hypersensitivity to metals in orthodontics. *Am J Orthod Dentofacial Orthop.* 2004; 126: 58-64.

[497] Koster, R., Vieluf, D., Kiehn, M., Sommerauer, M., Kahler, J., Baldus, S.., Meinertz, T., and Hamm, C.W. Nickel and molybdenum contact allergies in patients with coronary in-stent restenosis. *Lancet*, 2000; 356: 1895-1897.

[498] Kawano, H., Koide, Y., Baba, T., Nakamizo, R., Toda, G., Takenaka, M., and Yano, K. Granulation tissue with eosinophil infiltration in the restenotic lesion after coronary stent implantation. *Circ J.* 2004; 68: 722-723.

[499] Iijima, R., Ikari, Y., Amiya, E., Tanimoto, S., Nakazawa, G., Kyono, H., Hatori, M., Miyazawa, A., Nakayama, T., Aoki, J., Nakajima, H., and Hara, K. The impact of metallic allergy on stent implantation. Metal allergy and recurrence of in-stent thrombosis. *Int J Cardiol.* 2005; 104: 319-325.

[500] Lhotka, C.G., Szekeres, T., Fritzer-Szekeres, M., Schwarz, G., Steffan, L., Maschke, M., Dubsky, G., Kremser, M., and Zweymuller, K. Are allergic reactions to skin clips associated with delayed wound healing? *Am J Surg.* 1998; 176: 320-323.

[501] Federmann, M., Morell, B., Graetz, G., Wyss, M., Elsner, P., von Thiessen, R., Wuthrich, B., and Grob, D. Hypersensitivity to molybdenum as a possible trigger of ANA-negative systemic lupus erythematosus. *Ann Rheum Dis.* 1994; 53: 403-405.

[502] Svedman, C., Tillman, C., Gustavsson, C.G., Moller, H., Frennby, B., and Bruze, M. Contact allergy to gold in patients with gold-plated intracoronary stents. *Contact Dermatitis*, 2005; 52: 192-196.

[503] Mosseri, M., Tamari, I., Plich, M., Hasin, Y., Brizines, M., Frimerman, A., Miller, H., Jafar, J., Guetta, V., Solomon, M., and Lotan, C. Short-and long-term outcomes of the titanium-NO stent registry. *Cardiovasc Revasc Med.* 2005; 6: 2-6.

[504] Ramade, S.V., Miller, K.M., Richard, R.E., Chan, A.K., Allen, M.J., and Helmus, M.N. Physical characterization of controlled release of paclitaxel from the TAXUS Express drug eluting stent. *J Biomed Mater Res.* 2004; 71A: 625-634.

[505] Hwang, C.W., Wu, D. and Edelman, E.R. Physiologic transport forces govern drug distribution for stent-based delivery. *Circulation*, 2001; 104: 600-605.

[506] Vetrovec, G.V., Rizik, D., Williard, C., Snead, D., Piotrovski, V., and Kopia, G. Sirolimus PK trial: a pharmacokinetic study of the sirolimus-eluting Bx velocity stent in patients with de novo coronary lesions. *Catheter Cardiovasc Interv.* 2006; 67: 32-37.

[507] Tesfamariam, B. Local vascular toxicokinetics of stent-based drug delivery. *Toxicol Lett.* 2007; 168: 93-102.

[508] Descotes, J. and Choquet-Kastylevsky, G. Gell and Coombs`s classification: is it still valid? Toxicology 2001;58: 43-49.

[509] Beeler, A., Engler, O., Gerber, B.O., and Pichler, W.J. Long-lasting reactivity and high frequency of drug-specific T cells after severe systemic drug hypersensitivity reactions. *J Allergy Clin Immunol.* 2006; 117: 455-462.

[510] Nemmar, A., Hoet, P.H.M., Vermylen, J., Nemery, B., and Hoylaerts, M.F. Pharmacological stabilization of mast cells abrogates late thrombotic events induced by diesel exhaust particles in hamsters. *Circulation*, 2004; 110: 1670-1677.

[511] Chitkara, K., Hogrefe, K., Vasa-Nicotera, M., Swanson, N., and Gershlick, A.H. Eptifibatide-stent as an antiproliferative and antithrombotic agent: in vitro evaluation. *J Invasive Cardiol.* 2006; 18: 417-422.

[512] Camici, G.G., Steffel, J., Akhmedov, A., Schafer, N., Baldinger, J., Schulz, U., Shojaati, K., Matter, C.M, Yang, Z., Luscher, T.F., and Tanner, F.C. Dimethyl sulfoxide inhibits tissue factor expression, thrombus formation, and vascular smooth muscle cell activation. A potential treatment strategy for drug-eluting stents. *Circulation*, 2006; 114: 1512-1521

[513] Blindt, R., Vogt, F., Astafieva, I., Fach, C., Hristov, M., Krott, N., Seitz, B., Kapumiotu, A., Kwok, C., Dewor, M., Bosserhoff, A.K., Bemhagen, J., Hanrath, P.,

Hoffmann, R., and Weber, C. A novel drug-eluting stent coated with an integrin-binding cyclic Arg-Gly-Asp peptide inhibits neointimal hyperplasia by recruiting endothelial progenitor cells. *J Am Coll Cardiol.* 2006; 47: 1786-1795.

[514] Aoki, J., Serruys, P.W., van Beusekom, H., Ong, A.T., McFadden, E.P., Sianos, G., van der Giessen, W.J., Regar, E., de Feyter, P.J., Davis, H.R., Rowland, S., and Kutryk, M.J. Endothelial progenitor cells capture by stents coated with antibody against CD34: the HEALING-FIM (Healthy Endothelial Accelerated Lining Inhibits Neointimal Growth-First In Man) Registry. *J Am Coll Cardiol.* 2006; 45: 1574-1579

[515] Joner, M., Farb, A., Cheng, Q., Finn, A.V., Acampado, E., Burke, A.P., Skorija, K., Creighton, W., Kolodgie, F.D., Gold, H.K., and Virmani, R. Pioglitazone inhibits in-stent restenosis in atherosclerotic rabbits by targeting transforming growth factor-β and MCP-1. *Arterioscl Thromb Vasc Biol.* 2007; 27: 182-189.

[516] Sebakh, R.J., Sheller, J.R., Oates, J.A., Roberts, L.J., and FitzGerald, G.A. Inhibition of eicosanoid biosynthesis by glucocorticoid in humans. *Proc Natl Acad Sci USA* 1990; 87:6974-8.

[517] Theoharides, T.C. and Bielory, L. Mast cells and mast cell mediators as targets of dietary supplements. *Arm Allergy Asthma Immunol.* 2004; 93 (2 Suppl 1):S24-34.

[518] Leung, D.Y.M., Sampson, H.A., Ynginger, J.W., et al. Effect of anti-IgE therapy in patients with peanut allergy. *N Engl J Med.* 2003; 348: 986-93.

[519] Finkelman, F.D., Rothenberg, M.C., Brandt, E.B., Morris, S.C., and Strait, R.T. Molecular mechanisms of anaphylaxis: lessons from studies with murine models. *J Allergy Clin Immunol.* 2005; 115:449-57.

[520] Suissa, S., Assimes, T., Brassard, P., Ernst, P., Inhaled corticosteroids in asthma and the prevention of myocardial infarction. *Am J Med* 2003; 115: 377-81

[521] Takagi, S., Goto, Y., Terashima, M., Sakuragi, S., Suzuki,S., et al. Successful traetment of refractory vasospastic angina with corticosteroids: Coronary arterial hyperactivity caused by local inflammation? *Cic J* 2004; 68: 17-22

In: Angina Pectoris: Etiology, Pathogenesis and Treatment   ISBN: 978-1-60456-674-1
Editors: A. P. Gallo, M. L. Jones   © 2008 Nova Science Publishers, Inc.

Chapter IV

Atherosclerosis, Understanding Pathogenesis - Challenge for Treatment

Slavica Mitrovska[*,1], *Silvana Jovanova*[2], *Inge Matthiesen*[3], *and Christian Libermans*[4]

[1]Military Hospital, Department of Cardiology, Skopje, Macedonia
[2]Institute for Heart Disease, Clinical Center, Skopje, Macedonia
[3]Karolinska Institute, Solna, Sweden
[4]Hospital San Carlos, Emergency Department, Costa Rica, Central America

Abstract

Atherosclerosis is a chronic inflammatory disease that affects medium and large-sized arteries. It begins after birth and the progression depends on several factors – traditional triad: hypertension, hyperlipidemia and diabetes mellitus, then age, sex, smoking and sedentary life-style. At the beginning atherosclerosis is asymptomatic and we cannot estimate appropriately its frequency, but its complications – coronary artery diseases, cerebrovascular diseases, peripheral arterial diseases, which occur late, are responsible for more than half of the yearly mortality in the world. Unfortunately, sudden cardiac death may be the first clinical manifestation.

The incipient event is endothelial dysfunction, as a result of injury, caused by high level of cholesterol [especially low-density-lipoprotein LDL], hyperglycemia, hypertension, smoking, infectious agents, and toxins. Endothelial cells overexpress adhesion molecules – vascular cell adhesion molecule–1 [VCAM-1] and increases recruitment of inflammatory cells– monocytes [Mo], T-cells and subsequent release of monocyte chemo–attractant protein–1 [MCP-1] that results in additional leucocytes recruitment. Injured endothelium allows migration of inflammatory cells that release cytokines and lipids into the intima. That leads to cytokine-mediated progression of atherosclerosis and oxidation of LDL. Macrophages [MP] take up oxi-LDL and form foam-cell. They have metabolic activity and produce cytokines, proliferation of smooth

[*] Address for correspondence: Mitrovska Slavica M.D. Mr.Sci.Med,Ul.Sole Stojcev br.1-2-8, 1000 Skopje, Macedonia, Tel: 0038971634494, E-mail: mitrovska2000@yahoo.com.

muscle cells and formulate athero-fibrose plaque. Atherosclerotic plaque is composed of superficial layer – fibrose cap and lipid core, that consists of foam cells, extracellular lipid and necrotic cellular debris. It progresses as a result of accumulation of lipid and proliferation of smooth muscle cells and results in luminal narrowing of the arteries which leads to compromised blood and oxygen supply to the tissues. The gradually growing atherosclerotic plaques have thick fibrose cap and are stable. They cause symptoms of stable angina. Rapidly growing plaques cause unstable coronary artery disease. These plaques are mainly composed of lipids and have tiny fibrose cap that is prone to fissuring or rupture. Intraplaque hemorrhage from microvessels in plaque initiate platelet adhesion and activation of coagulation cascade that leads to platelet thrombus formation, i.e. promote thrombogenesis.

Knowledge of the pathogenesis of the atherothrombosis modifies the diagnostic and therapeutic approach.

Conclusion: Our attention should be focused on the management of three points:

1. Endothelial dysfunction [correction of modified risk factors: hypertension, hyperlipidemia, diabetes mellitus, life-style-smoking, physical activity and food],
2. Atherosclerosis [modification of the inflammatory cascade, i.e. elimination of inflammatory pathways and inhibition of oxidation of LDL],
3. Thrombogenesis [inhibition of platelet adhesion, activation and aggregation].

Keywords: *atherosclerosis, endothelial dysfunction, inflammatory pathways, thrombogenesis.*

Introduction

Atherosclerosis is a chronic inflammatory disease that affects medium and large-sized arteries. It begins after birth, initially it is a silent process but it progresses during the person's life. The atherosclerotic lesions are a result of continuum molecular and cellular interaction between vessel wall and blood constituents, release of number of signaling pathways and activation of the inflammatory and coagulation cascades that lead to structural changes. At the beginning atherosclerosis is asymptomatic and we cannot estimate appropriately its frequency. But, in some people atherosclerosis has rapid progress and triggers a vicious circle that leads to clinical manifestations of coronary artery diseases, cerebrovascular diseases, and peripheral arterial diseases. Unfortunately, sudden cardiac death may be the first clinical manifestation. The increasing incidence makes the atherosclerosis a leader of morbidity and mortality in the developing world.

According to the American Heart Association, more than 11 million people suffer from coronary artery disease [CAD] in USA, 30% have carotid artery disease, 1.5 million myocardial infarctions per year, more than 200,000 deaths per year caused by cerebrovascular diseases [1].

The other thing that should be a concern is the increasingly younger age group having onset of symptoms, as early as 35 years old. The progress of atherosclerosis depends on several factors – traditional triad: hypertension, hyperlipidemia and diabetes mellitus, than age, sex, stress, smoking and sedentary life-style [2].

Impaired Endothelial Function

The incipient changes occur in the endothelium and the earliest step is impaired endothelial function. Endothelium is an inner layer of the vessel wall that has an active role to respond to various stimuli. It acts as an endocrine organ that has secretory role and it takes place in the process of inflammation, hemostasis and fibroproliferative process. Also, endothelium regulates the vessel wall tonus by release endothelium derived relaxing [EDRF] and constrictive factors. The vasodilatation is providing by EDRF – nitric oxide [NO], produced by NO synthase enzyme [type III eNOS], whereas vasoconstriction is mediated by endothelin-1 [ET-1] and thromboxane A_2. The imbalance between vasodilatative and vasoconstrictive substances leads to the impairment of endothelial cell function. This is the first stage of atherosclerotic process – lack of activity of endothelium derived NO and impaired vascular relaxation. In the setting of hypertension, hyperlipidemia [especially high level of LDL-C], diabetes mellitus, genetic alterations, smoking, toxins, infectious agents, the blood flow became turbulent and provoked a number of insults to the endothelium [3].

Inflammatory Pathways Promote Atherosclerosis

As a "response to injury" the endothelium becomes active and initiates a cascade of subsequent events, which are compensatory mechanisms to keep the homeostasis. If the influence of provocative agents continues excessively, than these mechanisms overdrive normal properties of the endothelium and lead to the development of atherosclerotic plaque. The activated endothelium over expresses adhesion molecules, as vascular cell adhesion molecule-1 [VCAM-1] and increases recruitment of inflammatory cells - monocytes [Mo], T-cells and subsequent release of monocytchemo-attractant protein-1 [MCP-1] that results in their differentiation into macrophages [MP] [4].

In the acute phase, the inflammatory cells secrete a number of cytokines, mostly interleukins – IL-1ß, IL-6, IL-8, than tumor necrosis factor- α [TNF-α], interferon-γ [IFN-γ] and transforming growth factor-ß [TFG-ß] [5]. They increase permeability of the endothelium to lipoproteins, especially low-density-lipoproteins [LDL-C] and they have enhanced migration through the endothelial membrane into subendothelium. LDL deposit initiates additional induction of numbers MP and release of cytokines [especially IL-1], hydrolytic enzymes and chemokines, growth factors and a vicious circle of inflammation starts [6]. Increased accumulation of MP is associated with increased level of fibrogen and C-reactive protein [CRP]. It is believed that CRP helps the MP in the process of phagocytosis.

Intra intimal LDL undergoes oxidation [oxidant stress] by oxidant mechanisms that involve hydrogen peroxide and free radicals. MP recognizes and phagocyte oxidized low-density-lipoproteins [oxi-LDL] through scavenger receptors [7]. Accumulation of oxi-LDL and cholesterol esters in MP leads to formation of foam cells. Oxidized LDL have toxic effects. They produce free radicals that reduce activity of NO-synthase and inactivation of NO leads to vasoconstriction [8].

The foam cells have metabolic activity, secrete TGF-ß, stimulating the proliferation of smooth muscle cells, fibroblasts, collagen and elastin and form fibrous cap over the lipid collection. Thus, the atherofibrous plaque is formed [9].

The Composition of the Atherosclerotic Plaque

Atherosclerotic plaque progresses as a result of the progressive accumulation of lipids and proliferation of smooth muscle cells. As long as injurious agents persist, the affected endothelium reacts with abnormal inflammatory and fibroproliferative response, triggering the progression of atherosclerotic plaque, as well as the disease progression. Development of plaque deforms the arterial wall.

The gradually growing plaques cause thickening of the artery wall. The arterial wall becomes rigid. At the beginning they do not compromise arterial circulation. These plaques are angiographically invisible and according to the American Heart Association, are classified as type IV and V-a [10]. At that stage, the lumen of the artery remains unaltered due to "remodeling," compensatory dilatation of the wall, termed – Glagov phenomenon. Further enlargement of the lesion results in luminal narrowing and compromising of the blood and oxygen supply [11].

The gradually growing atherosclerotic plaques have a thick fibrous cap. They are stable and when the narrowing of the lumen is more than 50%, cause the symptoms of chronic stable angina. Clinicians note that these patients have better prognosis despite critical diminution of the coronary artery flow. Contrary, potentially dangerous lesions are usually nonocclusive. Thus, retrospective analyses of angiographic observations revealed that almost 2/3 of patients with acute coronary syndromes [unstable angina and myocardial infarction] have low-grade stenosis less than 70% [mostly < 50%]. Morphologic examinations have shown that these plaques are composed mainly of lipids and have a tiny fibrous cap [12].

These findings lead our attention to the other direction, to the composition of the atherosclerotic plaque, as an important predictor of adverse cardiac events.

In 1992, James Muller introduces the term "vulnerable" plaque. It is a morphologic description and concerns the cellular and molecular characteristics of the atherosclerotic plaques that are prone to rupture [13].

Peter Libby et al. describe vulnerable plaque as a lesion consisting of a central lipid-rich core, surrounded by a tiny fibrous cap [14]. Davies et al. estimate that the lipid core is 30-40% of the vulnerable plaque volume [15].

Lipid-rich core is composed of lipid-laden foam cells, necrotic cellular debris, extracellular lipid, free and esterified cholesterol and cholesterol esters.

The thickness of the fibrous cap is a second condition for stability/instability of the plaque. The tiny cap is collagen-deficient and also contains less proteoglicans. These things make the cap much more susceptible to destroying enzymes – matrix metalloproteinase (MMPs) that include collagenase and gelatinase and prone to disruption. Burne et al. define the fibrous cap as vulnerable if its thickness is less than 65 μm [16].

Several results from coronary atherectomy have shown that the culprit lesion in patients with unstable angina has increased neovascularization. These vasa vasorum that proliferate within the plaque are fragile and cause intraplaque hemorrhage with secondary rupture [17].

Concerning the mechanism of instability of atherosclerotic plaque, most of the theories accentuate the imbalance between presences of normal and inflammatory cells [18]. Thus, inflammatory cells, especially T-Ly, have a tendency to localize in the "shoulders" of the plaque. These sites are lesion prone sites. T-Ly produce cytokine, CD40 ligand, IFN-γ that impairs collagen synthesis and IL-1β and IL-4 stimulate MP to produce MMP that degrade the fibrous cap. The result of this activity is plaque rupture or plaque erosion and exposition of thrombogenic substances of the core to the blood [19].

Thrombogenesis

Normal endothelium maintains the platelets in a resting state by producing prostacyclin and NO. Loss of endothelium exposes the subendothelium to the blood constituents and initiates the activation of coagulation cascade [20]. Thus, the procoagulant milieu favors thrombus formation. The subendothelium releases von Willebrand factor and other adhesive proteins that bind to glycoprotein receptor Ib [GP Ib] on the platelet surface and provoke platelet adhesion to the subendothelial collagen. Furthermore, adhered platelets became active, secrete adenosine-diphosphate [ADP] and number of mediators-cytokines, Thrombocyte derived growth factor, Thrombocyte factor-4, C-reactive protein, TGF- β, Placental growth factor [PlGF] and together with thrombin promote platelet aggregation [21].

Final step in the process of thrombogenesis is the activation of the GP IIb/IIIa receptors of the platelet surface, and together with fibrinogen make tight connection between platelets. That leads to thrombus formation [22]. This is a defensive mechanism, to protect the organism from bleeding. Activation of platelets involves triggering of internal signaling pathways, as a releasing of adenosine diphosphate [ADP], serotonin, calcium and recruitment of more platelets. But sometimes those triggers became uncontrolled and thrombus formation culminates in thrombosis. The final outcome is occlusion of the artery and consecutive events – stable, unstable angina or myocardial infarction.

Thus thrombogenesis has become the second most important process in pathogenesis of acute coronary syndrome [23].

Therapeutic Approaches

The base of human physiology is to keep the balance between restoring and destroying processes. For this purpose, each process in the human body consists of pro and contra mechanisms [proinflammatory and anti-inflammatory, procoagulant and anticoagulant elements]. The aim is to maintain the equilibrium and to provide normal function for each organ.

The nature of the processes of atherosclerosis and thrombogenesis, as well as their alterations and signaling pathways, are a challenge for observation and action [24].

[5]   Ohji T, Urano H, Shirahata A et al: Transforming growth factor beta 1 and beta 2 induce down regulation of thrombomodulin in human umbilical vein endothelial cells. *Thromb. Haemost.* 1995; 73:812-818

[6]   Rajavashisth TB, Liao JK, Galis ZS, et al: Inflammatory cytokines and oxidized low-density lipoproteins increase endothelial cell expression of membrane type 1-matrix metalloproteinase. *J. Biol. Chem.* 1999; 274: 11924-11929.

[7]   Vieira O, et al: Oxidized LDLs alter the activity of the ubiquitin-proteasome pathway: Potential role in oxidized LDL-induces apoptosis, *Faseb. J.* 2000;14:532-542

[8]   Weinbrenner T, Cladellas M, Isabel Covas M et al: High oxidative stress in patients with stable coronary heart disease. *Atherosclerosis.* 2003; 168 [1]: 99-106

[9]   Galis ZS, Sukhova GK, Kranzhofer R, et al: Macrophage foam cells from experimental atheroma constitutively produce matrix-degrading proteinases. *Proc. Natl .Acad .Sci .USA* 1995; 92:402-406.

[10] Stary HC, Chandler AB, Dinsmore RE, Fuster V, Glagov S, Insull WJr, Rosenfeld ME Schwartz CJ, Wagner WD, Wissler RW: A definition of advanced types of atherosclerotic lesions and a histological classification of atherosclerosis. A report from the Commitee on Vascular Lesions of the Council on Atherosclerosis. American Heart Association. *Circulation* 1995; 92:1355-1374.

[11] Davies MJ: A macro and micro view of coronary vascular insult in ischemic heart disease. *Circulation* 1990;82 [suppl II]: II-38-II46.

[12] Stary HC: Natural history and histological classification of atherosclerotic lesions: An update. *Arterioscler. Thromb. Vasc. Biol.* 2000; 20:177-178.

[13] Muller JE, Tofler GH: Triggering and hourly variation of onset of arterial thrombosis. *Ann. Epidemiol.* 1992; 2:393-405

[14] Libby P: Current concepts of the pathogenesis of the acute coronary syndromes. *Circulation* 2001; 104:365-372.

[15] Davies MJ: The composition of coronary artery plaque. *N. Engl. J .Med.* 1997; 336:1312-13.

[16] Burke AP, Farb A, Malcolm GT, et al: Coronary risk factors and plaque morphology in men with coronary disease who died suddenly. *N. Engl. J. med.* 1997; 336:1276-1282

[17] Kwon HM, et al: Enhanced coronary vasa vasorum neovascularization in experimental hypercholesterolemia. *J. Clin. Invest.* 1998; 101:1551-1556

[18] Assoian RK, Marcantonio EE: The extracellular matrix as a cell cycle control element in atherosclerosis and restenosis. *J. Clin. Invest.* 1996; 98:2436-2439

[19] Davies MJ, Gordon JL, Gearing AJ, et al: The expression of the adhesion molecules ICAM-1, VCAM-1, PECAM, and E- selectin in human atherosclerosis. *J. Pathol.* 1993; 171:223-229

[20] Massberg S, Brand K, Gruner S, et al: A critical role of platelet adhesion in the initiation of atherosclerotic lesion formation. *J. Exp. Med.* 2002;196:887-896.

[21] Kroll M, Sullivan R: Mechanisms of platelet activation, in Loscalzo JA, Schafer A [eds]: Thrombosis and Haemorrhage. Philadelphia PA, Williams and Wilkins, 1998;261-291.

[22] Lefcovits J, Plow EF, Topol EJ: Platelet glycoprotein IIb/IIIa receptors in cardiovascular medicine. *N .Engl .J. Med .*1995;332:1553-1559

[23] Arbustini EDBB, Morbini P, Burke AP, Bocciarelli M, Specchia G, Virmani: Plaque erosion is a major substrate for coronary thrombosis in acute myocardial infarction. *Heart* 1999; 82:269-72

[24] Ross R. Atherosclerosis-An Inflammatory Disease.*Atherosclerosis.*1999;340:115-126.

[25] Falk e. Pathogenesis of atherosclerosis. *J. Am. Coll. Cardiol.* 2006;47:7-12

[26] Libby P, Theroux P: Pathophysiology of Coronary Artery Disease. *Circulation* 2005;111:3481-3488.

[27] Smith S, Blair S, Bonow R, et al: AHA/ACC Guidelines for Preventing Heart Attack and Death in Patients With Atherosclerotic Cardiovascular Disease: 2001 Update. *Circulation* 2001;104: 1577-1579.

[28] Ambrosioni E, Bacchelli S, Esposti DD, Borghi C:Anti-ischemic effects of angiotensin-converting enzyme inhibitors: a future therapeutic perspective. *J. Cardiovasc. Pharmacol.* 2001;37 [Suppl 1]:S3-9.

[29] Curzen NP, Fox KM: Do ACE inhibitors modulate atherosclerosis?. *Eur. Heart J.* 1997;18[10]:1530-5.

[30] Wannamethee S, Lowe G, Shaper A et al: The metabolic syndrome and insulin resistance: relationship to haemostatic and inflammatory markers in older non-diabetic men. *Atherosclerosis.* 2005; 181[1]:101-108.

[31] Pedersen, T.R., L.Wilhelmsen, O.Faergeman, et al.: Follow-up study of patients randomized in the Scandinavian Simvastatin Survival Study [4S] of cholesterol lowering. *Am. J. Cardiol.* 2000;86:257-262

[32] Ascer E, Bertolami M, Venturinelli M et al: Atorvastatin reduces proinflammatory markers in hypercholesterolemic patients. *Atherosclerosis.* 2004; Vol.177 [1]: 161-166

[33] Yusuf S. Clopidogrel in unstable angina to prevent recurrent ischemic events [CURE]. Program and abstracts of the American College of Cardiology 50-th Annual Scientific Session; March 18-21,2001;Orlando Florida, Presentation 9, Session 405.

[34] EPILOG Investigators. Platelet glycoprotein IIb/IIa receptor blockade and low-dose heparin during percutaneous coronary revascularization. *N. Engl. J. Med.* 1997;336:1689-96.

In: Angina Pectoris: Etiology, Pathogenesis and Treatment   ISBN: 978-1-60456-674-1
Editors: A. P. Gallo, M. L. Jones   © 2008 Nova Science Publishers, Inc.

Chapter V

The Role of Psychosocial Factors in Determining Cardiac Rehabilitation Attendance by Coronary Artery Disease Patients Following Surgery

Michael O'Connor[1,*], Guy D. Eslick[2] and Natasha Koloski[3]

[1] School of Psychology, The University of Queensland
Brisbane, Queensland, Australia
[2] School of Public Health, The University of Sydney, Sydney,
New South Wales, Australia
[3] School of Psychology ,The University of Queensland,Brisbane,
Queensland, Australia

Abstract

Background/Aims: Despite the reported benefits of cardiac rehabilitation, attendance at these programs is particularly poor among coronary artery disease patients following surgery. Very little is known about the role that psychosocial factors may play in patients' decision to attend a cardiac rehabilitation program post surgery. In a prospective study, we aimed to determine if psychosocial factors are independent predictors of cardiac rehabilitation attendance.

Methods: A consecutive sample of private hospital cardiac patients (n=146) with angina who had undergone surgical intervention including either angioplasty (n=61) or coronary artery bypass surgery (n=25) were invited to participate (response rate 58.9%; n=86). Patients were classified according to confirmed rehabilitation records into attendees (n=56) and non-attendees (n=30). Patients completed a self report valid questionnaire on anxiety, depression, social support, coping, illness perceptions, neuroticism, optimism and quality of life (QOL).

Results: Patients who decided to attend rehabilitation were significantly different compared with non-attenders with regards to having greater trait anxiety (P=0.01) and

* Tel: +617 3346-9521, Fax: +617 3365-4466, e-mail: michaelo@psy.uq.edu.au.

use of self blame as a coping mechanism (P=0.05). Attenders were more likely to label their condition as unpredictable (*P< .01*), perceived greater subsequent effects from their illness (*P = .01*), reported difficulty emotionally dealing with the circumstances (*P = .04*), and had less understanding of their illness (*P = .02*). In terms of QOL, attenders reported significantly greater emotional interference (*P = .04*), and subsequently greater impairment to their mental health (*P = .04*), compared with non-attenders. None of these factors however were independently associated with attendance. Depression, social support, coping, optimism and neuroticism did not significantly differentiate between the two groups.

Conclusions: Psychosocial factors including trait anxiety, a maladaptive coping style, impaired illness perceptions and poorer quality of life may play a role in patient's decision to attend a cardiac rehabilitation program following surgery, although other factors are likely to be more important.

Introduction

Cardiac rehabilitation is an important adjunct to the medical and surgical treatment for cardiovascular disease including angina. Although the physical [1] and psychological [2] benefits of cardiac rehabilitation are well established these programs generally evidence poor utilization rates. This chapter will provide an overview of the sociodemographic, practical and clinical barriers, as well as the psychosocial reasons for non-attendance at cardiac rehabilitation programs. Moreover this chapter will describe a study that was conducted specifically to explore potential risk factors for cardiac rehabilitation attendance among patients with angina who underwent surgical intervention for their condition.

Cardiac Rehabilitation

While surgical intervention often prolongs the life of patients with cardiovascular disease, lifestyles changes and risk factor modification are crucial components towards secondary prevention, which take the form of cardiac rehabilitation [3-4]. Cardiac rehabilitation services promote a safe and friendly atmosphere for exercise, guide and teach patients the skills necessary to maintain optimal heart/general health and functional independence, and provide support to patients at a crucial and often difficult time in their lives [5-6]. Major findings suggest that cardiac rehabilitation has amicable effects in terms of reductions in clinical events and hospital readmission rates, improvement in symptoms of angina and dyspnoea and an estimated reduction of between 20 to 25% in cardiac mortality [7-10]. Psychological improvements in terms of reduced anxiety and depression [2] have also been reported among patients attending a cardiac rehabilitation program. Despite these reported benefits, however, uptake of cardiac rehabilitation programs is particularly poor [3,11]. Understanding the reasons behind non attendance at cardiac rehabilitation programs is crucial in light of the potential for significant improvements in the health status of people with cardiovascular disease.

Definition of Adherence

Adherence in the literature has been defined in a number of ways [12]. Some researchers have operationalised cardiac rehabilitation adherence as: attendance of at least one session [13-14], attendance of at least 50% of sessions [15], or participation throughout the entire program [16]. For consistency throughout this chapter, adherence will broadly refer to the extent to which cardiac patients' adhere with agreed upon medical recommendations to attend (at any level) a structured cardiac rehabilitation program following hospital discharge.

Uptake of Cardiac Rehabilitation

Cardiac rehabilitation uptake across all studies cited in this chapter ranges from 10% to 65% [12,17], largely because of varying definitions of attendance. The majority of studies have looked at 50% attendance or full participation [15-16], with few looking at initial intention by the patient to attend. There is also a heavy reliance on self report indicators of rehabilitation attendance in studies, with only one study measuring attendance by actual records at the rehabilitation centre [15].

Sociodemographic Variables and Non-Attendance

The majority of research into cardiac rehabilitation attendance has focused on identifying sociodemographic variables that influence participation rates, as these factors are easily identifiable to health professionals, and now the focus of interventions towards those 'at risk' of non-attendance [16]. In general, females are less likely to attend in comparison to males, and one possible reason may be linked with the practical issue of transportation, as women are generally diagnosed and treated much later in life, many are no longer driving, and often widowed [14,18]. Older patients [19], patients from lower socioeconomic positions [20] and lower education levels [21], and those without current employment [15] also appear to display higher rates of non-attendance. Finally, patients who are married evidence greater uptake rates [22], and one reason for this may be linked with spousal support towards rehabilitation [21].

Practical/ Clinical Barriers and Non-Attendance

Qualitative evidence suggests practical or clinical barriers to cardiac rehabilitation adherence are important [14]. Practical barriers include availability to transportation, especially for elderly woman, and surgery patients who are prohibited from driving for six weeks post-operatively [23], distance to rehabilitation centre [16], lack of medical insurance and family obligations [11], inconvenient session times [7] and work commitments [20]. Poor physician referral rates, especially amongst elderly women [24] and among patients undergoing angioplasty [14] are also considered clinical barriers to rehabilitation. Moreover patients who have undergone coronary artery bypass surgery have a higher rate of attending a cardiac rehabilitation program (53.1%) compared with 10.3% of patients who have had angioplasty [17].

Psychological Factors and Adherence

A limited amount of research has been conducted into the relationship between psychosocial factors and cardiac rehabilitation adherence with mixed results.

Psychological Distress

The evidence for psychological distress in terms of anxiety and depression as predictors of attendance at a cardiac rehabilitation program is mixed. In one of the first studies conducted by Harlan et al. (1995) [18], baseline measures of psychological status were obtained in a sample of 393 patients who were recruited during the acute recovery period for coronary artery bypass surgery to participate in a three week outpatient rehabilitation program. Psychological status was assessed via four subscales from the General Well-Being Schedule (health concerns, depression, anxiety and energy level) [18]. The anxiety and depression subscales failed to differentiate between attenders and non-attenders [18]. Although, a strength of this study was that the cost of the program was wavered for those unable to afford it, serving to reduce any bias. Only 13% attended the program. Thus, making it difficult to draw conclusions as insufficient power may have been an issue. Another study that recruited patients with myocardial infarction within 24 hours of hospital admission also found no significant differences between cardiac rehabilitation attenders and non attenders on measures of anxiety and depression [24].

In contrast, Lane et al. (2001) conducted baseline assessments of myocardial infarction patients while in hospital, on average six days after their cardiac event [15]. A sample of 283 patients (25% female) recruited from two hospital sites in England, completed psychological measures including the Beck Depression Inventory and both scales of the State-Trait Anxiety Inventory. Adherence to cardiac rehabilitation was also determined from records held at the respective rehabilitation centre [15]. They found non-attenders demonstrate significantly higher mean depression (8.6) and trait-anxiety (33.4) scores in comparison to attenders (6.4 and 29.9) respectively [15].

The opposite, however, was found in a study by Whitmarsh et al. (2003) [12]. They assessed anxiety and depression levels in a rehabilitation sample of 93 patients with myocardial infarction from the United Kingdom (mean age 63.9 years; 27.3% female), via the Hospital Anxiety and Depression Scale after discharge, but prior to the commencement of the cardiac rehabilitation program [12]. Non-attenders reported significantly lower depression and anxiety levels, although these were not independent predictors of attendance. Reasons for these inconsistencies between studies remain unclear.

Social Support

The evidence for the role of social support in determining cardiac rehabilitation attendance is unequivocal. Johnson et al. (1998) investigated perceived social support in terms of patient adherence to cardiac rehabilitation services, in a sample of 254 patients with a mean age of 64 years, who had recently experienced an acute myocardial infarction, coronary artery bypass surgery or angioplasty [13]. Only 28% of the sample participated in at least one session of rehabilitation, and the response rate to all questionnaires was reported to be 54% [13]. They found patients with low social support were less likely to attend cardiac rehabilitation sessions [13], although patients were limited to those living in a rural location, limiting the generalisability of the findings. King et al. (2001), however, found no support for an association between perceived 'benefit' of sources of social support and rehabilitation adherence two weeks after hospital discharge [16]. One possible reason for this null finding may be that the social support instrument used in this study was very brief (i.e. five items). Further research assessing specific types of available social support is needed before social support can be ruled out as a potential predictor of rehabilitation adherence.

Coping

Whitmarsh et al (2003) evaluated attenders and non-attenders on their coping style using the COPE measure [12]. They found non-attenders were less likely to adopt adaptive coping styles such as emotion focussed or problem focused styles to manage their stressful situation [12]. Instead the use of more frequent maladaptive coping styles such as venting of emotions, denial, and both mental and behavioural disengagement were considered to be independent predictors of non-attendance. Thus, coping appears to be an important factor in determining attendance at cardiac rehabilitation, although confirmation of these findings is now needed.

Health Beliefs

The beliefs or perceptions one holds about their health has received more attention in the cardiac rehabilitation adherence literature. Cooper et al. (1999) were among the first to assess the role of specific illness beliefs in cardiac rehabilitation attendance [19]. The prospective design captured the beliefs of 152 acute myocardial infarction and coronary artery bypass surgery patients during hospitalisation, as measured by the Illness Perception Questionnaire. They found that non-attenders reported significantly less control over their condition, were older, and were less likely to believe that lifestyle factors may have contributed towards their illness, compared with attenders [19]. A similar finding was reported by Whitmarsh et al, 2003 who also assessed the role of illness perception using the Illness Perception Questionnaire among 93 myocardial infarction patients [12]. They found non-attenders reported significantly less symptoms and fewer consequences from their illness in terms of physical, social or psychological functioning [12]. Multivariate analyses revealed that the strongest predictors of non-attendance were fewer symptoms and greater perceived control

[12]. Moreover a recent meta-analysis of 8 methodologically sound studies showed support for a predictive role for illness perception and cardiac rehabilitation adherence [24].

The exception, however, was reported by French et al. (2005) who evaluated myocardial infarction patients during hospitalisation [25]. They found no significant differences between attenders and non-attenders on any measure of illness perceptions [25]. One possible explanation for this null finding could lie in the recruitment method, such that patients were recruited within the first 24 hours of hospital admission, a method that differs greatly from other research where patients are recruited whilst in hospital, but some time later prior to discharge [25]. Patients' may not have had sufficient time to psychologically adjust to the trauma of experiencing a heart attack.

Personality

No studies have directly assessed the role of personality on cardiac rehabilitation attendance. One study by Glazer et al. (2002) found that dropouts enrolled in a cardiac rehabilitation program had significantly higher levels of depression, neuroticism and trait anxiety but were significantly lower on optimism in comparison to attenders [26]. It must be noted that there are important conceptual differences between dropouts and non-attenders. Although this study provides preliminary evidence for a role of personality in cardiac rehabilitation attendance, future research employing earlier assessments of patient's intention or initial attendance are needed to confirm these observations.

Quality of Life

No studies have specifically examined quality of life in relation to attendance at a cardiac rehabilitation program, but it is hypothesised that reduced quality of life may contribute to the decision to attend a cardiac rehabilitation program

Summary

Attendance at cardiac rehabilitation programs is crucial for patients with cardiovascular disease including angina symptoms. Nonetheless most patients with these conditions do not attend these programs. Understanding the reasons behind this non attendance is important for identifying 'at risk' patients. While sociodemographic and practical and clinical barriers are among some of the reasons that patients do not attend, there are limited or conflicting findings regarding the role of psychological factors such as anxiety and depression, social support, coping, illness perception and personality. Further research is necessary to determine the relative contribution of these psychosocial factors to cardiac rehabilitation attendance.

Aims:

Therefore we aimed to determine whether demographic, psychosocial and quality of life factors are associated with non attendance at a cardiac rehabilitation program. We hypothesise that non-attenders will be more likely to express lower levels of depression, anxiety, social support and impairment in quality of life. Moreover non-attenders will use more adaptive coping strategies and have better illness perceptions compared with attenders.

Methods

Participants

A sample of 146 consecutive cardiac patients from the Wesley hospital, 37 females and 109 males, with an age range from 33 to 89 years ($M = 62.27$ years, $SD = 10.14$ years) were invited to participate in this study between June and September 2007. Any patient with confirmed coronary artery disease through angiographic techniques, which required a surgical intervention (either angioplasty or coronary artery bypass surgery), who was over 18 years of age and English speaking with standard literacy skills, was eligible to participate. The majority of these patients had experienced symptoms of angina ranging from mild to severe. The exclusion criteria were any persons without a telephone ($n=1$). Of the total sample, 106 agreed to participate, 13 refused to participate, 18 could not be contacted, four were still in hospital for various reasons, two returned uncompleted questionnaires, and three were excluded (i.e. non-English speaking). Of the remaining sample, 58 were returned on time and 46 reminder letters were sent out, of which 28 questionnaires were then returned completed, 18 were never received, and one was returned uncompleted (final $N=86$). A final response rate of 58.9% was achieved. Attenders were defined as those patients who attended cardiac rehabilitation at least once: ($n=56$). Non- attenders were defined as those patients who never attended any cardiac rehabilitation sessions. This was based on self report but confirmed via actual medical records.

Measures

Demographic Variables

Demographic information was provided on the hospital labels (age, date of birth, gender, martial status). Additional information on education level and employment status was obtained at follow up.

Clinical Variable

A clinical indicator of stress: a life threatening myocardial infarction (MI) prior to their procedure was obtained via hospital records.

Self-reported Psychological Measures

The questionnaire used in this study was comprised of eight well validated self-report psychological measures.

Beck Depression Inventory (BDI-II)[27].

The BDI-II is a widely used, valid and reliable instrument for measuring depressive symptomology. The BDI-II consists of 21 items which assess affective (e.g. irritability), cognitive (e.g. self-dislike), somatic (e.g. loss of energy) and behavioural features (e.g. changes in sleeping pattern) of depression, and respondents are asked to rate each item by choosing the statement which most accurately reflects how they have been feeling during the past two weeks.

State-Trait Anxiety Inventory (STAI – Form Y) [28]

The STAI is a frequently used measure of anxiety in health populations, which contains 40 items [28]. This instrument was originally designed to differentiate between anxiety as a 'momentary condition' (state anxiety), and anxiety as a 'stable characteristic' (trait anxiety). Half of the items measure *state* anxiety (e.g. I feel frightened), while the remaining items measure *trait* anxiety (e.g. I feel satisfied with myself). Respondents are asked to rate their agreement using a four-point Likert scale (*state* anxiety, 1 = *not at all*; 4 = *very much so*; *trait* anxiety, 1 = *almost never*; 4 = *almost always*).

Medical Outcome Study Social Support Scale (Mos-Ss) [29]

The MOS-SS scale is a multidimensional instrument used to assess perceived levels of availability of social support [29]. The MOS-SS scale consists of 19 items and measures four dimensions of social support: emotional/informational, tangible, and affectionate social support, in addition to positive social interactions.

Brief Coping Orientation to Problems Experienced (Brief COPE) [30]

Specific coping strategies and responses to certain stressful situations were assessed via the Brief COPE [30]. The brief COPE is a short-form of the 60-item full inventory originally developed by Carver, Scheier and Weintraub (1989), and consists of 28 items to assess coping reactions when faced with adversity. The authors state that minor changes can be made to item formats, so a more dispositional coping style was chosen (e.g. I *do* work or other activities to take my mind off things), and scales can be used selectively (i.e. 13 of the 14 original scales have been used). The scales are presented and explained in Table 1. Respondents are asked to respond using a four-point Likert scale (0 = *I haven't been doing this at all*; 3 = *I have been doing this a lot*) and possible scores for each scale range from zero to six, with higher scores represent more frequent use of a particular coping strategy.

Table 1. Scales defined for the Brief COPE

Scale dimension	Definition
Active coping	Taking active steps to remove/ameliorate effects of stressor
Planning	Coming up with action strategies to handle stressor
Positive reframing	Efforts aimed towards managing the emotions of the stressor
Acceptance	Person accepts the reality of the situation
Humour	Using jokes to ameliorate effects, or making fun of the situation
Using emotional support	Seeking moral support, sympathy, or understanding
Using instrumental support	Seeking advice, assistance, or information
Self-distraction	Using alternative activities to take one's mind off the problem
Venting	Tendency to focus on distress and ventilate these feelings
Substance use	Coping through means of alcohol and drugs to remove stressor
Behavioural disengagement	Reducing the effort required to deal with the stressor
Self-blame	Criticizing or placing blame internally for the situation
Denial	Reports of refusal to believe that the stressor exists/acting as though stressor is not real

Table 2. Explanations of illness dimensions

Illness dimension	Describes beliefs surrounding...
Identity	Symptoms they attribute to their disease
Timeline - acute/chronic	Expected duration of their illness
Timeline – cyclical	Predictability of their illness/symptoms
Consequences	Expected outcome of illness and subsequent effects
Personal control	Self-efficacy concerning control over their illness
Treatment control	Confidence in treatment methods to control illness
Illness coherence	Degree of understanding of their illness
Emotional representations	Emotional responses generated by their illness
Causal attributions	Potential factors that may have lead to their illness

Revised Illness Perception Questionnaire (IPQ-R) [31]

The IPQ-R is a widely used measure of cognitive and emotional dimensions surrounding illness beliefs [41] (Table 2). Agreement to each item is rated using a five-point Likert scale (1 = *strongly disagree*; 5 = *strongly agree*), with the exception of the identity scale which requires dichotomous (*yes/no*) responses.

Eysenck Personality Questionnaire Revised – Neuroticism scale (EPQ-R) [32]

The 12 item neuroticism scale of the EPQ-revised version was used. This scale was designed to assess the individual's tendency to experience negative or distressing emotions (e.g. does your mood often go up and down), and respondents are asked to rate their agreement to each item using a yes/no format. Higher scores indicate a greater tendency towards neuroticism.

Life Orientation Test Revised (LOT-R) [33]

The LOT-R consists of ten items designed to assess an individual's tendency to anticipate positive versus negative outcome expectancies from life events [33]. Three items are framed in a positive direction (e.g. in uncertain times, I usually expect the best), three are worded in a negative direction (e.g. if something can go wrong for me, it will), and four additional items are fillers (e.g. it's easy for me to relax). Respondents are asked to rate their agreement to each statement on a five-point Likert scale (1 = *strongly disagree*; 5 = *strongly agree*). Higher scores reflect a greater tendency to expect positive outcomes in life [33].

Medical Outcome Study 36 Item Short-Form Health Survey (SF-36) [34]

The SF-36 is a comprehensive assessment of an individual's current health status or quality of life (QOL). The measure consists of 36 items and eight scale dimensions: physical functioning, general mental health, general health concepts, vitality, role limitations due to physical problems and emotional problems, social functioning and bodily pain [34]. Response scales used are not systematic, ranging from yes/no formats, to other three-, five- and six-point rating scales. While some questions are quite general, others direct the responder to rate how they have been feeling during the past four weeks.

Follow Up Telephone Interview

All patients who returned the questionnaire were contacted again over the phone for follow up (*M* = 37.15 days, *SD* = 7.86 days). Follow up questions related to demographic (educational level and employment status), active referral (hospital staff vs. cardiologist), and medical issues (visits to GP). Importantly, patients were asked whether they attended rehabilitation, and if so to name the facility. Qualitative responses were recorded on issues surrounding attendance or non-attendance at rehabilitation.

Procedure

This study received ethical approval from the School of Psychology at the University of Queensland, and the Uniting Healthcare Human Research Ethics committee from the Wesley hospital prior to commencement. Hospital labels were used to contact eligible participants. Patients who met eligibility criteria were contacted over the phone (approximately five days after an angioplasty procedure, or 10 ten days after coronary artery bypass surgery) and invited to participate voluntarily in the study. An attempt was made to capture their level of psychological status at home as soon as possible after discharge, which explains this difference in time. Every effort was made to contact participants, although patients who could not be contacted within five separate phone attempts made by the researcher were excluded from the study (*n* = 18). Those who agreed to participate were then sent out a questionnaire package including participant information sheet, 22-page cardiac questionnaire, and consent form, and were asked to return the completed questionnaire and consent form in the reply paid envelope supplied within two weeks. A reminder letter was sent out to patients who failed to return the questionnaire within this time. A follow up telephone call was then given to all remaining patients.

Cross Check of Self-Reported Information

As an additional check, self-reported attendance at a nominated cardiac rehabilitation program was verified against actual cardiac rehabilitation records.

Results

Statistical Analyses

All data analyses were conducted through SPSS (critical value of <.05 was used). All dichotomous categorical, demographic and clinical variables were analysed through 2x2 chi-square analyses. Univariate differences between groups on all continuous variables were analysed through independent sample t tests. A power analysis was conducted using G*Power 3 and to detect a large effect size (0.75), with p = .05, 80 participants were required [35]. The multivariate method chosen was logistic regression.

Comparing Responders and Non-Responders

Responders and non-responders were not significantly different with respect to age (64.58 years vs. 66.14 years), $P=0.39$, martial status (80.2% vs. 77.6% married or living in defacto relationship), P= 0.70, or gender (75.6% vs. 74.1% males), P= 0.84. However significantly more non-responders had experienced a myocardial infarction prior to their procedure compared with responders (90.0% vs. 11.6%), $P < .01$.

Sample Characteristics

Demographics

The mean age of the sample was 64.58 years (SD = 9.22), and the majority were male (75.6%). While most were married or living in a defacto relationship (80.2%), only half reported an education level of grade 12 or higher (51.2%). The majority of the sample was now retired (52.3%), however 40.7% also reported working in some capacity (casual, part-time, full-time).

Psychological Variables

Of the total sample, approximately 82% met classification for 'nil or minimal' depression, 9% with 'mild' depression, and 8% with 'moderate' depression. Mean state and trait anxiety scores were similar to those presented by Speilberger et al. (1983) for working adults aged 50 to 69 years. Overall, the most commonly used coping strategies among patients were acceptance, active coping and planning.

Rates of Attendance, Referral, GP Consultations

The overall uptake rate of rehabilitation within the sample was 65.1%. There was no significant difference in attendance rates between the angioplasty (60.7%) and coronary artery bypass surgery (76.0%) samples, $P = 0.18$. In terms of referral rates, results showed that one patient was unaware of cardiac rehabilitation, 56 patients (65.1%) reported being referred by only heartwise hospital staff, while 29 patients (33.7%) stated active referrals from both heartwise staff and their respective cardiologist. Finally, a greater percentage of attenders (89.3%) than non-attenders (73.3%) had visited their general practitioner post-procedure, however this difference marginally failed to reach significance $P =0 .06$.

Verification of Self-Reported Attendance

Of the 57 self-reported attendees at cardiac rehabilitation, 56 patients (98.2%) were confirmed against official records.

Univariate Associations Regarding Attendance

Demographics

The sociodemographic characteristics of both attenders and non-attenders are presented in Table 3. The only significant difference was that significantly more attenders were male. In terms of age, attenders ($M = 64.31$, $SD = 7.48$) and non-attenders ($M = 66.77$, $SD = 11.63$) were not significantly different $P =0 .16$. Seven of the ten myocardial infarction patients in the total sample attended rehabilitation.

Psychological Variables

The psychological characteristics of the total sample as a function of attendance type are presented in Table 4. There were eight significant differences found between attenders and non-attenders. First, attenders demonstrated significantly higher trait anxiety than did non-attenders. Second, attenders reported significantly greater use of self-blame to cope with their circumstances in comparison to non-attenders. Third, attenders were significantly more likely to label their condition as unpredictable, expected significantly greater consequences from their condition, reported significantly less understanding of their condition, and had significantly more trouble emotionally dealing with their condition than did non-attenders respectively.

Table 3. Descriptive characteristics of the attenders and non-attenders samples

Characteristic	Attenders ($n = 56$)	Non-attenders ($n = 30$)	χ^2	p
Gender (% males)	82.1	63.3	3.75	.05*
Marital status (% married or in defacto relationship)	83.9	73.3	1.38	.24
Employment (% working in some capacity	35.7	50.0	1.65	.20
Education levels (% achieved grade 12 or higher)	53.6	46.6	0.37	.54

* $p < .05$.

Table 4. Psychological characteristics by attendance group

Measure	Attendance group		t	p
	Attenders ($n = 56$)	Non-attenders ($n = 30$)		
STAI				
State anxiety	34.43 *(11.74)*	31.03 *(10.78)*	-1.32	.19
Trait anxiety	36.04 *(10.42)*	31.00 *(7.28)*	-2.52	.01*
BDI-II	8.35 *(6.84)*	5.44 *(5.16)*	-1.88	.06
MOS-SS				
Tangible	71.11 *(15.54)*	67.71 *(19.01)*	-0.89	.38
Affectionate	66.46 *(15.09)*	70.22 *(13.48)*	1.14	.26
Positive social interaction	65.36 *(15.92)*	66.07 *(15.33)*	0.20	.84
Emotional/informational	74.54 *(18.14)*	73.39 *(15.51)*	-0.29	.77
Brief COPE				
Active coping	4.60 *(1.36)*	4.00 *(1.71)*	-1.76	.08
Planning	4.58 *(1.36)*	4.00 *(1.98)*	-1.60	.11
Positive reframing	4.35 *(1.57)*	4.10 *(1.78)*	-0.64	.52
Acceptance	4.82 *(1.25)*	4.63 *(1.40)*	-0.63	.53
Humour	3.19 *(1.90)*	3.10 *(2.24)*	-0.18	.86
Using emotional support	4.06 *(1.67)*	3.93 *(1.72)*	-0.32	.75
Using instrumental support	3.87 *(1.54)*	3.14 *(1.83)*	-1.93	.06
Self-distraction	3.43 *(1.75)*	3.27 *(1.98)*	-0.38	.71
Denial	0.80 *(1.05)*	0.63 *(1.07)*	-0.68	.50
Venting	1.91 *(1.34)*	1.86 *(1.88)*	-0.13	.90
Substance use	0.63 *(1.20)*	0.13 *(0.57)*	-0.34	.74

Table 4. (Continued)

Measure	Attendance group		t	p
	Attenders (n = 56)	Non-attenders (n = 30)		
Behavioural disengagement	0.70 (1.08)	0.60 (0.97)	-0.41	.68
Self-blame	1.65 (1.46)	1.00 (1.36)	-2.02	.05*
IPQ-R	M (SD)	M (SD)		
Timeline acute/chronic	19.32 (5.18)	18.38 (5.36)	-0.75	.45
Timeline cyclical	10.46 (2.94)	8.97 (2.06)	-2.73	.01**
Consequences	20.83 (4.21)	18.30 (3.61)	-2.65	.01*
Personal control	23.82 (2.74)	23.36 (1.85)	-0.81	.42
Treatment control	18.95 (2.25)	18.81 (1.94)	-0.27	.79
Illness coherence	18.25 (3.49)	19.86 (2.93)	2.10	.04*
Emotional representations	16.80 (4.80)	14.83 (2.87)	-2.37	.02*
Causal items				
Psychological attributions	15.04 (4.41)	14.07 (3.47)	-1.03	.31
Risk Factors	29.50 (5.69)	27.25 (5.00)	-1.77	.08
Immunity	5.95 (1.92)	6.37 (1.84)	0.95	.34
Chance	2.38 (1.11)	2.20 (0.96)	-0.75	.45
Accident	1.76 (0.86)	1.90 (0.62)	0.82	.42
EPQ-R (Neuroticism)	3.89 (4.16)	2.30 (2.87)	-1.62	.11
LOT-R	12.22 (3.42)	12.69 (2.27)	0.67	.51

* $p < .05$, ** $p < .01$.

Quality of Life

Table 5 present the findings regarding attenders and non-attenders across all QOL scales. There were two significant differences between attendance groups across the subscales. Attenders reported significantly greater impairment to their work or regular daily activities from the emotional problems associated with their condition and significantly greater impairment to their general mental health than non-attenders respectively.

Qualitative Responses Surrounding Non-attendance

Qualitative responses for non-adherence with cardiac rehabilitation related to issues surrounding distance to facility, family obligations, work commitments, and interestingly, 11% commented that rehabilitation was unnecessary for them personally.

Table 5. Quality of life scale scores by attendance type

Measure SF-36	Attendance group			
	Attenders	Non-attenders	t	p
	($n = 56$)	($n = 30$)		
	M (SD)	M (SD)		
Physical functioning	63.21 (24.38)	68.04 (26.64)	0.82	.41
Role Physical	21.08 (35.49)	33.93 (40.38)	1.47	.15
Role Emotional	48.08 (43.99)	69.05 (42.48)	2.06	.04*
Social Functioning	60.71 (27.22)	65.00 (31.04)	0.66	.51
Mental Health	71.78 (16.55)	80.14 (18.55)	2.08	.04*
Vitality	48.33 (20.19)	56.17 (23.66)	1.60	.11
Pain	56.35 (24.62)	52.76 (27.50)	-0.61	.54
General Health	62.00 (20.82)	68.40 (18.57)	1.41	.16
Summary scores				
Physical	38.67 (8.92)	37.78 (10.68)	-0.37	.72
Mental	45.00 (9.89)	49.77 (11.77)	1.78	.08

* $p < .05$.

Multivariate Associations

A logistic regression model that included attendance type as the dependent variable, and the univariate significant variables including timeline cyclical, consequences, illness coherence, emotional representations, self-blame, trait anxiety, role emotional, mental health, age, gender, MI status and revascularisation technique as the independent variables. None of the psychosocial variables in the model were significantly independently related to rehabilitation attendance.

Discussion

This study was the first of its kind to comprehensively and prospectively assess the role of a range of psychosocial characteristics in cardiac rehabilitation adherence. We found some support for the role of psychosocial factors in distinguishing between attenders and non attenders to cardiac rehabilitation.

The rehabilitation uptake rate in the present study was considerably higher than most of the reported research [15,18], although it was identical to the 65% uptake rate among patients reported by Whitmarsh et al. (2003) [12]. Moreover we believe this figure to be accurate as it was cross checked with actual attendance records from respective rehabilitation centres. Reasons for the higher uptake rate may be due to the fact that we asked patients if they had attended any cardiac rehabilitation sessions. We did not obtain any information on whether all participants completed the full program. Also the higher rate observed in this study could reflect differences in health care system and cardiac treatment practices in Australia compared with overseas. For example these patients were attending a private hospital. While a nurse educator is responsible for making sure all patients receive brochures and an appointment to attend cardiac rehab, only 33% of patients reported a referral to rehabilitation from both hospital staff and their respective cardiologist. Although this appeared to have little impact on uptake in the present study, other research suggests that active referrals from medical specialists are crucial for patient adherence [36]. Additionally, while the researcher introduced themselves independent of the Wesley hospital, the nature of the initial phone call two weeks after discharge may have served to remind the patient about rehabilitation after their procedure, although this is unlikely to have greatly affected the uptake rate.

In terms of sociodemographic characteristics we did not confirm previous findings that non-attenders were more likely to be older, unemployed, less well educated and not presently married or living in a defacto relationship [do refs]. Although we found a significantly greater percentage of non-attenders were female, in comparison to attenders, which is consistent with the findings of Worcester et al. (2004) [14]. One possible reason for these findings may be that the present sample consisted of private patients compared with previous research and thus are more likely to be affluent (i.e. private health insurance), which may serve to reduce the influence of sociodemographic or practical barriers to rehabilitation [11]. We did find uptake to be slightly higher among coronary artery bypass surgery versus angioplasty patients, although this difference was smaller than that reported by Bunker et al. (1999) [17]. The practical reasons given by patients for non-attendance such as distance to facility and work commitments were similar to those presented in previous research [11,16, 23].

The findings regarding the role of depression and anxiety in determining rehabilitation adherence in the literature have been inconsistent [12,15]. The results of the present study showed that depression just failed to be significantly associated with adherence, however, patients who had a natural tendency to perceive stressful situations as dangerous and threatening (i.e. high trait anxiety) were more likely to involve themselves with rehabilitation. This is along the lines of Whitmarsh et al. (2003) who suggest that high levels of psychological distress are characteristic of attenders [12]. However we did not find anxiety or depression to be independent predictors of rehabilitation attendance and with insufficient power to detect a moderate effect size, future research with larger and equal sample sizes is needed to clarify any potential association.

Additionally, there have also been inconsistent findings in terms of the role of social support in rehabilitation adherence [13,16]. The present results were found to be more consistent with those of King et al. (2001), suggesting that perceived levels of available social support have no association to whether a patient decides to attend rehabilitation [16]. However the majority of the total sample were married or in a relationship and thus this may have contributed to the lack of differences in social support seen between the two groups.

In terms of coping, prior research by Whitmarsh et al. (2003) suggested that non-attenders displayed significantly lower levels of adaptive coping strategies [12]. We found the opposite in that those who decided to attend rehabilitation were more likely to criticize themselves and place the blame internally for their current situation, than were non-attenders.

However, this specific coping strategy was one of the least frequently used and therefore should be interpreted with caution.

Nonetheless we did find support for the role of illness perceptions in patient adherence with rehabilitation which is in line with others [12,19]. This study however extends upon these previous findings, by using the full revised version of the IPQ and reveals additional significant associations between attenders and non-attenders. In the present study, patients who attended rehabilitation had less understanding of their condition, were more likely to describe their condition as unpredictable, perceived greater consequences and expressed problems emotionally handling the present situation, than did non-attenders. However these variables were not independently associated with attendance.

Without prior research in terms of optimism and neuroticism, it was expected based on a related study by Glazer et al. (2002) [26] that non-attenders would demonstrate significantly higher neuroticism and significantly lower optimism scores compared with attenders. There was however no support for this prediction, which seems to suggest that the differences found between dropouts and attenders do not generalise to differences between initial attenders/non-attenders to cardiac rehabilitation.

While quality of life associations have not been previously used to predict initial rehabilitation adherence, we found that patients who actively choose to participate in cardiac rehabilitation were significantly more likely to report a high level of emotional interference with their work or daily tasks over the past four weeks from their condition, a finding that is consistent with what was found on the emotional representations subscale of the IPQ-R.

Although there were a number of univariate significant associations between attendance types, the logistic regression model accounted for just 26% of the variance and revealed no independent psychosocial predictors of rehabilitation adherence. It could be that other psychological constructs that were not assessed may be more important in this relationship, the most obvious being locus of control and self efficacy [37-38]. For example, one study showed that heart patients receiving psychological preparation before surgery who have a high external locus of control and high self efficacy experience less psychological distress post surgery [38]. There was however a crude measure of LOC in the present study (i.e. personal control subscale of IPQ-R) which revealed little difference between groups, although future research employing a more comprehensive measure of LOC is needed to determine the importance of this variable in rehabilitation adherence.

Strengths and Weaknesses

There were a number of strengths of this study including the response rate of 58.9%, which was reasonable considering the special population used and the circumstances surrounding their participation (e.g. just had surgery), and is comparable to other research that contacted patients over the telephone two weeks after hospital discharge [16]. Also we used a combined recruitment method (i.e. structured telephone calls and self-report questionnaires), which is generally considered more reliable in research than self-report measures alone. In addition the vast majority of self-reported attendance by patients at rehabilitation was confirmed with official records, which has been lacking in past research.

The most notable limitation was that the present sample consisted of private patients only, although they were recruited from one of the largest private cardiac tertiary referral centres in Queensland, the results cannot be generalised to patients attending public hospitals. Another problem with the sample was that females were underrepresented, making up only 30% of the total sample raising concerns about the generalisability of findings to females with cardiovascular disease. However the incidence rate for coronary artery disease is higher among men and this proportion is consistent with previous research using coronary artery disease patients [15]. Other limitations include the failure to adjust for multiple comparisons using a Bonferroni adjustment, which may affect some of the univariate significant associations. Finally, only a crude measure of clinical severity, namely presence of a myocardial infarction prior to surgery was used. It is possible that other clinical factors may have confounded the present study, including the presence of comorbid conditions, number of coronary arteries treated (i.e. disease severity), time since diagnosis and the number of previous interventions.

Implications

The results from this study have important implications for cardiac rehabilitation staff by helping them to target patients 'at risk' of not attending cardiac rehabilitation following surgery despite its reported physical and psychological benefits [1-2]. With more research it is hoped that a sociodemographic and psychosocial profile of non-attenders can be made and with appropriate screening early after surgery those 'at risk' patients can be targeted and encouraged to attend cardiac rehabilitation. This will help to reduce the enormous personal and economic costs associated with higher mortality and hospital readmission rates associated with non adherence with cardiac rehabilitation.

Future Research

Future research in this area should endeavour to recruit a larger sample using a multi-centre approach, including private and public patients and a greater number of females, to increase the potential generalisability of these findings. Also additional clinical and other psychosocial factors such as locus of control should be investigated.

Conclusion

In conclusion, this study revealed a modest role for stable (i.e. trait anxiety and coping) and current (i.e. illness perceptions and quality of life) psychological states in distinguishing between cardiac rehabilitation attenders and non-attenders post surgery. Future research employing larger sample sizes from both the private and public sectors should evaluate the contribution of these and other psychosocial factors in addition to clinical indicators of disease as a means to improving our understanding behind what drives patients to attend or not attend cardiac rehabilitation post surgery.

References

[1]   Yoshida, T., Kohzuki, M., Yoshida, K., Hiwatari, M., Kamimoto, M., Yamamoto, C., et al. Physical and psychological improvements after phase II cardiac rehabilitation in patients with myocardial infarction. *Nursing and Health Sciences 1999; 1:* 163-170.

[2]   Milani, R. V., Lavie, C. J., and Cassidy, M. M. Effects of cardiac rehabilitation and exercise training programs on depression in patients after major coronary events. *American Heart Journal 1996; 132:* 726-732.

[3]   Graves, K. D., and Miller, P. M. Behavioral medicine in the prevention and treatment of cardiovascular disease. *Behavior Modification 2003; 27:* 3-25.

[4]   National Health and Medical Research Council. (1996). *A consumer's guide: Angioplasty and Bypass Surgery*: Australian Government Publishing Service.

[5]   American Association of Cardiovascular and Pulmonary Rehabilitation. (1999). *Guidelines for Cardiac Rehabilitation and Secondary Prevention Programs* (3rd ed.). United States of America: Human Kinetics Publishers, Inc.

[6]   Williams, M. A., Ades, P. A., Hamm, L. F., Keteyian, S. J., LaFontaine, T. P., Roitman, J. L., et al. Clinical evidence for a health benefit from cardiac rehabilitation: An update. *American Heart Journal 2006; 152:* 835-841.

[7]   Grace, S. L., Abbey, S. E., Shnek, Z. M., Irvine, J., Franche, R.-L., and Stewart, D. E. Cardiac rehabilitation II: Referral and participation. *General Hospital Psychiatry 2002; 24:* 127-134.

[8]   Lerman, A., and Zeiher, A. M. Endothelial function: cardiac events. *Circulation 2005; 111:* 363-368.

[9]   Oldridge, N., Guyatt, G., Fischer, M., and Rimm, A. Cardiac rehabilitation after myocardial infarction. Combined experience of randomized clinical trials. *Journal of the American Medical Association 1988;* 260: 945-950.

[10]   Williams, M. A., Ades, P. A., Hamm, L. F., Keteyian, S. J., LaFontaine, T. P., Roitman, J. L., et al. Clinical evidence for a health benefit from cardiac rehabilitation: An update. *American Heart Journal 2006; 152:* 835-841.

[11]   Jackson, L., Leclerc, J., Erskine, Y., and Linden, W. Getting the most out of cardiac rehabilitation: a review of referral and adherence predictors. *Heart 2005; 91:* 10-14.

[12]   Whitmarsh, A., Koutantji, M., and Sidell, K. Illness perceptions, mood and coping in predicting attendance at cardiac rehabilitation. *British Journal of Health Psychology 2003; 8: 209-221.*

[13]   Johnson, J. E., Weinert, C., and Richardson, J. K. (1998). Rural residents' use of cardiac rehabilitation programs. *Public Health Nursing 1998; 15:* 288-296.

[14]   Worcester, M. U. C., Murphy, B. M., Mee, V. K., Roberts, S. B., and Goble, A. J. (2004). Cardiac rehabilitation programmes: predictors of non-attendance and drop-out. *European Journal of Cardiovascular Prevention and Rehabilitation, 2004;11:* 328-335.

[15] Lane, D., Carroll, D., Ring, C., Beevers, D. G., and Lip, G. Y. Predictors of attendance at cardiac rehabilitation after myocardial infarction. *Journal of Psychosomatic Research 2001; 51: 497-501.*

[16] King, K. M., Humen, D. P., Smith, H. L., Phan, C. L., and Teo, K. K. Psychosocial components of cardiac recovery and rehabilitation attendance. *Heart 2001; 85:* 290-294.

[17] Bunker, S., McBurney, H., Cox, H., and Jelinek, M. Identifying participation rates at outpatient cardiac rehabilitation programs in Victoria, Australia. *Journal of Cardiopulmonary Rehabilitation 1999; 19: 334-338.*

[18] Harlan, W., Sandler, S., Lee, K., Lam, L., and Mark, D. Importance of baseline functional and socioeconomic factors for participation in cardiac rehabilitation. *American Journal of Cardiology 1995; 76*: 36-39.

[19] Cooper, A., Lloyd, G., Weinman, J., and Jackson, G. Why patients do not attend cardiac rehabilitation: role of intentions and illness beliefs. *Heart, 1999; 82:* 234-236.

[20] Cooper, A. F., Jackson, G., Weinman, J., and Horne, R. Factors associated with cardiac rehabilitation attendance: A systematic review of the literature. *Clinical Rehabilitation 2002; 16:* 541-552.

[21] Evenson, K. R., Rosamond, W. D., and Luepker, R. V. Predictors of outpatient cardiac rehabilitation utilization: the Minnesota Heart Surgery Registry. *Journal of Cardiopulmonary Rehabilitation 1998; 18: 192-198.*

[22] Farley, R. L., Wade, T. D., and Birchmore, L. Factors influencing attendance at cardiac rehabilitation among coronary heart disease patients. *European Journal of Cardiovascular Nursing : Journal of the Working Group on Cardiovascular Nursing of the European Society of Cardiology 2003; 2: 205-212.*

[23] Thorogood, M., Coulter, A., Jones, L., Yudkin, P., Muir, J., and Mant, D. Factors Affecting Response to an Invitation to Attend for a Health Check. *Journal of Epidemiology and Community Health 1993; 47:* 224-228.

[24] French, D. P., Cooper, A., and Weinman, J. Illness perceptions predict attendance at cardiac rehabilitation following acute myocardial infarction: A systematic review with meta-analysis. *Journal of Psychosomatic Research 2006; 61:* 757-767.

[25] French, D. P., Lewin, R. J. P., Watson, N., and Thompson, D. R. Do illness perceptions predict attendance at cardiac rehabilitation and equality of life following myocardial infarction? *Journal of Psychosomatic Research 2005; 59:* 315-322.

[26] Glazer, K. M., Emery, C. F., Frid, D. J., and Banyasz, R. E. Psychological predictors of adherence and outcomes among patients in cardiac rehabilitation. *Journal of Cardiopulmonary Rehabilitation 2002; 22: 40-46.*

[27] Beck, A., Steer, R., and Brown, G. (1996). *Beck depression inventory II test manual.* San Antonio: Harcourt Brace and Company.

[28] Spielberger, C., Gorsuch, R., Lushene, R., Vagg, P., and Jacobs, G. (1983). *Manual for the state-trait anxiety inventory (Form Y).* California: Consulting Psychologists Press, Inc.

[29] Sherbourne, C. D., and Stewart, A. L. The MOS social support survey. *Social Science and Medicine 1991; 32:* 705-714.

[30] Carver, C. S. You want to measure coping but your protocol's too long: Consider the Brief COPE. *International Journal of Behavioral Medicine 1997; 4:* 92-100.

[31] Moss-Morris, R., Weinman, J., Petrie, K. J., Horne, R., Cameron, L. D., and Buick, D. The revised illness perception questionnaire (IPQ-R). *Psychology and Health 2002;, 17:* 1-16.

[32] Eysenck, S. B., Eysenck, H. J., and Barrett, P. A revised version of the Psychoticism scale. *Personality and Individual Differences 1985; 6:* 21-29.

[33] Scheier, M. F., Carver, C. S., and Bridges, M. W. Distinguishing optimism from neuroticism (and trait anxiety, self-mastery, and self-esteem): A reevaluation of the Life Orientation Test. *Journal of Personality and Social Psychology 1994; 67:* 1063-1078.

[34] Ware, J. E., and Sherbourne, C. D. The MOS 36-item short-form health survey (SF-36): I. Conceptual framework and item selection. *Medical Care 1992; 30:* 473-483.

[35] Faul, F., Erdfelder, E., Lang, A.-G., and Buchner, A. G*Power 3: A flexible statistical power analysis program for the social, behavioural, and biomedical sciences. *Behaviour Research Methods 2007; 39: 175-191.*

[36] Ades, P. A., Waldmann, M. L., Polk, D. M., and Coflesky, J. T. Referral Patterns and Exercise Response in the Rehabilitation of Female Coronary Patients Aged Greater-Than-or-Equal-to-62 Years. *American Journal of Cardiology 1992; 69:* 1422-1425.

[37] Wallston, K., Wallston, B., and DeVellis. Development of the Multidimensional Health Locus of Control (MHLC) scales. *Health Education Monographs 1978; 6:* 161-170.

[38] Shelley M, Pakenham K. The effects of preoperative prepartations on postoperative outcome. The moderating role of control appraisals. Health Psychology 2007;26: 183-191.

In: Angina Pectoris: Etiology, Pathogenesis and Treatment ISBN: 978-1-60456-674-1
Editors: A. P. Gallo, M. L. Jones © 2008 Nova Science Publishers, Inc.

Chapter VI

Important Role of Rho-Kinase in the Pathogenesis of Coronary Artery Disease

Yoshihiro Fukumoto[*]

Department of Cardiovascular Medicine, Tohoku University Graduate School of
Medicine 1-1 Seiryo-machi, Aoba-ku Sendai 980-8575, JAPAN

Abstract

Rho-kinase has been identified as one of the effectors of the small GTP-binding
protein Rho. In a series of experimental and clinical studies, it has been demonstrated
that Rho-kinase is substantially involved in the pathogenesis of coronary spasm.
Intracoronary administration of fasudil or its metabolite, hydroxyfasudil, both of which
are Rho-kinase inhibitors, markedly inhibited coronary spasm in animal models.
Importantly, the inhibition of Rho-kinase with fasudil/hydroxyfasudil was associated
with the suppression of enhanced myosin light chain (MLC) phosphorylations at the
spastic coronary segments in those models. The activity and the expression of Rho-
kinase were enhanced at the inflammatory/arteriosclerotic coronary lesions, thereby
suppressing myosin phosphatase through phosphorylation of its myosin-binding subunit
with a resultant increase in MLC phosphorylations and coronary spasm. In patients with
vasospastic angina, intracoronary fasudil markedly inhibited acetylcholine-induced
coronary spasm and related myocardial ischemia, demonstrating that Rho-kinase pathway
is substantially involved in the pathogenesis of coronary spasm in humans as well.
Fasudil was also effective in treating patients with microvascular angina, indicating an
involvement of Rho-kinase-mediated hyperreactivity of coronary microvessels.
Intracoronary administration of fasudil was effective in reducing tachypacing-induced
myocardial ischemia even in patients with stable effort angina without changing heart
rate or blood pressure, suggesting that inappropriate coronary microvascular
vasoconstriction is involved in the pathogenesis of effort angina. Intracoronary fasudil
also was effective for the treatment of intractable coronary spasm resistant to maximal

---

[*] (Tel) +81-22-717-7153, (Fax) +81-22-717-7156 (EM) fukumoto@cardio.med.tohoku.ac.jp.

vasodilator therapy with calcium channel blockers and nitrates after coronary artery bypass surgery. These lines of evidence indicate that Rho-kinase is an important therapeutic target for the treatment of the spasm.

Introduction

Recent advances in molecular biology have demonstrated the substantial involvement of intracellular signaling pathways mediated by small GTP-binding proteins (G proteins), such as Rho, Ras, Rab, Sarl/Arf, and Ran families.[1, 2] In mid 1990s, 2 Japanese groups and 1 Singapore group independently identified one of the effectors of Rho and termed it as Rho-kinase.[3] The Rho/Rho-kinase pathway has recently attracted much attention in various research fields, especially in the cardiovascular research field.[4] First, the Rho/Rho-kinase pathway plays an important role in various cellular functions that are involved in the pathogenesis of cardiovascular disease.[5] Second, this intracellular signaling pathway is substantially involved in the effects of many vasoactive substances that are implicated in the pathogenesis of cardiovascular disease.[5] Third, the so-called pleiotropic effects of statins are mediated, at least in part, by their inhibitory effects on Rho with a resultant inhibition on Rho-kinase.[6] In this article, the recent progress in the treatment of angina pectoris will be reviewed with a special reference to Rho-kinase inhibitors.

Pathophysiological Role of Rho-Kinase in Angina Pectoris

Shimokawa et al. have demonstrated that Rho-kinase is a novel therapeutic target in ischemic heart disease and essential hypertension.[5] Rho-kinase reduces myosin phosphatase activity by phosphorylating the myosin-binding subunit of the enzyme and thus augments vascular smooth muscle cell (VSMC) contraction at a given intracellular calcium concentration.[7, 8] It has been demonstrated that the Rho-kinase pathway is associated with the myosin light chain (MLC) phosphorylations at the hyperconstrictive artery segments in animals.[4]

Animal Studies

Several animal studies have demonstrated that Rho-kinase is substantially involved in the pathogenesis of coronary vasospasm.[9-13] The activity and the expression of Rho-kinase are enhanced at these inflammatory/arteriosclerotic coronary lesions, thereby suppressing myosin phosphatase through phosphorylation of its myosin binding subunit (MBS) with resultant increase in MLC phosphorylations and coronary spasm.[4] Recently, it also has been demonstrated that sustained elevation of serum level of cortisol, one of the important stress hormones, causes coronary hyperreactivity through activation of Rho-kinase in pigs in vivo.[14]

The porcine model of coronary vasospasm/arteriosclerosis with interleukin-1β (IL-1β) is characterized by constrictive remodeling,[18, 19] which is also an important mechanism for restenosis after coronary intervention.[20] Importantly, the long-term inhibition of Rho-kinase by either a Rho-kinase inhibitor or in vivo gene transfer of dominant-negative Rho-kinase induces a marked regression of the constrictive remodeling in this porcine model in vivo.[21, 22] The regression of constrictive remodeling is associated with functional inhibition of ERM family (ezrin, radixin, and moesin) and adducin, suggesting that these effectors of Rho-kinase may be involved in the development and maintenance of the vascular remodeling.[21, 22]

Both in vivo gene transfer of dominant-negative Rho-kinase and long-term treatment with a Rho-kinase inhibitor suppress balloon injury-induced neointimal formation in animals in vivo.[15-17] Long-term treatment with monocyte chemotactic protein-1 (MCP-1), oxidized low-density lipoproteins (ox-LDL), and remnant lipoproteins (from patients with sudden cardiac death) causes vascular lesions characterized by neointimal formation and constrictive remodeling in porcine coronary arteries in vivo.[11, 13] Long-term oral treatment with fasudil, a Rho-kinase inhibitor, significantly suppressed this vascular lesion formation, which is caused, at least in part, by the inhibition of macrophage migration in vivo.[11]

VSMC hypercontraction mediated by activated Rho-kinase plays a key role in coronary artery spasm in macro- and micro-vessels of coronary arteries.[4, 5, 23-26] Rho-kinase inhibition may be preferable to calcium channel blockers because of its selective spasmolytic effect on vascular hyperconstrictive segments.[5, 24] Moreover, it has been recently demonstrated that Rho-kinase inhibition increases endothelial nitric oxide synthase (eNOS) expression and decreases inflammatory cell migration or anigiotensin II-induced mRNA expression of MCP-1 and plasminogen activator inhibitor-1 in vivo or in vitro.[5] Because these cascades occur in the development of arteriosclerosis, Rho/Rho-kinase pathway may play an important role in the development of ischemic heart disease.

Rho-Kinase as a Novel Therapeutic Target of Angina Pectoris

The goal of the management of angina pectoris is to improve myocardial ischemia in daily life by pharmacological and/or interventional treatment and to improve long-term prognosis.[27] It also has been recently demonstrated that Rho-kinase inhibition with a specific Rho-kinase inhibitor, fasudil, reduces myocardial ischemia in patients with epicardial coronary artery spasm, coronary microvascular spasm, or even stable effort angina pertoris.[24-26] The anti-anginal effects of fasudil are caused by the suppression of the up-regulated Rho-kinase in patients with ischemic heart disease, because Rho-kinase pathway in coronary microcirculation is not functional in normal hearts, but is up-regulated under pathological conditions including stable effort angina.[24-26] It also has been demonstrated that the long-term oral treatment with fasudil exerts anti-anginal effects in patients with stable effort angina.[5, 28] The direct demonstration of the beneficial effects of fasudil on myocardial ischemia has been also examined, in which Rho-kinase activation is functionally involved in the increased coronary vascular resistance in stable effort angina, both under control conditions and in response to increased myocardial oxygen demand.[26].

Fasudil as a Specific Rho-Kinase Inhibitor

Fasudil is a potent and selective inhibitor of Rho-kinase, with the inhibitory effect on Rho-kinase being 10 and 100 times more potent than on protein kinase C and myosin light chain kinase, respectively.[7, 10, 29, 30] The 15-min intracoronary infusion of 300 µg/min of fasudil reaches the peak concentrations to 3.7±0.4 µmol/L in the coronary circulation in humans.[24] Fasudil potently inhibits the Rho-kinase activity in a dose-dependent manner (IC_{50} 1.9 µmol/L) in vitro,[10, 29] the achieved concentrations (mean value, 3.7 µmol/L) are considered to be high enough to effectively inhibit Rho-kinase activity.

Rho-Kinase and Coronary Hyperconstriction

Accumulating evidence indicates that Rho-kinase is substantially involved in the pathogenesis of coronary vasospasm.[4] The activity and expression of Rho-kinase are enhanced at the inflammatory/arteriosclerotic coronary lesions.[4, 12] Thus, intracoronary administration of fasudil or hydroxyfasudil markedly inhibits coronary vasospasm in a porcine model treated with IL-1β,[9, 10] MCP-1,[11] and remnant lipoproteins obtained from patients with sudden cardiac death.[9-11, 13] Furthermore, it has been also demonstrated that Rho-kinase inhibition by fasudil also is quite effective in suppressing epicardial coronary vasospasm,[24] microvascular spasm,[25] and intractable severe coronary spasm resistant to intensive conventional vasodilator therapy.[24, 25, 31] Actually, we have experienced some cases with severe coronary artery spasm as a serious complication of coronary artery bypass grafting (CABG),[31] who showed severe myocardial ischemia resistant to intensive therapy with intravenous conventional vasodilators, including isosorbide dinitrate (ISDN), diltiazem, and nicorandil after CABG. The administration of fasudil (1.5 mg/min for 15 minutes) into the spastic arteries successfully resolved the spasm and improved myocardial ischemia without any systemic adverse effects.[31]

Therefore, the Rho-kinase inhibition can be a useful and favorable strategy to treat abnormal coronary circulation caused by the macro- and micro-vessels of coronary artery dysfunction, especially fatal coronary spasm resistant to intensive conventional vasodilator therapy in patients with angina pectoris.

Future Directions and Conclusions

It has been demonstrated that fasudil is an effective anti-anginal drug for effort angina pectoris and coronary vasospasm, confirming our notion that Rho-kinase is a novel therapeutic target for the treatment of ischemic heart disease.[4, 12] Since Rho-kinase activation is also associated with the development and progression of atherosclerosis, the long-term treatment with fasudil could inhibit the process of atherosclerosis or even causes regression of the process. [4, 12] It is expected that clinical trials with long-term oral treatment with Rho-kinase inhibitors will elucidate their effectiveness and safety for the treatment of patients with angina pectoris.

References

[1]   Fukata Y, Amano M, Kaibuchi K. Rho-Rho-kinase pathway in smooth muscle contraction and cytoskeletal reorganization of non-muscle cells. *Trends Pharmacol Sci.* Jan 2001;22(1):32-39.

[2]   Takai Y, Sasaki T, Matozaki T. Small GTP-binding proteins. *Physiol Rev.* Jan 2001;81(1):153-208.

[3]   Ishizaki T, Maekawa M, Fujisawa K, et al. The small GTP-binding protein Rho binds to and activates a 160 kDa Ser/Thr protein kinase homologous to myotonic dystrophy kinase. *Embo J.* Apr 15 1996;15(8):1885-1893.

[4]   Shimokawa H, Takeshita A. Rho-kinase is an important therapeutic target in cardiovascular medicine. *Arterioscler Thromb Vasc Biol.* Sep 2005;25(9):1767-1775.

[5]   Shimokawa H. Rho-kinase as a novel therapeutic target in treatment of cardiovascular diseases. *J Cardiovasc Pharmacol.* 2002;39(3):319-327.

[6]   Takemoto M, Liao JK. Pleiotropic effects of 3-hydroxy-3-methylglutaryl coenzyme a reductase inhibitors. *Arterioscler Thromb Vasc Biol.* Nov 2001;21(11):1712-1719.

[7]   Uehata M, Ishizaki T, Satoh H, et al. Calcium sensitization of smooth muscle mediated by a Rho-associated protcin kinase in hypertension. *Nature.* 1997;389(6654):990-994.

[8]   Somlyo AP, Somlyo AV. Signal transduction by G-proteins, rho-kinase and protein phosphatase to smooth muscle and non-muscle myosin II. *J Physiol.* 2000;522 Pt 2:177-185.

[9]   Katsumata N, Shimokawa H, Seto M, et al. Enhanced myosin light chain phosphorylations as a central mechanism for coronary artery spasm in a swine model with interleukin-1beta. *Circulation.* Dec 16 1997;96(12):4357-4363.

[10] Shimokawa H, Seto M, Katsumata N, et al. Rho-kinase-mediated pathway induces enhanced myosin light chain phosphorylations in a swine model of coronary artery spasm. *Cardiovasc Res.* 1999;43(4):1029-1039.

[11] Miyata K, Shimokawa H, Kandabashi T, et al. Rho-kinase is involved in macrophage-mediated formation of coronary vascular lesions in pigs in vivo. *Arterioscler Thromb Vasc Biol.* 2000;20(11):2351-2358.

[12] Kandabashi T, Shimokawa H, Miyata K, et al. Inhibition of myosin phosphatase by upregulated rho-kinase plays a key role for coronary artery spasm in a porcine model with interleukin-1beta. *Circulation.* 2000;101(11):1319-1323.

[13] Oi K, Shimokawa H, Hiroki J, et al. Remnant lipoproteins from patients with sudden cardiac death enhance coronary vasospastic activity through upregulation of Rho-kinase. *Arterioscler Thromb Vasc Biol.* May 2004;24(5):918-922.

[14] Hizume T, Morikawa K, Takaki A, et al. Sustained elevation of serum cortisol level causes sensitization of coronary vasoconstricting responses in pigs in vivo: a possible link between stress and coronary vasospasm. *Circ Res.* Sep 29 2006;99(7):767-775.

[15] Eto Y, Shimokawa H, Hiroki J, et al. Gene transfer of dominant negative Rho kinase suppresses neointimal formation after balloon injury in pigs. *Am J Physiol Heart Circ Physiol.* 2000;278(6):H1744-1750.

[16] Sawada N, Itoh H, Ueyama K, et al. Inhibition of rho-associated kinase results in suppression of neointimal formation of balloon-injured arteries. *Circulation.* May 2 2000;101(17):2030-2033.

[17] Shibata R, Kai H, Seki Y, et al. Role of Rho-Associated Kinase in Neointima Formation After Vascular Injury. *Circulation.* 2001;103(2):284-289.

[18] Shimokawa H, Ito A, Fukumoto Y, et al. Chronic treatment with interleukin-1 beta induces coronary intimal lesions and vasospastic responses in pigs in vivo. The role of platelet-derived growth factor. *J Clin Invest.* Feb 1 1996;97(3):769-776.

[19] Fukumoto Y, Shimokawa H, Ito A, et al. Inflammatory cytokines cause coronary arteriosclerosis-like changes and alterations in the smooth-muscle phenotypes in pigs. *J Cardiovasc Pharmacol.* Feb 1997;29(2):222-231.

[20] Andersen HR, Maeng M, Thorwest M, et al. Remodeling rather than neointimal formation explains luminal narrowing after deep vessel wall injury: insights from a porcine coronary (re)stenosis model. *Circulation.* May 1 1996;93(9):1716-1724.

[21] Shimokawa H, Morishige K, Miyata K, et al. Long-term inhibition of Rho-kinase induces a regression of arteriosclerotic coronary lesions in a porcine model in vivo. *Cardiovasc Res.* 2001;51(1):169-177.

[22] Morishige K, Shimokawa H, Eto Y, et al. Adenovirus-mediated transfer of dominant-negative rho-kinase induces a regression of coronary arteriosclerosis in pigs in vivo. *Arterioscler Thromb Vasc Biol.* 2001;21(4):548-554.

[23] Masumoto A, Hirooka Y, Shimokawa H, et al. Possible involvement of Rho-kinase in the pathogenesis of hypertension in humans. *Hypertension.* 2001;38(6):1307-1310.

[24] Masumoto A, Mohri M, Shimokawa H, et al. Suppression of coronary artery spasm by the Rho-kinase inhibitor fasudil in patients with vasospastic angina. *Circulation.* 2002;105(13):1545-1547.

[25] Mohri M, Shimokawa H, Hirakawa Y, et al. Rho-kinase inhibition with intracoronary fasudil prevents myocardial ischemia in patients with coronary microvascular spasm. *J Am Coll Cardiol.* Jan 1 2003;41(1):15-19.

[26] Fukumoto Y, Mohri M, Inokuchi K, et al. Anti-ischemic effects of fasudil, a specific Rho-kinase inhibitor, in patients with stable effort angina. *J Cardiovasc Pharmacol.* Mar 2007;49(3):117-121.

[27] Gibbons RJ, Abrams J, Chatterjee K, et al. ACC/AHA 2002 guideline update for the management of patients with chronic stable angina--summary article: a report of the American College of Cardiology/American Heart Association Task Force on practice guidelines (Committee on the Management of Patients With Chronic Stable Angina). *J Am Coll Cardiol.* Jan 1 2003;41(1):159-168.

[28] Vicari RM, Chaitman B, Keefe D, et al. Efficacy and safety of fasudil in patients with stable angina: a double-blind, placebo-controlled, phase 2 trial. *J Am Coll Cardiol.* Nov 15 2005;46(10):1803-1811.

[29] Davies SP, Reddy H, Caivano M, et al. Specificity and mechanism of action of some commonly used protein kinase inhibitors. *Biochem J.* 2000;351(Pt 1):95-105.

[30] Sward K, Dreja K, Susnjar M, et al. Inhibition of Rho-associated kinase blocks agonist-induced Ca2+ sensitization of myosin phosphorylation and force in guinea-pig ileum. *J Physiol.* 2000;522 Pt 1:33-49.

[31] Inokuchi K, Ito A, Fukumoto Y, et al. Usefulness of fasudil, a Rho-kinase inhibitor, to treat intractable severe coronary spasm after coronary artery bypass surgery. *J Cardiovasc Pharmacol.* Sep 2004;44(3):275-277.

In: Angina Pectoris: Etiology, Pathogenesis and Treatment   ISBN: 978-1-60456-674-1
Editors: A. P. Gallo, M. L. Jones

Chapter VII

Angina

William H. Wehrmacher
Loyola University Medical Center, Stritch School of Medicine
Maywood, IL, USA

Identification of the specific cause for pain or distress in the chest in clinical practice is ordinarily more difficult than the specific treatment for it becomes after proper recognition. At least 100 different disorders have been identified that produce pain or discomfort in the chest. The diagnosis is certain to be overlooked if that disorder is not considered. Such oversight has been responsible for most of the treatment failures that have come to my attention is consultation practice.

With broad perspective and recognition that pain felt to be within the chest may actually originate in the wall of the chest or from disorders in the head, neck, or abdomen, diagnosis may ordinarily be fairly simply established when the significant details from the clinical history taking, from physical examination, and from laboratory investigation are adequately evaluated. Sometimes, special investigations, ordinarily available in university and diagnostic centers become essential although details of readily available diagnostic facilities ordinarily are more important safeguards for correct diagnosis than are the reports from specialized facilities.

Detailed analysis of the pain itself provides the best guide through the perplexing maze of its more than a hundred possible causes. Unfortunately the patient readily abandons his leadership through this maze if he is forced into a rigid question-answer mold prematurely. With skill and experience, however, the patient can be enticed to go all the way through it.by a physician who appreciates the diagnostic revelations of the trip and the patient will ordinarily take the physician almost directly to the correct diagnosis even when personally mistaken, often fearfully mistaken, about the real significance of his own symptoms.

I have found seven characteristics of the pain -- location, radiation, quality, duration, intensity, fluctuation and periodicity, and the circumstances of its occurrence and subsidence essential not only for proper diagnosis but also for the patient's own appreciation of the problem and the assurance that I actually understand it too..

The characteristics often emerge from the patient-physician encounter in variable order and detail. To keep the record straight and free from interruption until the patient has done his best, I have found a grid on my note pad listing these characteristics useful during the inquiry. After the patient has done his best, I can complete the record with a minimum of direct questions. Ordinarily the information fills in rather well and promptly when one is equipped to deal with it as it spills forth from the distraught patient.

As one listens to a patient with Angina pectoris describe symptoms, one hears words describing deep sub-sternal pain, perhaps inclined slightly to the left, perhaps radiating into the anterior cords of the neck or down the medial surface of the left or both arms. The patient may say that the pain is pressing or crushing quality , but ordinarily experiences difficulty finding appropriate .words to describe it. The pain almost always lasts less than 30 minutes and ordinarily only 1-3 minutes after the end of the provocative exertion. To the patient, and particularly if fearful, it may seem to last much longer. The pain of myocardial infarction ordinarily does last longer. Timing is best done with a watch and the patient will use it if recognizing the importance of its duration. The severity of the pain is variable and of relatively little value either diagnostically or as a measure of the seriousness of the illness but perhaps of considerable importance in determining the amount of disability. If one were to insist upon finding pain commensurate with the seriousness of the illness, he would miss more cases of angina than he would find. Angina is ordinarily precipitated by exercise, not by movement as of the chest or arms. It is aggravated by anything that increases the work of the heart, including emotional disturbances and fear. It is ordinarily relieved by rest or nitroglycerin.

Diurnal variations in angina are related to eating, walking, working and other habits of daily living. Eating predisposes to anginal attacks: (1) by reflex coronary constriction. (2) by increasing the work demand upon the heart called forth by the digestive process, and (3) by alterations in blood viscosity resulting from agglutination of the red cells following ingestion of the fats in the meal. Ingestion of food decreases the time required to produce anginal attacks by 20 to 40% under stressful con-ditions. On the other hand. some protection against anginal at- tack is afforded after eating for those patients who benefit from resulting greater concentrations of sugar in the blood. Angina decubitus occurs during recumbency, usually at night when nocturnal increase of the blood volume results from hydrostatic pressure changes.. A regimen which induces dehydration or a semirecumbant position may prevent the attacks of pain.

As one listens to a patient with one of the innocent pains of the chest wall, such as Tietze's syndrome, slipping rib, or tussive fracture of a rib, one will hear complaints of pain directly over the offending lesion and of radiation into the same sclerotome rather than into the classical distribution of angina pectoris. Usually the pain is sharp, but depending upon the nature of the lesion, it may resemble a muscular pain or rheumatic pain. It is not so difficult for the intelligent patient to describe as the pain of angina is. Innocent chest wall pain may come and go in a flash or be a catch-in-the-side like pleurisy. It may be prolonged and resemble rheumatic pain but rarely exactly duplicates the pattern of the pain of coronary artery disease. Referred pain to the chest wall that sometimes complicates coronary artery disease, on the other hand, and may exactly simulate other chest wall pain because it is a chest-wall pain and related to pectoral and intercostal muscular spasm. Severity varies and is often commensurate with the disturbance responsible. Chest wall pains are likely to be brought on by movement of the chest, particularly by deep breathing, coughing, sneezing, or stretching and are relieved by immobilizing the involved area. Many pains of chest wall origin and particularly that pain resulting from tussive fracture of the rib may be called pleurisy erroneously because they may feel so much like a stitch-in-the-side. Pericarditis does. All these pains have much in common with one another and each must be considered along with diseases of the underlying pleura and pericardium in making a differential diagnosis whenever the characteristic pain appears.

As one listens to a patient with pulmonary pain he may hear complaints suggesting the deep, difficult-to-describe pain of myocardial ischemia. As a pulmonary embolism lodges in the artery, the quality of the pain is likely to be deceptive until pulmonary infarction results and produces an overlying pleuritis or until the diagnostically helpful haemoptysis appears.

As the patient whose pain originates outside the chest as in the head, neck or abdomen relates his symptoms, the patient will ordinarily refer to some distress over the offending lesion even when most of the pain is felt within the chest. If suffering from Cervical Nerve Root Compression by spurs from the uncovertebral joint of Luschka or by other masses the patient should be expected to complain about his neck even when most of the pain is felt in his chest. The pain often exhibits a shooting character and extends into the anatomical distribution of the involved nerve roots. It may be shock-like and simulate the distress after hitting the ulnar nerve (the "crazy-bone") at the elbow

Summary

I have found seven characteristics of the pain -- location, radiation, quality, duration, intensity, fluctuation and periodicity, and the circumstances of its occurrence and subsidence --to be essential not only for accurate diagnosis but also for the patient's own appreciation of the problem and assurance that I actually understand it too..

References for Further Study

Wehrmacher, W.H. Unstable Angina Treatment. *2006 Update*. Comp Ther. 2006 32(3): 144-146.

Wehrmacher, W.H. Acute Myocardial Infarction 2000 Recognition. Comprehensive Therapy. Vol. 27, 2001, P. 140-143.

Wehrmacher, W.H. And K.A. Wetklo. Schmerzen Im Thoraxbereich. Diagnostik 9:38-40,

Wehrmacher, W.H. And C.A. Vera. Causa De Dolor De Pecho:: Pericarditis. La Prensa Medica, Argentina 55:1977, 1968.

Wehrmacher, W.H. Anterior Chest Pain. J.A.M.A. 194:217, 1965.

Wehrmacher, W.H. Pain In The Chest. Springfield:Charles C. Thomas Co., 403p, 1964. .

Wehrmacher, W.H. Musculo-Skeletal Pain Masquerading As Angina Pectoris. Sixth International Congress Of Internal Medicine, Basel, 1960.

Wehrmacher, W.H. The Painful Anterior Chest Wall Syndromes. Med. Clin. N. A. 1958; 42:111-118.

Wehrmacher, W.H. Significance Of Tietze's Syndrome In Differential Diagnosis Of Chest Pain. J.A.M.A. 1955; 157: 505-507.

Blonsky, E., P. Kezdi And Wehrmacher, W.H. Pain In The Chest Associated With Hypertension Of The Lesser Circulation.I.Mitral Valvular Disease. Quarterly Bulletin, Nw U Med School, 35 241-247, 1961.

Wehrmacher, W.H., K. Kuroda And P. Kezdi. Pain In The Chest Associated With Hypertension Of The Lesser Circulation. Ii. Congenital Heart Disease. Minn. Med. 44:347-379, 1961.

.Wehrmacher, W.H. Chest Pain-Significant Or Insignificant? Proceedings Of The 49th Annual Meeting Of The American Life Convention, Hot Springs, Virginia, 1961.

Wehrmacher, W.H. Clinical Clues In The Diagnosis Of Cardiac Disease. N:Therapeutic Advances In The Practice Of Cardiology, Chap.1. Eds., C.P. Bailey, A.G. Shapiro And S. Gollub, Ny: Grune And Stratton, 1970.

Wehrmacher, W.H. Pain In The Chest. In: Current Diagnosis, Chapter 4. Eds., H.F. Conn And R.B. Conn. Philadelphia: W. B. Saunders Company, 1974.

In: Angina Pectoris: Etiology, Pathogenesis and Treatment   ISBN: 978-1-60456-674-1
Editors: A. P. Gallo, M. L. Jones   © 2008 Nova Science Publishers, Inc.

Chapter VIII

Angina Pectoris: Character and Location among those Presenting to Emergency Departments with Acute Chest Pain

Guy D. Eslick[1,2,5] *and Maria Chiu*[3,4]

[1] Department of Medicine, The University of Sydney, Nepean Hospital,
Penrith, New South Wales, Australia
[2] School of Public Health, The University of Sydney, Sydney,
New South Wales, Australia
[3] Institute for Clinical Evaluative Sciences, Toronto, Ontario, Canada
[4] Institute of Medical Science, University of Toronto, Ontario, Canada

Abstract

Aims: The aim of this study was to determine how the location and symptoms of angina pectoris differed among those presenting with acute chest pain.

Methods: The sample consisted of individuals who presented to Nepean Hospital Emergency Department with acute chest pain. At initial presentation, patients who elected to undergo further diagnostic tests were assessed according to a standard protocol. All patients were asked to fill out the Chest Pain Questionnaire (CPQ). A cluster analysis was undertaken to determine any pattern in the angina pectoris location and symptoms described by patients.

Results: This study recruited 212 subjects with acute chest pain (aged 21-90, mean 57, SD: 14). The prevalence of angina pectoris was 39% (n=75). Cluster analysis identified three distinct angina pectoris locations: 1) mid-left chest; 2) central chest and left arm; and 3) central and upper left chest.

[5] Address for correspondence: Dr. Guy D. Eslick, Program in Molecular and Genetic Epidemiology Harvard School of Public Health 677 Huntington Ave Bldg II, 2nd Floor Boston, MA 02115 U.S.A.Tel: +1 617-432-5896 Fax: +1 617-525-2008, E-mail: geslick@hsph.harvard.edu.

Conclusions: Angina pectoris is a heterogenous condition. There is significant overlap of chest pain symptoms and locations among angina pectoris, thus making differentiation from other 'causes' difficult.

Introduction

Historical Background

Ancient physicians made little mention of chest pain and its possible relationship with the heart [1]. The Bible makes the earliest possible mention of angina/cardiac arrest in 1 Samuel 25:37-38 [2], "Then in the morning, when Nabal was sober, his wife told him all these things, and his heart failed him and he became like a stone. About ten days later, the Lord struck Nabal and he died." However, the first published description of angina pectoris and it's differentiation from other types of chest pain was made by William Heberden in 1772 [3], this work which was read at the College of Physicians in 1768 has been reported as "one of the greatest milestones in the history of cardiology", and it was later referred to as 'Heberden's angina' [4,5]. This resulted in a subsequent publication in Medical Transactions in 1785 [6] by Heberden where an anonymous physician who had read an abstract of Heberden's description realized that it described his own symptoms. The anonymous physician wrote to Heberden describing his condition:

"I have often felt, when sitting, standing, and at times in my bed, what I can best express by calling it a universal pause within me of the operations of nature for perhaps three or four seconds; and when she had resumed her functions, I felt a shock at the heart, like that which one would feel from a small weight being fastened to a string to some part of the body, and falling from the table to within a few inches of the floor…If it please God to take me away suddenly, I have left directions on my will to send an account of my death to you, with permission for you to order such an examination of my body, as will shew the cause of it; and perhaps tend at the same time to a discovery of the origin of that disorder, which is the subject of this letter, and be productive of means to counteract and remove it."

Surprisingly, within three weeks the writer had died, and as per his letter to William Heberden an autopsy was conducted by John Hunter who after a thorough examination could find no obvious cause for his death.

21st Century

It has been 240 years since Heberden's original description of angina and much has changed in terms of the understanding of the clinical history, diagnosis, pathophysiology, management and therapy of angina pectoris [7]. One in five acute chest pain patients who present to hospital will die within three years [8,9]. This is an important statistic since acute chest pain is the second most common presentation to hospital emergency departments [10]. Annually, in the United States there are approximately six million patients admitted to hospital for acute chest pain with an annual economic cost to the health care system of US$8 billion dollars [11]. Moreover, the annual economic burden in terms of direct and indirect costs for coronary heart disease and associated acute myocardial infarction is US$142 billion [12] Despite the large numbers presenting with chest pain, obtaining an accurate diagnosis as to the cause of the chest pain continues to be a major challenge [13, 14].

Chest pain is a fairly non-specific symptom and is associated with a wide variety of conditions [13]. Acute chest pain can indicate an acute coronary syndrome and because of the potentially fatal consequences of chest pain as a result, it is vital to find ways to quickly and accurately determine the source and thus the significance of a patient's chest pain. Traditionally, assessment of each patient is based on the history of the presenting symptoms including a description of the pain, the overall clinical picture, electrocardiogram (ECG), and cardiac enzymes including troponin levels [15].

Individuals present with varying angina symptoms which makes a definitive diagnosis difficult even with a diagnostic work-up. Previous studies have been conducted to determine if manual gestures, verbal descriptions, facial descriptions and pain radiation are reliable indicators of myocardial infarction [16-23]. One study reported that reliance on Heberden's original features of angina-retro-sternal location, strangling quality, relation to exertion, and accompaniment by mental anxiety – is inadequate due to the overlap between cardiac and non-cardiac causes of chest pain [24].

The aim of this study was to determine how clusters (groups) of individuals with respect to chest pain locations/symptoms compare to a clinical diagnosis of angina pectoris. The hypothesis is that angina pectoris characteristics alone are not useful in differentiating cardiac from non-cardiac chest pain.

Patients and Methods

Subjects

This study was approved by the Wentworth Area Health Service (WAHS) Ethics Committee. A consecutive sample of patients with chest pain, who presented to Nepean Hospital Emergency Department (a tertiary teaching and referral hospital) over a 12-month period were enrolled in this cross-sectional methodological study. Patients were followed through to general admission or to the chest pain clinic at Nepean Hospital. All admissions to these centers were monitored to capture patients referred from other sources. The baseline characteristics of this cohort have been described elsewhere [25].

Patients come from the WAHS catchment area which consists of a population of 307,787 (7.7% of the Sydney population) and is socio-demographically very similar to the Australian population according to 2001 Census data, except that its inhabitants are slightly younger (30 vs 35 median years) and it has a slightly higher socioeconomic status based on income ($450 vs $350 median individual income per week), respectively. Ethnic status was not obtained, but the majority would be Caucasian based on Australian Bureau of Statistics data (www.abs.gov.au).

On presentation, all subjects were invited to participate in the study. An information package was provided. This included the Chest Pain Questionnaire (CPQ), a letter describing the study, and a patient consent form (requiring a signature), which gives permission to access the patient's medical records. The CPQ measures symptoms over the previous 12-month pre-survey period, with individual items assessing the prevalence, frequency and severity of chest pain, possible causes of chest pain, and other chest pain characteristics. This instrument has been previously described and validated [26,27]. The Chest Pain Questionnaire incorporates several existing validated and widely used instruments including the SF-36 (used to assess general health status) [28], Rose Angina Questionnaire [29], Hospital Anxiety and Depression Scale (used to assess anxiety and depression) [30], Gastroesophageal Reflux Questionnaire [31], Beck Anxiety Inventory (used to assess panic disorder) [32], Seattle Angina Questionnaire [33], and the Eysenck Personality Questionnaire (used to assess neuroticism) [34].

All patients were asked to fill out the Chest Pain Questionnaire including those who did not wish to undergo further diagnostic procedures. At initial presentation, patients who elect to undergo further diagnostic tests were assessed according to a standard protocol. This is based on National Health and Medical Research Council (NHMRC) guidelines and is used for assessment of chest pain in the Nepean Hospital Emergency Department [35,36]. The NHMRC guidelines are based on the American College of Cardiology and American Heart Association guidelines, which were updated in 2002 [37]. A detailed history and physical examination were included in these initial procedures. More specialized diagnostic tests, which are dependent on the origin of the pain (eg. gastrointestinal, cardiac), were determined by the individual characteristics of each case presenting. No clinical data on medications, electrocardiograms, additional risk factors (i.e., obesity, history of cerebrovascular disease, family history of coronary heart disease) was collected or available for this particular study.

Definitions

Angina pectoris: Chest pain associated with coronary heart disease.
Diabetes: Blood sugar level >7.8mmol/L.
Smoking status: Non-smoker, current smoker, never smoked.
High cholesterol: Total cholesterol >5.5mmol/L.
High blood pressure: Blood pressure >140/90mmHg.

Statistical Analysis

Cluster Analysis

Cluster analysis is a generic term, which describes a subset of statistical procedures that can be used to create a classification [38-42]. These procedures start with a data set, which contains information (e.g., chest pain locations) about a sample of entities (e.g., individuals with chest pain) and attempts to sort these entities into relatively homogenous and mutually exclusive groups (or clusters). In this article cluster analysis is used to sort individuals into "angina pectoris" clusters or groups, based on similarities in the symptoms that they have reported.

The term cluster and cluster membership are synonymous with more common epidemiological terms group and group membership. Indeed, these terms can be used interchangeably in the current setting. I have elected to use the term cluster in lieu of group to maintain consistency with earlier literature that has reported these techniques.

Cluster analysis: A k-means cluster analysis was applied (which involves first specifying the number of clusters desired (k)), using factors extracted from the principal components analysis as the basis for forming the cluster solution [37-42]. The analysis commenced with a two-cluster solution and proceeded by generating increasingly complex cluster solutions (i.e., three, four, five, six clusters). We based the initial choice of two clusters as a starting point on the literature of "angina pectoris" reporting at least two symptom locations [e.g., retrosternal chest pain and left arm pain] [43,44].

Three criteria were used to cease forming increasingly complex cluster solutions. First, when comparing the cluster membership of a simpler and a more complex solution, if the more complex solution appeared to systematically break up a large cluster into substantive sub-clusters the more complex solution was adopted, whereas if the more complex solution appeared simply randomly to draft small numbers of members of several clusters into a new cluster or clusters, the simpler solution was adopted. Second, the Euclidean distance (a measure of distance for two observations) method was used to judge whether the within-cluster homogeneity was enhanced by moving to a more complex cluster solution. If the average Euclidean distance was substantively reduced with a more complex solution, the more complex solution was favored. Third, in order to preserve reliability of within-cluster estimates, no cluster could be made up of less than 5% of the entire sample. Thus, no sample size calculations were required for this study. In the current study, items with factor scores equal to or greater than 40 were used in describing the clusters.

The clinical interpretation of each cluster was aided by describing a cluster profile that comprised the mean score per factor per cluster. Hence, for each cluster there is a series of mean scores centered about zero. A mean of or close to zero indicates that cluster is average, i.e. undistinguished, on that particular factor. The unit of measurement is the standard deviation (due to the unit normal distribution of factor scores). Thus a score of +2.0 indicates the cluster is within the top 5% in terms of that factor. The scores of <-1.0 or >+1.0 were interpreted as indicating clear differentiation, and scores between 0.5 and 1.0 (either positive or negative) as indicating possible differentiation.

General Statistics

Patient demographic and clinical characteristics have been reported as mean and standard deviation or confidence interval for numeric-scaled features and percentages for discrete characteristics. Chi-square tests were used to compare univariate groups with odds ratios and 95% confidence intervals. All p-values calculated were two-tailed and the alpha level of significance was set at 0.05.

Results

Demographic

This study recruited 212 (84 females: 128 males) acute chest pain patients (aged 18-90, mean 57 years, SD: 14). Overall, there was no significant difference with respect to age or gender. There were 75 individuals with angina pectoris (50 male: 25 female) (aged 39-89 years; mean age 64 years, SD: 12 years).

Angina Pectoris and Age

Figure 1 shows that there were few cases of angina under the age of 40 years. There is a skewed bimodal distribution where the prevalence of angina is higher among those in the 60-69 and 70-79 year age groups.

Angina Pectoris and Gender

The prevalence of angina pectoris among males and females was 67% (95% CI: 55-77%) and 33% (95% CI: 23-45%), respectively (p=0.20). Males were four times more likely to suffer from angina pectoris compared to females (OR=4.00, 95% CI: 1.92-8.36, p<0.0001).

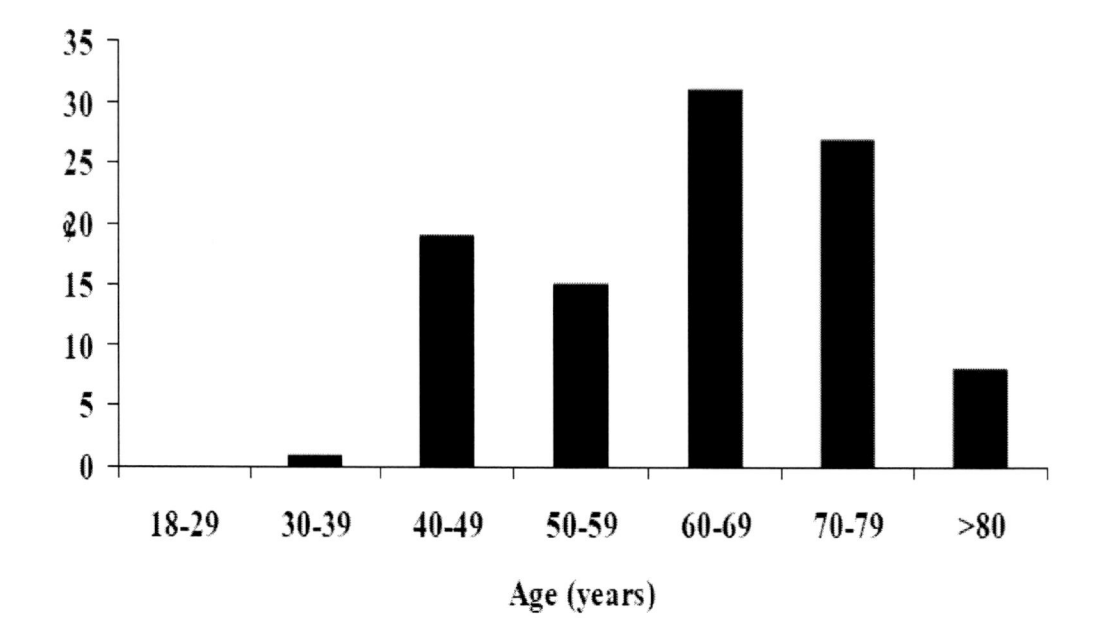

Figure 1. Type of chest pain by age.

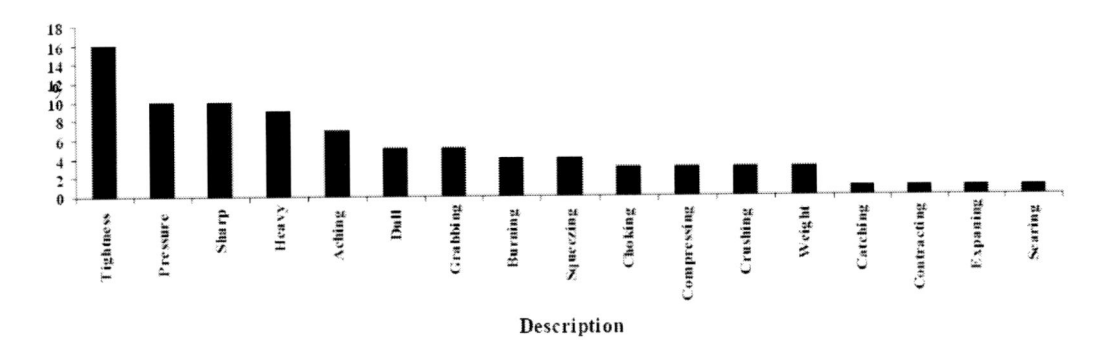

Figure 2. Descriptions of angina pectoris pain.

Table 1. Cluster analysis of factors identified in the patient sample (mean factor scores by cluster)

Chest pain location	Mid-left chest	Central chest and left arm	Central and upper left chest
A	0.12	0.14	0.28
B	0.29	0.34	0.28
C	0.18	0.31	0.47
D	0.29	0.46	0.02
E	0.68	0.68	0.40
F	0.56	0.73	0.03
G	0.24	0.00	0.00
H	0.85	0.00	0.02
I	0.35	0.02	0.00
J	0.12	0.05	0.02
K	0.06	0.44	0.11
	0.00	0.22	0.03

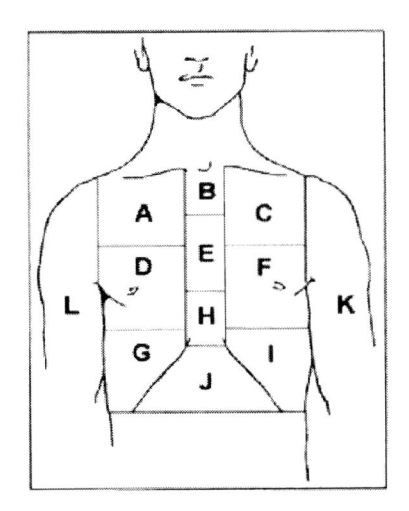

Dysphagia

Those with angina reported lower rates of dysphagia (OR=0.92, 95% CI: 0.45-1.87, p=0.81).

Gastroesophageal Reflux

Angina pectoris did not differ significantly with respect to gastroesophageal reflux compared with those who had no angina pectoris (OR=0.74, 95% CI: 0.38-1.43, p=0.34).

Chest pain groups

Results of the K-means analysis appear in Table 1. The sample yielded a complex cluster structure with three groupings of locations. These were mid-left chest, central chest and left arm, and central and upper left chest (Figure 4). The majority of clusters represented single anatomical chest locations, however, there was overlap of the locations.

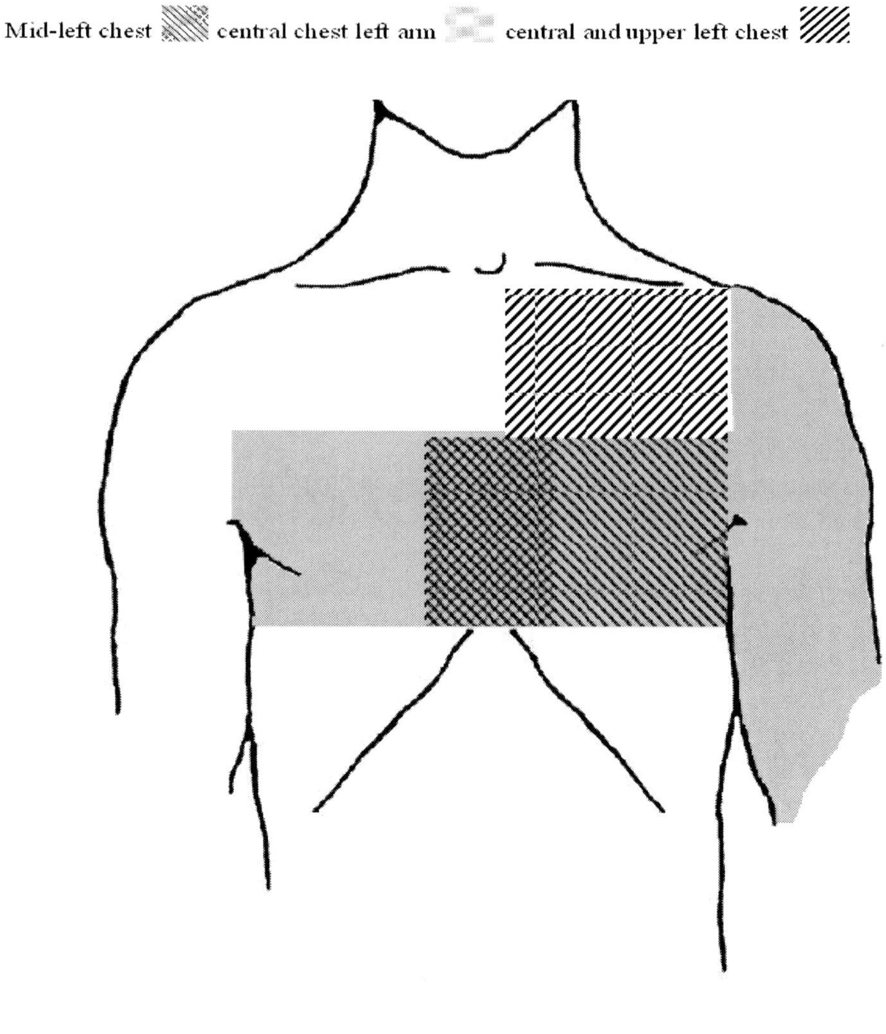

Mid-left chest ▨ central chest left arm ▨ central and upper left chest ▨

Figure 4. Cluster locations of angina pectoris.

Discussion

The present study suggests that characteristics of angina pectoris such as pain location and patient description may not be useful in differentiating acute coronary syndromes from non-cardiac chest pain. This study used a cluster analysis technique to determine how patients' chest pain locations group and the likely clinical interpretations of such groupings. There were three clusters of chest pain location among this acute chest pain patient sample, which included the mid-left chest, central chest and left arm and central and upper left chest.

The scientific methodology involved using a K-means (non-hierarchical) cluster analysis. Cluster analysis is not entirely new to medicine, however, this methodology is rarely used to assess symptoms in a clinical cardiology patient setting. This is somewhat surprising considering the advantages of this technique in interpreting patterns among patients with symptoms (e.g., acute chest pain) [38-42].

Previous studies have reported various differences in chest pain symptoms, whether it be differences due to gender, race, socio-economic status, or education level. These sociodemographic factors/characteristics have all been shown to affect how an individual perceives and describes their chest pain when presenting to a hospital Emergency Department. Moreover, studies have reported acute myocardial infarction symptom comparisons between males and females with conflicting results [22,23,45]. In Goldberg et al.'s multi-center hospital study [45], males (n=810) and females (n=550) with acute myocardial infarction were compared in terms of their symptom presentation. Males were more likely to have diaphoresis and less likely to have nausea, jaw, back and neck pain associated with their presentation. This study had several limitations including no socio-economic/educational data collected and there was no examination of symptom severity between genders. A patient-based study comparing males (n=1395) and females (n=601) acute myocardial infarction patients found that females were more likely to report arm pain, neck pain, back pain, jaw pain, headache, nausea, and dyspnoea compared to males. However, males were more likely to report sweating, belching and hiccups [23]. Milner et al.[22] in a community-based study comparing males (n=276) and females (n=246) with acute myocardial infarction found that females were more likely to report arm pain, neck pain, back pain. A recent hospital-based study assessed the occurrence of patient symptoms relating to acute myocardial infarction site. The patients were grouped according to the site of infarction, anterior (n=731), inferior (n=719), and lateral (n=96) [23]. Patients who had anterior infarctions were more likely to present with multiple symptoms which included chest, shoulder and arm pain, whereas, those with a lateral infarction were more likely to have left arm, left shoulder and back pain.

It should be noted that all of the above mentioned studies had no non-cardiac chest pain comparison group. However, a recent study among 267 acute chest pain patients (118 with an acute myocardial infarction; 149 without an acute myocardial infarction) reported that it was difficult to draw any conclusions about reliable indicators for acute myocardial infarction [47]. The possible reasons for the lack of conclusions may relate to the qualitative and descriptive nature of the study.

Traditionally, chest pain associated with pain travelling down the left arm has generally been considered more suggestive that the patient is having an acute myocardial infarction

[43,45]. In contrast, a prospective study consisting of 278 consecutive patients admitted to an emergency ward for chest pain where patients were assessed for numerous clinical indicators at the time of admission reported that the highest positive predictive value associated with acute myocardial infarction was right arm involvement (Positive Predictive Value=80.4%) [16]. However, in the present study there was no relationship between cardiac chest pain and right arm involvement (p=0.56), nor did right arm involvement support any relationship with non-cardiac chest pain. Furthermore, when looking at the general prevalence rates for the "left chest and arm" (which has traditionally been seen as an indicator for an acute coronary syndrome), cluster it suggests that because this particular cluster is lowest amongst the non-cardiac chest pain group and highest among the cardiac chest pain group that it likely makes sense from a clinician's point of view. However, when comparing the cardiac and non-cardiac chest pain groups we see that there is a large amount of overlap between the two groups for the "left chest and left arm" cluster.

In addition, it must not be forgotten that there remains a sub-group of acute myocardial infarction and angina pectoris patients who present without chest pain symptoms [48,49]. Furthermore, a majority of these patients delay health care seeking due to a lack of "obvious" warning signs and as a consequence have worse outcomes [50].

There are limitations of this study. Firstly, it should be mentioned that the patients who participated in this study came from a single Emergency Department, however, it should be noted that this large tertiary referral hospital serves a catchment area that is representative of the Australian population in terms of age, socio-economic status, and ethnic background. Secondly, there may be possible misclassification bias by younger and less experienced physicians in ascertaining the cause of the chest pain. In addition, some of the cardiovascular risk factors were not associated with angina, this may have been because of a lack of statistical power to detect a difference between groups.

Conclusion

In summary, the data suggest that patients who present to hospital emergency departments with acute chest pain suggestive of angina pectoris show considerable symptom overlap. Angina pectoris appears to be a heterogeneous symptom. Traditional diagnostic clues for an acute coronary syndrome, such as pain down the left arm should not be emphasized as being associated with acute ischemic event nor should this type of presentation by patients be regarded as anything other than non-cardiac chest pain until further investigations are completed.

References

[1]   Eslick GD. Chest pain: a historical perspective. *International Journal of Cardiology* 2001;77:5-11.
[2]   The Holy Bible [New International Version (NIV)]. 1 Samuel 25:37-38.

[3]   Heberden W. Some account of a disorder of the breast. *Medical Transactions of the Royal College of Physicians of London* 1772;2:59-67.

[4]   Heberden E. (1989). *William Heberden: Physicoan of the Age of Reason.* Royal Society of Medicine Services Limited. London, United Kingdom. pp. 124-126.

[5]   Bradford E. William Heberden's contribution to cardiology. *Journal of the Royal College of Physicians* 1968;2.

[6]   Heberden W. A letter to Dr Heberden concerning the angina pectoris; and Dr Heberden's account of the dissection of one who had been troubled with the disorder. *Medical Transactions of the Royal College of Physicians of London* 1785;3:1.

[7]   Kelemen MD. Angina pectoris: Evaluation in the office. *Medical Clinics of North America* 2006;90:391-416.

[8]   Fleischmann KE, Goldman L, Robiolio PA, et al. Echocardiographic correlates of survival in patients with chest pain. *Journal of the American College of Cardiology* 1994;23:1390-1396.

[9]   Herlitz J. Karlson BW. Lindqvist J. Sjolin M. Predictors and mode of death over 5 years amongst patients admitted to the emergency department with acute chest pain or other symptoms raising suspicion of acute myocardial infarction. *Journal of Internal Medicine* 1998;243:41-48.

[10]   Eslick GD, Couldshed DS, Talley NJ. Diagnosis and treatment of noncardiac chest pain. *Nature Clinical Practicce: Gastroenterology and Hepatology* 2005;2:463-472.

[11]   Eslick GD, Coulshed DS, Talley NJ. Review article: the burden of illness of non-cardiac chest pain. *Alimentary Pharmacology and Therapeutics* 2002;16:1217-1223.

[12]   American Heart Association/American Stroke Association-Heart Disease and Stroke Statistics. 2006.

[13]   Boie ET. Initial evaluation of chest pain. *Emergency Medical Clinics of North America* 2005;23:937-957.

[14]   Kelly BS. Evaluation of the elderly patient with acute chest pain. *Clinics in Geriatric Medicine* 2007;23:327-349.

[15]   Bhatheja R, Mukherjee D. Acute coronary syndromes: Unstable angina/non-ST elevation myocardial infarction. *Critical Care Clinics* 2007;23:709-735.

[16]   Berger JP, Buclin T, Haller E, Van Melle G, Yersin B. Right arm involvement and pain extension can help differentiate coronary diseases from chest pain of other origin: a prospective emergency ward study of 278 consecutive patients admitted for chest pain. *Journal of Internal Medicine* 1990;227:165-172.

[17]   Alban Davies H, Jones DB, Rhodes J, Newcombe RG. Angina-like esophageal pain: differentiation from cardiac pain by history. *Journal of Clinical Gastroenterology* 1985;7:477-481.

[18]   Edmondstone WM. Cardiac chest pain: does body language help the diagnosis? *BMJ* 1995;311:1660-1661.

[19]   Everts B, Karlson BW, Wahrborg P, Hedner T, Herlitz J. Localization of pain in suspected acute myocardial infarction in relation to final diagnosis, age and sex, and site and type of infarction. *Heart and Lung* 1996;25:430-437.

[20]   Zerwic JJ. Symptoms of acute myocardial infarction: expectations of a community sample. *Heart and Lung* 1998;27:75-81.

[21] Dalton JA, Brown L, Carlson J, McNutt R, Greer SM. An evaluation of facial expression displayed by patients with chest pain. *Heart and Lung* 1999;28:168-174.

[22] Milner KA, Funk M, Arnold A, Vaccarino V. Typical symptoms are predictive of acute coronary syndrome. *American Heart Journal* 2002;143:283-288.

[23] Čulić V, Eterović D, Mirić D, Silić N. Symptom presentation of acute myocardial infarction: influence of sex, age, and risk factors. *American Heart Journal* 2002;144:1012-1017.

[24] Davies HA, Jones DB, Rhodes J. "Esophageal angina" as the cause of chest pain. *JAMA* 1982;248:2274-2278.

[25] Eslick GD, Talley NJ. Non-cardiac chest pain: predictors of health care seeking, the types of health care professional consulted, work absenteeism, and interruption of daily activities. *Alimentary Pharmacology and Therapeutics* 2004;20:909-915.

[26] Eslick GD, Jones MP, Talley NJ. Non-cardiac chest pain: prevalence, risk factors, impact and consulting - a population-based study. *Alimentary Pharmacology and Therapeutics* 2003;17:1115-1124.

[27] Eslick GD, Talley NJ. The development and validation of the Chest Pain Questionnaire (CPQ) for non-cardiac chest pain (NCCP). *Gastroenterology* 2004;126(Suppl 2):A-309.

[28] Ware JE, Kosinski M, Bayliss MS, McHorney CA, Rogers WH, Raczek A. Comparison of methods for the scoring and statistical analysis of SF-36 health profile and summary measures: summary of results from the medical outcomes study. *Medical Care* 1995;33:AS264-AS279.

[29] Rose GA. Chest pain questionnaire. *Milbank Memorial Fund Quarterly* 1965;43:32-39.

[30] Zigmond AS, Snaith RP. The Hospital Anxiety and Depression Scale. *Acta Psychatrica Scandinavia* 1983;67:361-370.

[31] Locke GR 3rd, Talley NJ, Weaver AL, Zinsmeister AR. A new questionnaire for gastroesophageal reflux disease. *Mayo Clinic Proceedings* 1994;69:539-547.

[32] Beck AT, Epstein N, Brown G, Steer RA. An inventory for measuring clinical anxietyL psychometric properties. *Journal of Consulting and Clinical Psychology* 1988;56:893-897.

[33] Spertus JA, Winder JA, Dewhurst TA, Deyo RA, Prodzinski J, McDonell M, Fihn SD. Development and evaluation of the Seattle angina questionnaire: A new functional status measure for coronary artery disease. *Journal of the American College of Cardiology* 1995;25:333-341.

[34] Eysenck SBG, Eysenck HJ, Barrett P. A revised version of the psychoticism scale. *Personality and Individual Differences* 1985;6:21-29.

[35] National Health and Medical Research Council [NHMRC] (1997). *Clinical Practice Guidelines: Diagnosis and Management of Unstable Angina.* Commonwealth Department of Health and Family Services, Australia.

[36] Aroney CN, Boyden AN, Jelinek MV, Thompson P, Tonkin AM, White H. Management of unstable angina guidelines – 2000. *Medical Journal of Australia* 2000;173(Suppl):S66-S88.

[37] Braunwald E, Antman EM, Besley JW, et al. ACC/AHA guidelines for the management of patients with unstable angina and non-ST-segment elevation

myocardial infarction: a report of the American College of Cardiology/American Heart Association Task Force on Practice Guidelines. *Journal of the American College of Cardiology* 2000;36:970-1062. Updated March 2002 at http//:www.acc.org and http//:www.americanheart.org

[38] Brusco M, Cradit JD. A variable-selection heuristic for k-means clustering. *Psychometrika* 2001;66:249-270.

[39] Coleman DA, Woodruff DL. Cluster analysis for large datasets: An effective algorithm for maximizing the mixture likelihood. *Journal of Computational and Graphical Statistics* 2000;9:672-688.

[40] McLachlan GJ. Cluster analysis and related techniques in medical research. *Statistical Methods in Medical Research* 1992;1:27-48.

[41] Milligan GW, Cooper MC. Methodology review: Clustering methods. *Applied Psychology and Measurement* 1987;11:329-354.

[42] Eslick GD, Howell SC, Hammer J, Talley NJ. Empirically derived symptom sub-groups correspond poorly with diagnostic criteria for functional dyspepsia and irritable bowel syndrome. A factor and cluster analysis of a patient sample. *Alimentary Pharmacology and Therapeutics* 2004;19:133-140.

[43] Pope JH, Selker HP. Diagnosis of acute cardiac ischemia. *Emergency Medical Clinics of North America* 2003;21:27-59.

[44] Boersma E, Mercado N, Poldermans D, Gardien M, Vos J, Simoons ML. Acute myocardial infarction. *Lancet* 2003;361:847-858.

[45] Panju AA, Hemmelharn BR, Guyatt GH, Simel DL. Is this patient having a myocardial infarction? *JAMA* 1998;280:1256-1263.

[46] Canto JG, Shlipak MG, Rogers WJ, et al. Prevalence, clinical characteristics, and mortality among patients with myocardial infarction presenting without chest pain. *JAMA* 2000;283:3223-3229.

[47] Albarran JW, Durham B, Chappel G, Dwight J, Gowers J. Are manual gestures, verbal descriptors and pain radiation as reported by patients reliable indicators of myocardial infarction? Preliminary findings and implications. *Intensive Critical Care Nursing* 2000;16:98-110.

[48] Stern S. Angina pectoris without chest pain. *Circulation* 2002;106:1906-1908.

[49] Conti RC. Silent cardiac ischemia. *Current Opinion in Cardiology* 2002;17:537-542.

[50] Lanza GA, Sciahbasi A, Sestito A, Maseri A. Angina pectoris: a headache. *Lancet* 2000;356:998.

In: Angina Pectoris: Etiology, Pathogenesis and Treatment   ISBN: 978-1-60456-674-1
Editors: A. P. Gallo, M. L. Jones   © 2008 Nova Science Publishers, Inc.

Chapter IX

Immunologic Mechanisms Involved in Ischemic Cardiopathy

Jorge Delgado[‡], Manuel Baños-González[†]
and Carlos Ramírez-Velázquez*
[‡]National University of Mexico,
[†]National Institute of Cardiology "Ignacio Chávez" and
*Allergology and Clinic Immunology Department, "20 de Noviembre"
Medical National Center, ISSSTE

Abstract

During the past decades, ischemic cardiopathy has been extensively studied. Nonetheless it has been an important advance in its diagnostics and its treatment; this illness is a currently public health challenge in developed countries. Moreover, in emerging economies, ischemic cardiopathy has also started to follow the same trend as in developed countries. Epidemiological studies on ischemic cardiopathy have shown important genetic and ambient risk factors. In particular, it is well recognized that atherosclerosis, a suffering of large arteries, is the primary cause of ischemic cardiopathy. Atherosclerosis is characterized by an immunologic mechanism; where adaptive and innate immune response are involved. One of the most common triggering events for this response is an accumulation of minimally oxidized LDL molecules. This event involves mainly the endothelial cells; which produce pro-inflammatory molecules. Other cells involved here and in progressive thrombosis are T and B cells. Lately, infection by cytomegalovirus and elevated homocysteine, have been also recognized as another triggering events for immune response activation. As a consequence, nowadays the atherosclerosis has been clearly recognized as a chronic inflammation that could promote severe clinical consequences due to atherosclerotic plaque and thrombosis. This is in high contrast with the previously understanding; where atherosclerosis and atherome were considered just as probable degenerative sufferings related with age. A thrombus can cause an abrupt diminishing of blood flow through the affected blood vessels as well as a complete blood flow interruption. As a result, the oxygen cell distribution is affected and an ischemic clinical condition is promoted. The ischemic cardiopathy diagnostic and prognostic can be done by several biomarkers. Some of them can also point out the future occurrence of ischemic cardiopathy. Although some pharmacological treatments have been focused on the acute ischemic cardiopathy, the importance of pharmacological treatments where the immunological modulation of inflammatory process plays an essential role has been recently increased. The recognition of immunologic mechanisms involved in ischemic cardiopathy is undoubtedly necessary. Drugs acting at this level enhance the possibilities for a good prognostic of ischemic cardiopathy.

1. Introduction

Nonetheless important advances in ischemic cardiopathy (IC) diagnostics and treatment during the past 30 years, IC continues being a main public health problem in developed countries. Moreover, in emergent economies, IC is becoming an important disease [1]. In EEUU, almost a million of patients suffer every year a disease related with IC, and more than a million get into coronary care units under IC suspect [2]. IC mortality has been diminished in the past decade. In contrast, people suffering IC are frequently in its most productive years: IC origins deep economic and psychosocial consequences.

Isquemia is produced by inadequate metabolite elimination and deficient oxygen supply: most of the times the blood flow thorough coronary arteries goes down because of a rupture of an unstable atherosclerotic plaque. As a consequence, the oxygen income equilibrium is lost and isquemia symptoms take place [3]. Despite coronary thrombosis could be clinically silent, symptoms of coronary thrombosis can be found in many forms: as a stable or unstable angina; or as a myocardium infarction (MI) with or without ST-segment elevation [4].

Atherosclerosis is a wide arterial disease and the main reason of IC. Nowadays it is clear that atherosclerosis is not a degenerative and an unavoidable consequence of growing, but a longstanding inflammatory condition[5]. In this disease, particular cells and cytokines play an important role in the innate immune response as well as in adaptive immune response. These immunological response mediators have been used in clinical practice for orient diagnostics and prognostics of IC [6]. Recently, the knowledge of immunological mechanism at molecular level has been really important because it has allowed looking at new therapeutic possibilities that modify the advance of IC disease.

In this work, we will focus on the immunologic process involved in IC and on the new therapeutics that have relevance for this mechanism. We will also review briefly general and well-known aspects of IC.

2. History

The pathologic diagnostics of a total coronary blocking was described in the middle of the 19th century by Quain [7]. He stated a relationship between the occlusive coronary disease and the heart fatty degradation. Moreover, in this time it was well known that a complete occlusion of a coronary artery was mortal. Nonetheless the antemortem diagnostics of MI started at the end of the 19th century, the relation between MI and coronary thrombosis has not been described until ~1910. In 1912, the classical work of Herrick [8] described clinical results about coronary thrombosis as a function of size and location of the occluded blood vessels. After Herrick´s work, coronary occlusion was synonymous of MI. Other works of that time claimed that the thrombus formation was the result but not the reason for MI. Brandwood et al [9] found some evidence of a coronary occlusive thrombus just in 36 of 61 patients died after MI. They also noticed that arterial thrombosis take place before MI does. Their conclusion was that the myocardium necrosis has taken place before arterial occlusion. In 1973, Erhardt et al [10] injected the radioactive fibrinogen in patients presenting MI before the decease. 6 of 7 patients after the decease have shown radiation emission from the entire regions where an occlusive thrombus has occurred. Unfortunately, they guess that the thrombi were formed after MI. In these studies, it was erroneously stated that the thrombus formation was related with a heart volume diminishing or with a coronary arterial severe occlusion. They have also guessed that the occlusive thrombus was a terminal manifestation; not related with IC beginning.

The nature of the thrombus was continued under discussion [11] and for the end of 70´s, pathologist believed that the thrombus was the main reason for transmural MI. For nontransmural MI, a pathologic analysis did not show frequently coronary thrombosis. In 1980, deWood et al [12] presented a classical result about angiography in patients with MI. These patients presented an elevation of the ST segment. Almost 90% of the patients, who underwent cardiac catheterization 4 hours after precordial pain, presented a complete arterial occlusion from MI. Most of them showed evidence of internal coronary formation of the thrombus. It was also shown that thrombolitic agents introduced by arterial or venom paths after MI open occluded arteries and avoid dead [13].

Another authors during 80´s, have suggested from angiography and angioscophy that thrombus formation was important during unstable angina and without ST-segment elevation MI. When unstable angina was possible to define in early stages, most of the patients have presented thrombotic lesions at internal coronary level. However, during this disorder, the blood vessel was not completely occluded as it was during MI [14].

3. Epidemiology

For an occurrence analysis of IC, official statistical data of mortality and prospective studies of general inhabitants are usually consulted. The latter ones give in general a good level of confidence. It is obvious the need of a definition standardization and classification in order to provide, for the data coming from different studies, the possibility of a comparison between them. Clinical history was standardized from questionnaires. It was also important the classification of electrocardiographic findings for a correct judgment between IC well established cases and non-IC occurrences. Nowadays, Gillum et al [15] have established a detailed IC diagnostic algorithm, based on "The Monitoring Trends and Determinants in Cardiovascular Disease Project" (MONICA Project). This algorithm incorporates electrocardiographic fluctuations in acute periods as well as blood levels of some enzymes as levels of creatinephosphokinase (CPK). Mortality, incident ratio, cumulated incidence, lethality and prevalence; as a function of percentage of inhabitants, are good indices for IC studies. They allow taking into account age, gender and race.

Today, IC is one of the most relevant pathologies because of its mortality and its defeat of life quality [16, 17]. In 1990 died in the world 6.3 millions of people because of IC. If the actual tendency in IC growing occurrences continues, for 2020, IC will continue being the first reason of dead in developed countries. It is also expected an increment of IC occurrences in old people and women, as well as an increment of IC occurrences in emergent economies [18].

In Mexico, deceases due to MI are approximately 11 % of total deceases of inhabitants between 15 and 64 years old. MI is the third reason for deceases between inhabitants during productive years. It is still more shocking the fact that for inhabitants older than 65 years, heart attacks is the main reason of decease; presenting 23% of total deceases. In 2001, 45402 deceases were attributed to IC: 20391 women and 25011 men. It was 10.3% of the total deceases and the second reason of mortality in Mexico [19]. In Latin American and Caribbean countries, chronic diseases are the main reason for deceases and earlier incapacity. In 2002, chronic diseases represented 44% of total deceases among inhabitants younger than 70 years old. These deceases represent two of every three deceases. The most common chronic diseases are cardiovascular diseases and the prevalent is the IC. During the first ten year of the 21 century, it will be 20.7 millions of people deceased by cardiovascular diseases. In 2005, 31% of the total deceases occurred in Latin America and the Caribbean could be attributed to these diseases [20]. It is also expected that in the next 20 years, the deceases in Latin America due to IC and vascular-brain accidents will growth three times [21].

In EEUU, it is estimated that 80,700,000 adult people (1 of 3) have one or more cardiovascular diseases. 38,200,000 of them are older than 60 years (See Table 1). 16,000,000 of them present IC; 8,100,000 present MI and 9,100,000 present chest angina. The incidence of new IC cases is of 770,000 and from here, 430,000 cases present several heart attacks. Another important estimated report is that 190,000 Americans present silent MI cases. The first MI occurrence for men is around 64 years old and for women is around 70 years old [22]. In 2004, IC was the reason for one of every five deceases (See Table 2 and 3).

At Europe, Spain presents 40% of deceases due to IC [23]. The REGICOR study has shown mortality ratios of 183 for 100,000 inhabitants as Table 4 and Table 5 presents [24].

During the first part of 20th century, epidemiological studies have established some relationships of IC occurrence among several countries and communities. It was the moment when cardiovascular epidemiology has born as a discipline. One of those ambitious studies was "The Seven Countries Multicentric Study" [25]. It established a relationship between plasmatic cholesterol concentration of inhabitants and IC geographical occurrence of 12,000 men studied in seven countries [26]. After this study, the aim of a lot of subsequent studies was to identify differences of IC occurrence among different populations; see for instance The Ni-Hon-San Study [27]. Another set of subsequent studies were focused on the different IC occurrence among persons of the same population; see for instance The Framingham study [28]. All those studies have helped to develop fundamental instrumentation for cardiovascular epidemiology [29]. However, it was until 1961 when the concept of cardiovascular risk factor was coined [30]. After this event, the planning of intervention studies was capable to probe that the lesser the occurrence of interventions, the lower the morbidity for IC.

Table 1. Cardiovascular Disease Statistics*

Population Group	Prevalence in 2005 for people older than 20 years. (Thousands of individuals)	Mortality in 2004. All ages	Hospital discharges in 2005. All ages. (Thousands of individuals)	Costs in 2008 (billions of dollars)
Both sexes	80,700 (37.1%)	869,724	6,159	448.5
Males	37,900 (37.5 %)	410,628 (47.2 %)	3,136	**
Females	42,700 (36.6%)	459,096 (52.8%)	3,023	**

* Taken and modified from "The Heart Disease and Stroke Statistics, 2008"
**No data available.

Table 2. Data for Ischemic Cardiopathy*

Population group.	Prevalence CHD in 2005 for people older than 20 years. (Thousands of people)	Prevalence of MI in 2005 for people older than 20 years. (Thousands of people)	New and recurrent MI and fatal IC for people older than 35 years. (Thousands of people)	New and recurrent MI for people older than 35 years. (Thousands of people)	IC mortality in 2004 for all ages.	MI mortality in 2004 for all ages.	IC cost, 2008 (Billions of dollars)
Both sexes	16,000 (7.3 %)	8,100 (3.7%)	1,200	920	451,326	156,816	156.4
Males	8,700 (8.9 %)	5,000 (5.1%)	710	555	233,538 (51.7%)	82,909 (52.9%)	**
Females	7300 (6.1%)	3,000 (2.5%)	490	365	217,788 (48.3%)	73,907 (47.1%)	**

* Taken and modified from "The Heart Disease and Stroke Statistics, 2008"
**No data available.

Table 3. Statistics for Angina Pectoris* (AP)

Population group	Prevalence in 2005 for people older than 20 years. (Thousands of people)	Stable AP incidence for people older than 45 years. (Thousands of people)	Hospital discharges in 2005 for all ages. (Thousands of people)
Both sexes	9,100 (4.1%)	500	44
Males	4,400 (4.4%)	320	18
Females	4,600 (3.9%)	180	25

* Taken and modified from "The Heart Disease and Stroke Statistics, 2008"

Table 4. International Death Rates (Revised 2007) in Men from 35 to 74 years old: Death Rates (Per 100 000 Population) for Total Cardiovascular Disease, Coronary Heart Disease, and Total Deaths in Selected Countries*

	CVD deaths	IC deaths	Total deaths
Russian Federation (2002)	1555	835	3187
Romania (2004)	770	314	1652
Poland (2003)	557	228	1484
Czech Republic (2004)	481	231	1248
China Rural (1999)	413	64	1260
Argentina (2001)	406	120	1262
China Urban (1999)	389	106	1003
Scotland (2002)	373	247	1084
Finland (2004)	334	211	921
Colombia (1999)	331	168	1021
Northern Ireland (2002)	322	217	876
England / Wales (2002)	301	196	811
United States (2004)	289	174	907
New Zealand (2000)	279	190	779
Germany (2004)	271	142	846
Portugal (2003)	253	97	967
Sweden (2002)	247	151	686
Republic of Korea (2002)	236	57	1085
Mexico (2001)	235	130	1056
Austria (2004)	226	131	818
The Netherlands (2004)	222	96	759
Italy (2002)	218	101	744
Norway (2003)	217	125	720
Canada (2002)	212	142	741
Spain (2003)	205	101	822
Australia (2002)	196	127	659
France (2002)	183	73	896
Switzerland (2002)	181	97	674
Israel (2003)	180	95	717
Japan (2003)	170	53	694

* Taken and modified from "The Heart Disease and Stroke Statistics, 2008"

International Death Rates (Revised 2007) in Women from 35 to 74 years old: Death Rates (Per 100 000 Population) for Total Cardiovascular Disease, Coronary Heart Disease, and Total Deaths in Selected Countries*

	CVD deaths	IC deaths	Total deaths
Russian Federation (2002)	659	288	1192
Romania (2004)	403	134	787
Poland (2003)	222	68	617

	CVD deaths	IC deaths	Total deaths
Czech Republic (2004)	213	82	594
China Rural (1999)	279	41	799
Argentina (2001)	174	35	617
China Urban (1999)	273	71	663
Scotland (2002)	183	98	649
Finland (2004)	104	48	412
Colombia (1999)	230	95	640
Northern Ireland (2002)	150	79	534
England / Wales (2002)	138	68	509
United States (2004)	150	73	575
New Zealand (2000)	136	71	498
Germany (2004)	111	45	426
Portugal (2003)	123	35	449
Sweden (2002)	107	51	422
Republic of Korea (2002)	133	24	452
Mexico (2001)	166	69	713
Austria (2004)	90	42	405
The Netherlands (2004)	102	34	466
Italy (2002)	92	29	372
Norway (2003)	88	38	430
Canada (2002)	92	48	452
Spain (2003)	79	26	343
Australia (2002)	85	43	390
France (2002)	66	16	389
Switzerland (2002)	71	27	362
Israel (2003)	83	31	431
Japan (2003)	69	16	302

* Taken and modified from "The Heart Disease and Stroke Statistics, 2008".

4. Risk Factors of Isquemic Cardiopathy

Epidemiological studies during the last 50 years have revealed a lot of risk factors for atherosclerosis. They can be classified in genetic and environmental factors. It is important to recognize IC environmental and heritage factors in patients. They can be detected in early stages of the suffering and as a consequence, early therapeutic actions must be applied.

The relative increment of some plasmatic lipoproteins seems to be of main importance because their increment is a prerequisite for most of the IC different forms. Multiple genes are also involved in each one of the risk factors. This complexity can be clearly observed in genetic studies of animals maintained under similar environmental conditions. In mice, genetic studies have revealed dozens of genetic loci involved in lipoprotein levels, body fats and other risk factors. Another level of complexity involves interactions among risk factors. Frequently, risk factors are not additive, for instance, effects of hypertension during IC are considerably amplified when cholesterol levels are high [31].

IC could be developed as a consequence of a lack of homeostasis in a physiological system. IC can also occur as a result of a failure in genetics (for instance, a failure in gene transcription) or due to environmental exposition (for instance, due to smoking). It is not common to observe IC as a result of a single mutation in a single important gene. More frequently, IC will occur as a consequence of several mutations in genes that control risk factors. These genes can control the expression of other genes or control the structure or function of the transcripted protein. These gene malfunctions explain the biological diversity of homeostatic systems. Without malfunctions, all the human beings would response identically to an environmental stimulus. As a consequence, the risk for a disease occurrence would be directly proportional to that stimulus; we know that this is not the case. For instance, only some individuals exposed to cigarette smoke will develop IC. From the precedent discussion, we can state that IC is actually considered as a multifactor illness; where environmental and genetic factors are involved [32].

Until now, genetic IC probes are poorly developed due to the multiple risk factors presented in the precedent paragraph. Single mutations have a low impact in IC occurrence but their relative risk can be as high as 40% (for instance, variations in E-apolipoprotein is a well documented case). The main objective in clinics is to weight the risk of a particular mutation in particular subsets of the population because it is clinically important to correlate several risk factors [33]. Conventional techniques are useful to identify several mutations that can be intrinsic from genetics or associated to genetic risk amplification factors (gene and environmental interaction). Environmental risk factors of IC are feeding, male sex, diabetes, obesity and smoking. The relationship between a mutated gene that codifies a protein or an enzyme is phenotypically represented in lipid levels as well as in other relevant proteins as coagulation factors or C-reactive protein (CRP). As expected, this relationship gives us a better comprehension about IC progress.

Familiar IC history is a significant risk factor [34] when IC has been observed in individuals less than 20 years old. However, this risk factor could be a product of familiar feeding. Figure 1 shows a survival diagram of Kaplan and Meier for IC incidence when IC familiar history is present. Studies in twins have helped to determine the IC genetic contribution. Marenberg et al [35] have shown a high correlation between IC starting in twins. Monozygotic twins presented 8.1 relative risk for IC occurrence under 55 years; compared with a 3.8 relative risk for dizygotic twins.

At molecular level, atherosclerosis is a time dependent process that implies the interaction between several metabolic pathways. These pathways involve lipoprotein metabolism, coagulation and inflammation. The mutation of a gene involved in those pathways could produce an incorrect protein quantity and, as a consequence, the lost of homeostasis. Some phenotypic identities as hypertension, diabetes or obesity, interact among them and increase a risk for atherosclerosis occurrence. Variations are polygenetic; a single mutation will provide only a small contribution to the risk. As previously described, gene-gene and gene-environmental interactions, can also modulate the risk. An important exception in polygenetic variations is the familiar hypercholesterolemia [36].

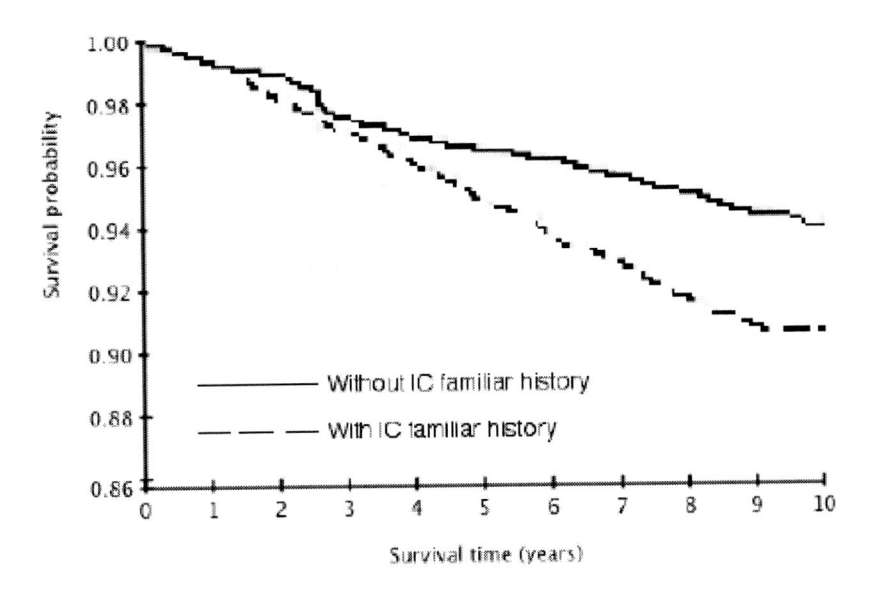

Figure 1. Survival Kaplan-Meier graph for men with IC familiar history. From "The Second Northwick Park Heart Study (NPHS-II)".

5. Inmunopathology of Isquemic Cardiopathy

As we have previously discussed, atherosclerosis is the main IC triggering and it has been increased during the last decades in the entire world. Epidemiological studies have revealed environmental and genetic factors related with atherosclerosis. However, the process for finding cellular and molecular interactions in these factors has become difficult as a consequence of IC etiologic complexity [37]. In the past decade, new research possibilities like genetic modification of a disease in murine media, have placed a better comprehension of molecular mechanism between cholesterol malfunction metabolism and atherosclerotic plaque growing. Actually, we know that inflammation plays an important roll in IC as well as in other atherosclerosis signs. Immune response cells in early lesions of atherosclerotic plaque growing impose celerity in lesion progression. As a consequence, an acute IC event, called acute coronary syndrome, take place. A lot of molecular mechanisms involved in atherosclerosis have been recently found. These mechanisms could, in a future, modify the actual evolution for this disease [6]. Hereupon, we will mention the immunologic bases in the atherosclerosis pathogenesis.

5.1. Atherosclerosis

Atherosclerosis is a progressive disease, mainly noted for lipid accumulation, cellular components and fibrous elements on large arterials [19]. Three different layers form a normal artery (see Figure 2): the layer in contact with blood is formed by a monolayer of endothelial cells, elastin fibers and connective tissue, the intermediate layer and the adventicious layer.

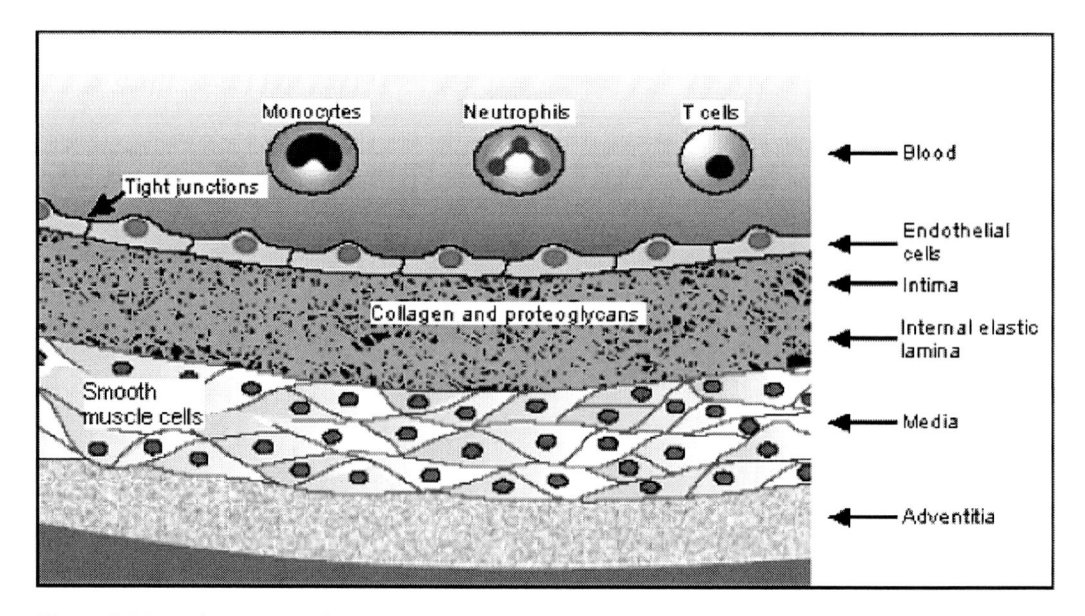

Figure 2. Normal structure of an artery.

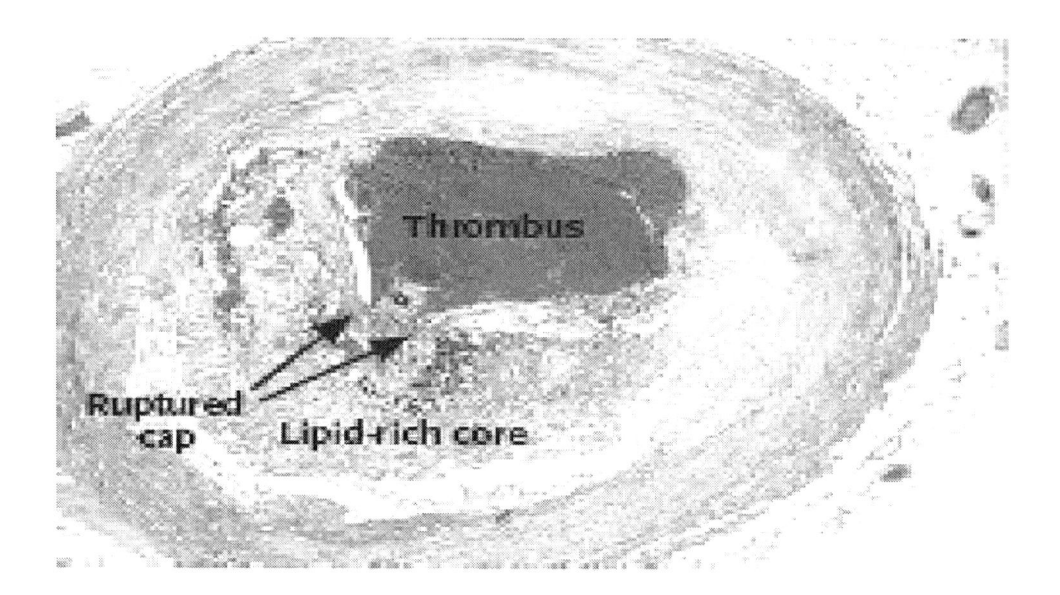

Figure 3. Atherosclerotic lesion in a human Artery.

Atherosclerotic lesions (atheromata) are asymmetric focal thickenings of the innermost layer of the artery, the intima (Figure 3). Blood-borne inflammatory and immune cells constitute an important part of an atheroma, the remainder being vascular endothelial and smooth-muscle cells. The atheroma is preceded by a fatty streak: an accumulation of lipid-laden cells beneath the endothelium. Most of these cells in the fatty streak are macrophages, together with some T cells. Fatty streaks are prevalent in young people, never cause symptoms, and may progress to atheromata or eventually disappear. In the center of an atheroma, foam cells and extracellular lipid droplets form a core region surrounded by a cap of smooth-muscle cells and a collagen-rich matrix. T cells, macrophages, and mast cells infiltrate the lesion and are particularly abundant in the shoulder region where the atheroma grows. Many of the immune cells exhibit signs of activation and produce inflammatory cytokines [38].

5.1.1. Lipoproteines Involved in Atherosclerosis

The cholesterol triggers an inflammatory response in the vascular tissue, and recent studies have found several reasons for high cholesterol concentrations as molecular mechanisms producing atherogenesis [39]. The experimental atherosclerosis induced by hypercholesterolemia has presented a well described relationship since early years of 20th century until now. After an atherogenic feeding, it has been observed a few quantities of leukocytes getting into the endothelial cells forming the intima monolayer. Under normal circumstances, this monolayer does not allow leukocyte adherence.

A lot of cellular and molecular mechanisms during atherogenesis have been observed in animal models. The beginning of atherogenesis is commonly observed as an innate immune response from an accumulation and modification of lipoproteins in the intima arterial layer [40, 41]. These modifications involve lipid and protein oxidation as well as nonenzymatic glycosylation of lipoproteins. In addition, during first stages of atherogenesis, the extracellular accumulation of lipids take place as a response of high levels of lipoproteins in blood [42]. In vitro evidence supports an important effect of modified lipoproteins and its components as a trigger mechanism of innate immune response mediator production. This response is very important for the activation of the adaptive immune response.

The platelet is the first blood cell to arrive at the scene of endothelial activation. Its glycoproteins Ib and IIb/IIIa engage surface molecules on the endothelial cell, which may contribute to endothelial activation. Inhibition of platelet adhesion reduces leukocyte infiltration and atherosclerosis in hypercholesterolemic mice [38]. Endothelial cell activation helps the expression of leukocyte adhesion molecules, in particular, on the surfaces where atherome is forming. Leukocyte adhesion molecules during early atherogenesis produced in mices, have the adhesion vascular-1 molecule (VCAM-1), the E and the P-selectine of the cell (See Figure 4). Moreover, lipidic components of modified lipoproteins can induce directly the expression of adhesion molecules, lysophosphatdylcholine and other kinds of phospholipids that are produced during lipid peroxidation. These expressed components act as proinflammatory stimulus [43].

5.1.2. Innate immune response during atherosclerosis

A cytokine or growth factor produced in the inflamed intima, a macrophage colony stimulating factor, induces monocytes entering the plaque to differentiate into macrophages (Figure 5). This step is critical for the development of atherosclerosis [44] and is associated with up-regulation of pattern-recognition receptors for innate immunity; including scavenger receptors and toll-like receptors. Scavenger receptors internalize a broad range of molecules and particles bearing molecules with pathogen-like molecular patterns [45, 46]. Bacterial endotoxins, apoptotic cell fragments, and oxidized LDL particles are all taken up and destroyed through this pathway. If cholesterol derived from the uptake of oxidized LDL particles cannot be mobilized from the cell to a sufficient extent, it accumulates as cytosolic droplets. Ultimately, the cell is transformed into a foam cell, the prototypical cell in atherosclerosis.

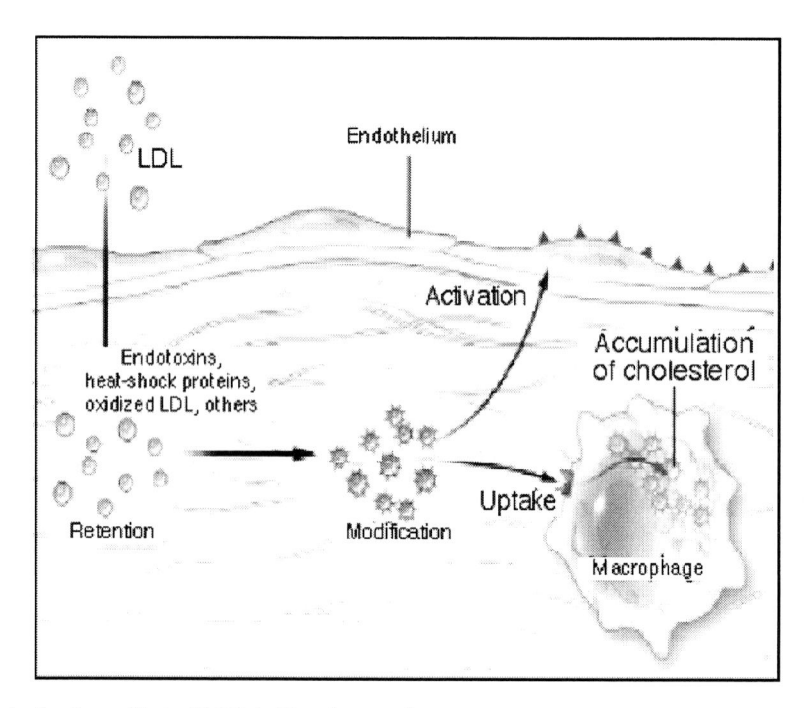

Figure 4. Activating effect of LDL infiltration on the artery.

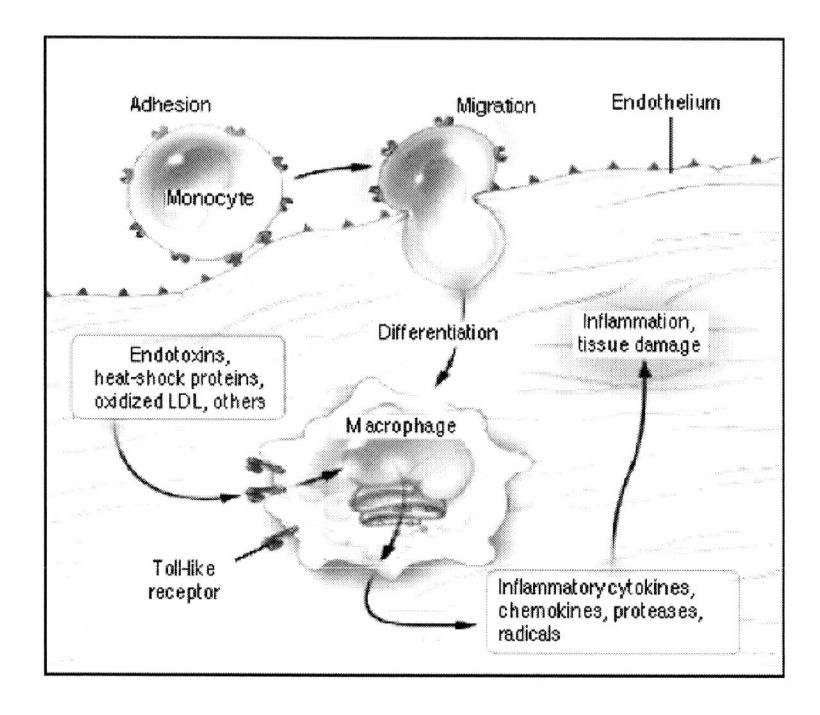

Figure 5. Role of the innate immune response in atherosclerosis.

Toll-like receptors also bind molecules with pathogen-like molecular patterns, but in contrast to scavenger receptors, they can initiate a signal cascade that leads to cell activation. The activated macrophage produces inflammatory cytokines, proteases, and cytotoxic oxygen and nitrogen radical molecules. Similar effects are observed in dendritic cells, mast cells, and endothelial cells, which also express toll-like receptors. Bacterial toxins, stress proteins, and DNA motifs are all recognized by various toll-like receptors [47]. In addition, human heatshock protein 60 and oxidized LDL particles may activate these receptors [48]. Cells in human atherosclerotic lesions display a spectrum of toll-like receptors [49], and plaque inflammation may partly depend on this pathway. In support of this notion, genetic removal of a molecule in the toll-like receptor signaling pathway inhibits atherosclerosis in apoE - knockout mice [50].

5.1.3. Adaptive immune response during atherosclerosis

Immune cells, including T cells, antigen-presenting dendritic cells, monocytes, macrophages, and mast cells, patrol several tissues (including atherosclerotic arteries) in search of an antigen. A T-cell infiltrate is always present in atherosclerotic lesions (Figure 6). Such infiltrates are predominantly CD4+ T cells, which recognize protein antigens presented to them as fragments bound to major-histocompatibility- complex (MHC) class II molecules. CD4+ T cells reactive to the disease-related antigens oxidized LDL, heat-shock protein 60, and chlamydia proteins have been cloned from human lesions [38].

A minor T-cell subpopulation, the natural killer T cell, is prevalent in early lesions. Natural killer T cells recognize lipid antigens, and their activation increases atherosclerosis in apoE-knockout mice [51]. CD8+ T cells restricted by MHC class I antigens are also present in atherosclerotic lesions [52]. These cells typically recognize viral antigens, which may be present in the lesions (see below). Activation of CD8+ T cells in apoE-knockout mice can cause the death of arterial cells and accelerate atherosclerosis [53].

When the antigen receptor of the T cell is ligated by antigen, an activation cascade results for the expression of a set of cytokines, cell-surface molecules, and enzymes. In inbred mice, two stereotypical responses can be elicited. The type 1 helper T (Th1) response activates macrophages, initiates an inflammatory response similar to delayed hypersensitivity, and characteristically functions in the defense against intracellular pathogens. The type 2 helper T (Th2) response elicits an allergic inflammation. Although the Th1–Th2 system is more plastic in humans, the general pattern is similar [54].

The atherosclerotic lesion contains cytokines that promote a Th1 response (rather than a Th2 response) [8, 38]. Activated T cells therefore differentiate into Th1 effector cells and begin producing the macrophage-activating cytokine interferon γ. Interferon γ improves the efficiency of antigen presentation and augments synthesis of the inflammatory cytokines tumor necrosis factor and interleukin-1 [54]. Acting synergistically, these cytokines instigate the production of many inflammatory and cytotoxic molecules in macrophages and vascular cells [52]. All these actions tend to promote atherosclerosis. Indeed, in apoE -knockout mice lacking interferon γ or its receptor, the development of atherosclerosis is inhibited. Similarly, the extent of the disease is reduced when the Th1 pathway is inhibited pharmacologically [35] or genetically in animals. Cytokines of the Th2 pathway can promote antiatherosclerotic immune reactions. However, they may also contribute to the formation of aneurysms by inducing elastolytic enzymes.

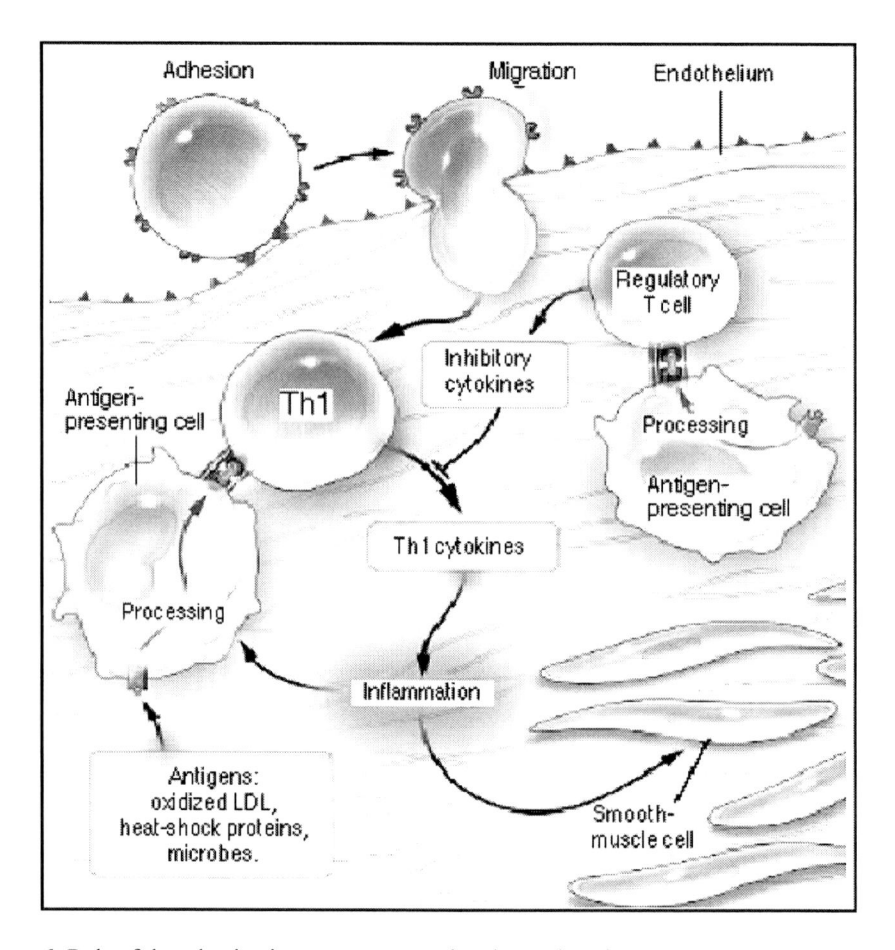

Figure 6. Role of the adaptive immune response in atherosclerosis.

Therefore, switching the immune response of atherosclerosis from Th1 to Th2 may not necessarily lead to reduced vascular disease [38]. T-cell cytokines cause the production of large amounts of molecules downstream in the cytokine cascade. As a result, elevated levels of interleukin- 6 and C-reactive protein may be detected in the peripheral circulation. In this way, the activation of a limited number of immune cells can initiate a potent inflammatory cascade, both in the forming lesion and systemically [19].

5.1.4. Infection as a Reason for Atherosclerosis

The potential pathogenic roll of infectious agents on the beginning and progression of atherosclerosis is still under discussion. Chlamydia pneumoniae and Cytomegalovirus (CMV) are the most frequent involved infectious agents. Studies in patients under heart surgery have found higher concentrations of antibodies against CMV than CMV antibodies in control patients. The same results were observed in patients with restenosis under coronary surgery. In these cases, 43% of seropositive and only 8% of seronegative patients have developed defined angiographically restenosis. As a consequence, restenosis risk was related with IgG antibody for CMV. Same kind studies have observed a relation between a seropositive result for C Pneumoniae and the coronary artery disease. High antibody concentrations have also been found in atherosclerotic lesions. Nonetheless those previous sero-epidemiologic discussed results, it is still unclear if infectious agents are a reason, a cofactor or an incidental element of pathological importance during coronary atherosclerosis and acute coronary syndromes [55, 56].

Several researchers suggest that microbial products can promote the growing or the activation of the plaque. Liposaccharides (LPS) and Thermal Shock Proteins can act on the DNA of vascular cells. These changes in the DNA can be detected in atheromatous lesions. In addition sero-epidemiological studies have found a correlation between antibody titling against microbes and the progression of the cardiovascular illness. Recently, it has been found the expression of the T-lymphocyte receptors in atherosclerotic plaques. This discovery offers a possible mechanism for an activation of the plaque cells due to microbes [57].

5.1.5. Atherosclerosis progression

When rupture or erosion of the unstable atherosclerotic plaque occurs, several phisiophatological processes arise and thrombus are formed in the place of the artery lesion. When the formation of the thrombus has as a consequence the abrupt reduction or the blocking of the blood flowing through affected vessels, the lack of equilibrium oxygen income promote the observation of clinical IC signs.

6. Clinical Presentation

The clinical symptomology of IC is diverse. It is important to make a distinction between clinical signs for IC stable disease and clinical signs for IC unstable disease. During IC stable disease, the thoracic pain (thoracic angina) is the most frequent symptom: the occlusion of the blood flow at coronary level promotes the presence of myocardial ischemia that takes place clinically as a pain. A typical pain can be described as a sensation of pushing or crushing. Some patients also describe a sensation of ardor or thoracic sleeping. The pain location uses to be retrosternal with irradiation to the left arm. It is not so common a pain irradiation to the right or both arms. Bread shortness, diaphoresis, nausea and vomiting can also take place. Physical and mental stresses are common triggering for angina. Less than 20 minutes is a normal interval for an angina. It uses to finish with resting or with a pharmacological nitrate healing (a coronary artery vasodilator). It is important to know that this suffering could be non-symptomatic. Silent angina can be only evidenced using laboratory tests or imaging methods. Unstable angina could observe the same symptomology described in this paragraph, but these symptoms are early observed often more frequently with higher intensity; they are present during rest or as a response to minimal stress.

On the other side, a more severe symptomology, including intense thoracic pain under resting, dead imminent feeling, nausea, vomiting and sweating during more than 30 minutes; suggest MI. MI is, in a lot of cases, the first symptom of isquemic cardiopathy (IC) and could be a reason of a sudden death. The presence of MI or unstable angina, commonly called acute coronary syndromes (ACS), need by force an urgent presence in a medical unit.

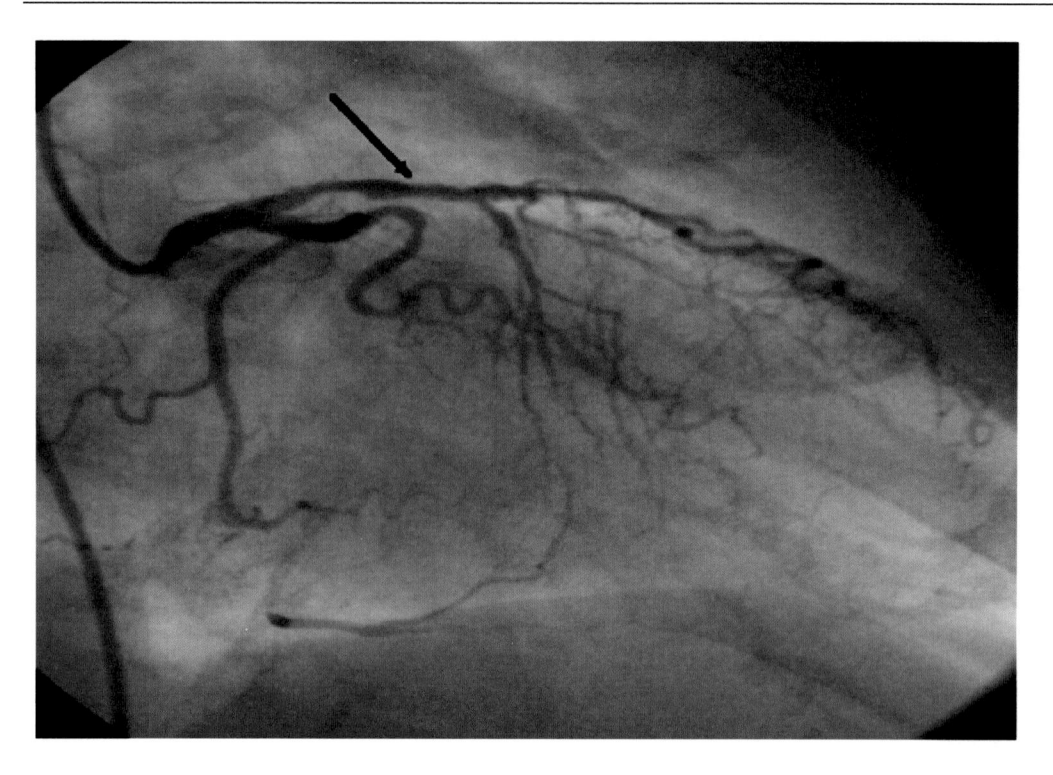

Figure 8. Coronary angiography took in a woman 59 years old. She had diabetes mellitus and arterial hypertension history with a symptomology of stable angina. It is observed an important lesion in the anterior left descendent artery in its proximal segment (arrow marked). Diffuse important suffering in the entire artery trajectory follows this lesion.

7.1. Specific Cardiac Markers

Biomarkers of myocardial damage could appear in blood after the death of myocites. The myoglobine, CK and LDH are not very specific markers of myocardial damage. Troponines are the most sensible biochemical marker because they react to myocardial damage due to ischemia. However, myocarditis, lung thromboembolia, cardiac contusion, cardiac shortage or kidney failure are pathologies where troponines could also be present.

The traditional marker CK-MB is being changed by more sensible markers like T and I cardiac troponines. Actually, troponines are the most specific biochemical marker for myocardial damage. They are present in blood flow 4 hours after an acute myocardial infarction; with a maximum peak after 12 to 24 hrs and with abnormal values for 4 to 10 days as Figure 9 describes [59]. Troponines have an aggregate prognostic value, independently of their importance as a criterion of diagnostics in MI: several studies have shown that a high level of troponines when the patient is getting into the medical unit, predicts the mortality in patients under clinical suspect of infarction. For instance, the study GUSTO IIA [60] has shown, measuring mortality at 30 days, a 5% of deceases in patients with normal values of troponin against 13% of deceases in patients with high values of troponin. Other studies have confirmed the valuable prognostic of troponines in patients with acute coronary syndromes [61, 62].

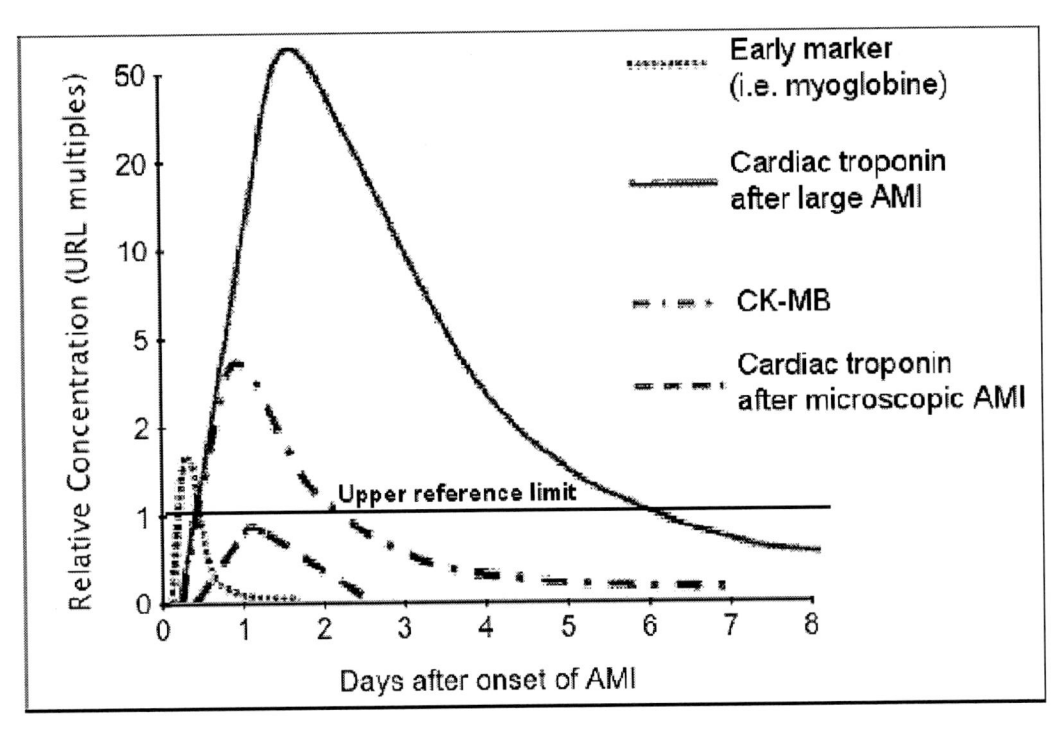

Figure 9. Increasing of cardiac markers as a function of time since an acute myocardial infarction (AMI) at t=0 days. (From Panteghine, M. Chest 2002, 122, 1428-1435.).

Recently, in morbidity prediction of IC, some biomarkers involved in atherosclerosis inflammation have been used.

8. Innflamatory Markers as Factors of Prediction in Ischemic Cardiopathy

The measuring of biological markers (biomarkers) is used as an indicator in a normal biological process, in a pathological process, or during a pharmacological response after a therapeutic treatment [63]. Multiple biomarkers have been described in IC. They have helped to the better understanding of atherosclerotic physiopathology and have enhanced the diagnostics and prognostics capacity during IC. They have also been useful for a better handling of the patients [19]. In the subsequent sections, some biomarkers of the best utility in clinical practice will be described.

8.1. C Reactive Protein (crp)

CRP is a pentameric protein linked to calcium. CRP subunits are not covalently linked and each one weights 23 kDa [64]. It was identified in 1930 by Tillet and Frances as a substance in serum of patients infected with Neumococica pneumonia. This substance reacted with C-polysaccharide of Streptococcus pneumoniae [65]. It was demonstrated that this protein could be present in high concentrations during infectious acute processes and acute and chronic inflammatory states. CRP levels in healthy people are under 1 mg/L. These values would be higher than 30 mg/L during several infectious processes [66]. An important community believes nowadays that CRP, far from being a spectator in atherosclerotic process, has a key role in atherosclerotic pathogenesis. CRP promotes a higher oxidized LDL caption for macrophages [67], induces the expression of capillary adhesion molecules [68], stimulates the tissue factor production [69] and changes the normal production of nitric oxide [70].

The first evidence about the prediction of an increment in cardiovascular death risk by CRP was showed in the MRFIT study [71]. This observational study was made in a population without cardiovascular disease that was clinically followed during 17 years: smokers with high values of CRP had 4.3 times higher a cardiovascular death risk than smokers with normal CRP values. After 1996, a lot of studies have confirmed the CRP role in the prediction of cardiovascular events among apparent healthy people [72, 73]. The PROVE-TIMI-22 study [74] has shown that patients with acute coronary syndromes and with a lower level of CRP 30 days after this event; had had a lower MI incidence and lower cardiovascular death during the next two years. This result was independent of LDL cholesterol levels.

The Center for Disease Control and Prevention (CDC), and the American Heart Association (AHA), recommend the use of the CRP for assessing the risk factor in IC. CRP values lower than 1 mg/L are considered of low risk. CRP values between 1.0 and 3.0 mg/L are considered as values of middle risk and more than 3.0 mg/L are high-risk values [75]. On the other hand, it has considered the redefinition of the Framingham prediction risk model. In order to do that, it has been used the CRP of patients with middle risk for cardiovascular events (risk to 10 years of 10 to 20%). According to this middle risk, it is possible to classify them like high or low risk [76]. High risk reclassified patients should have an intensive healing in their traditional risk factors.

8.2. Lipoprotein [a]

Lp[a] is a molecule presenting a LDL (apoB-100 surrounding cholesterol, triglycerides and phospholipids). It is linked to glycoprotein apo [a] through an apoB-100 by two disulphide bridges [77]. Lp[a] competes with plasminogen for union sites of lysine because of their similar structure. This competence helps to block fibrinolysis in blood vessels [78]. The antifibrinolytic mechanism depends on the high affinity from small Apo[a] isoforms in fibrin [79, 80, 81]. More than 25 inheritable forms of Lp[a] have been described and, as a consequence, coronary risk factors due to heritage factors in the population [82]. Lp[a] heterogeneity is given by apo[a]. Higher levels of Lp[a] and a higher degree of atherogenecity are related with the smaller iso-forms of apo[a] [83]. Plasmatic concentration of Lp[a] varies from 1 to 100 mg/dL. Levels of Lp[a] are higher in patients with kidney failure, nefrotic symptom, diabetes and postmenopausic state, but non-genetic mechanisms that control the levels of Lp[a] are not known [84].

Nonetheless, contradictory results of different prospective studies, a meta-analysis in asymptomatic people that studied 18 prospective studies with a 10 years of probing in average, has shown that individuals with higher levels of Lp[a] in the third upper level of the distribution had had a risk of cardiovascular events 1.7 larger than individuals in the third lower level of the same distribution [85]. For individuals with preexistence coronary suffering, the evidence that Lp[a] envisage new cardiovascular events is not so clear. The same meta-analysis done in 9 studies has shown a combined risk of previous cardiovascular events and new coming cardiovascular events predicted from high levels of Lp[a] of only 1.3.

8.3. Homocysteine

Homocysteine is a sulfured aminoacid, formed metabolically from the essential aminoacid methionine. After methionine ingestion, it is transformed to S-adenosylmethionine from which, homocysteine is formed [86]. The normal concentration of homocysteine goes from 5 to 15 μmol/L. The increment in homocysteine levels can arise with age, menopause, hipotiroidism, chronic kidney failure and with lack of B6, B12 and folate. Genetic variations of enzymes coming into homocysteine metabolism also increase homocysteine serum levels.

Two meta-analysis of prospective studies have shown that an increment in homocysteine concentration makes stronger the risk of cardiovascular events [87, 88]. It has been shown that a concentration of homocysteine larger than 15 mmol/L increases the risk of cardiovascular death in patients with preexistent cardiovascular pathologies [89]. Nonetheless the precedent evidence, maybe the most important reason for homocysteine studies is the possibility of helping young people with premature atherosclerosis and without cardiovascular risk factors: a large homocysteine increment, together with other risk factors, could be computed as a risk atherosclerosis increment. The risk for this increment is not as significant as the increment of CRP increment is.

8.4. Fibrinogen

It is a glycoprotein of 340 kDa formed by two identical subunits that are linked by a disulphide bond. It is synthesized in the liver and takes part in the final part of the coagulation cascade. During this cascade, fibrinogen is transformed to fibrin by thrombin. A normal fibrinogen concentration goes from 200 to 400 mg/dL. A high fibrinogen concentration takes place as a consequence of an increased hepatic production or a reduced flow depuration. Fibrinogen concentration is correlated with other cardiovascular risk factors like high LDL-cholesterol, low HDL-cholesterol and high Ld[a] concentrations. Hyper tense patients, smokers and patients suffering diabetes mellitus present a higher fibrinogen concentration.

Fibrinogen concentration predicts risk of cardiovascular events in asymptomatic patients and in patients with previous preexistent cardiovascular disease. Two meta-analysis in 12 prospective studies, one by Danesh et al [90] and another one by Maresca et al [91], have shown a relative risk of 1.8 for cardiovascular events. These meta-analysis have compared

350 mg/dL (third higher level) against 250 mg/dL (third lower level) in previously healthy people. In people with previous coronary disease and previous peripheral vascular or vascular brain diseases, the relative risk for recurrent events was 1.7.

8.5. Oxidized LDL

Since several decades ago, low density cholesterol (LDL-c) has been used as a biomarker because it presents an important correlation with coronary artery disease [92, 93]. Pharmacologic therapy for decreasing LDL-c using statins also reduces the cardiovascular risk [94].

One of the initial atherosclerotic stages is the lipidic oxidation, mainly of LDL (oxLDL). oxLDL is not only involved in the formation of foaming cells; it also activates endothelial cells, the expression of adhesion molecules and the acquiring and retention of leukocytes [95]. This is why oxLDL is a useful marker in recognition of patients with coronary artery disease [96, 97]. Holvoet et al [98] have determined the convenience of using the circulating oxLDL concentration as a sensible marker of the coronary artery disease that also enhances the prediction of cardiovascular risk. This study has compared patients with preexistent coronary disease and healthy patients: circulating oxLDL concentration has also correlated with other classical risk factors like hypercholesterolemia, diabetes mellitus, age and obesity. Other studies of unstable plaque showed that circulating oxLDL can stimulate the expression of metalloproteinase matrix (1 and 9 MMPs) in endothelial vascular human cells and in macrophages [99, 100].

9. Biomarkers of Unstability and Unstable Plaque Rupture

Inflammation has a main role during all atherosclerosis suffering. The final stage is characterized for unstable atherosclerotic plaque and erosion and rupture of the plaque. Nowadays, different biomarkers of instability in the atherosclerotic plaque were analyzed [101].

9.1. Metalloproteinases

Metalloproteinases (MMPs) are specialized enzymes that cooperate with degradation and reorganization of extracellular matrix. They are part of physiological and pathological vascular restructuring and are present in the atherosclerotic suffering. MMP are expressed in macrophages and are related with the fibrous layer degradation that triggers unstable plaque and a subsequent plaque rupture.

9.2. Cytokines

Cytokines have an important role in atherosclerosis inflammatory condition. A high concentration of cytokines can predict the risk for IC.

9.2.1. Interleukyn-6 (IL-6)

It is a simple chain glycoprotein of 26 kDa; produced by a lot of cells like macrophages/activated monocytes, endothelial cells and lipid tissue. IL-6 is capable of stimulate macrophages for promote smooth-muscle cells abundance. IL-6 also favors the expression of adhesion molecules from endothelial cells [102]; but the main function of IL-6 is the amplification of the inflammatory cascade on the wall of the artery. Using the receptor type 1 of angiotensine II (AT-1), large quantities of IL-6 have been found in atherosclerotic plaques [103]. The presence of larger quantities of IL-6 in the region where atherosclerotic plaque is broken, suggests a main role of IL-6 in unstable plaque [104]. IL-6 is the main stimulus for hepatic CRP release: high concentrations of IL-6 correlate with larger CRP concentrations. In previous healthy patients, IL-6 acts as predictor for cardiovascular events [105, 106, 107]. In patients with acute coronary syndrome, high concentrations of IL-6 are related with hospital morbidity and mortality [108]. The FRISC II study suggests that patients with acute coronary syndromes and high concentrations of IL-6 could obtain additional benefits from an invasive earlier therapy in contrast with benefits from a conservatory therapy [109].

9.2.2. Interleukyn-18 (IL-18)

Several observational studies have described that the IL-18 concentration is higher in patients presenting acute coronary syndrome. IL-18 is a strong advisor of cardiovascular death in patients with preexistent coronary disease [50].

9.3. Cd 40 / Cd 40 Ligand

Both are members of the TNF super-family. They are expressed together by T-lymphocytes, endothelial cells and macrophages. Interaction between these molecules favors the expression of another proatherogenic-like adhesion molecules; MCP-1, cytokines and growing factors. Studies in patients suffering carotid atherosclerosis have showed that CD40 ligand high concentrations are related with a high lipid concentration inside the plaque and with a risk increment for cardiovascular events in apparently healthy population [110].

10. Treatment

A lot of inspections are effective for decreasing the cardiovascular risk in previous healthy patients and in IC established patients. A low saturated-lipid diet, aerobic exercise and non-smoking habits are adequate for all the patients. The control of risk factors is important: systemic arterial hypertension, diabetes mellitus, dislipidemy, etc. Previous advises reduce inflammation. Other actions, like hormonal replacement, decrease fibrinogen and other inflammation markers; but it has no evidence of lowering cardiovascular risk in these cases [111]. A lot of drugs are used in the acute state of IC. Some of them do not have an important significance in inflammatory processes. Some others can be used manly to prevent new IC events; most of them have important implications for the IC immunological state.

10.1. Statins

These are drugs that inhibit the 3-hydroxy-3-methylglutaryl-coenzime A (HMG-CoA) reductase. This enzyme is the key for choloesterol biosynthesis. Statins reduce the containing of cellular cholesterol in hepatocytes. Hepatic cells have a response for depletion of steroids through activation of the nuclear sterol regulator. The latter promotes the overregulation of key gene transcription from cholesterol metabolism; including HMG-CoA reductase and LDL receptor. It conduces to the increment of atherogenic lipoproteins in liver that contain Apo-B (VLDL, IDL, LDL). In addition, a small, but significant elevation of antiatherogenic HDL cholesterol can be observed. In addition, statines have biological effects on inflammation, thrombogenesis and artery motility [pleiotropic effects; ref 112] A therapy based on statin reestablish the antiatherogenic / atherogenic lipoproteins equilibrium and favors the reversal cholesterol transport. This is why; statins guide benefits in composition, structure and atherosclerotic plaque stability (See Figure 10). An intensive therapy based on statins is nowadays under study because it reduces the advance of atherosclerotic disease and enhances the clinical prognostics [113, 114, 115, 116].

Anti-inflammatory properties of statins are firmly stated [117]. A reduced cholesterol concentration in membrane cells exposed to statines can interfere with the grouping of antigen receptors of T-cells during the immune activation [118]. Also an immune modulation effect has been observed [119]. This effect on T-cells could explain the benefit of statins in other pathologies that present inflammatory and/or immunologic stages like encephalitis [120] and rheumatoid arthritis. The REVERSAL study [121], has compared a therapy with high statin doses (atorvastatine, 80 mg) against moderate statin doses (pravastatine, 40 mg) in cholesterol, CRP levels and atherosclerotic disease tested by intra-vessel ultrasound. It has found that a reduction in atherosclerosis progression is associated with higher reduction concentrations of LDL and CRP, but not significant correlation exists between them.

About the risk during statin use, evidence suggests its reduction in proportional ratio of cholesterol concentration. On the other hand, statin reduces maturation and functions in dendritic cells as well as in cells capable of beginning an immune primary response for some antigens from activating T-lymphocytes. These data support the use of statins as an anti-inflammatory and immune-modulated therapy in IC [122, 123]

10.2. Thiazolidinediones

They are part of the group of the agonists of Peroxisome-Proliferator-Activated-Receptors (PPAR-y). The latter is mainly involved in adipocyte differentiation, lipid storage and glucose homeostasis. In recent years, it has been shown that PPAR-y has specific anti-atherogenic functions through anti-inflammatory events [124]. The treatment with these drugs has drastically reduced inflammatory markers like CRP, tumor necrosis factor-alpha (TNF-α), MMPs and others [125]. The treatment with rosiglitazone, a thiazolidinedione, has shown to decrease significantly the expression of some pro-inflammatory cytokines like TNF-α and IL-8 (both present since initial atherosclerosis states) from monocytes [126].

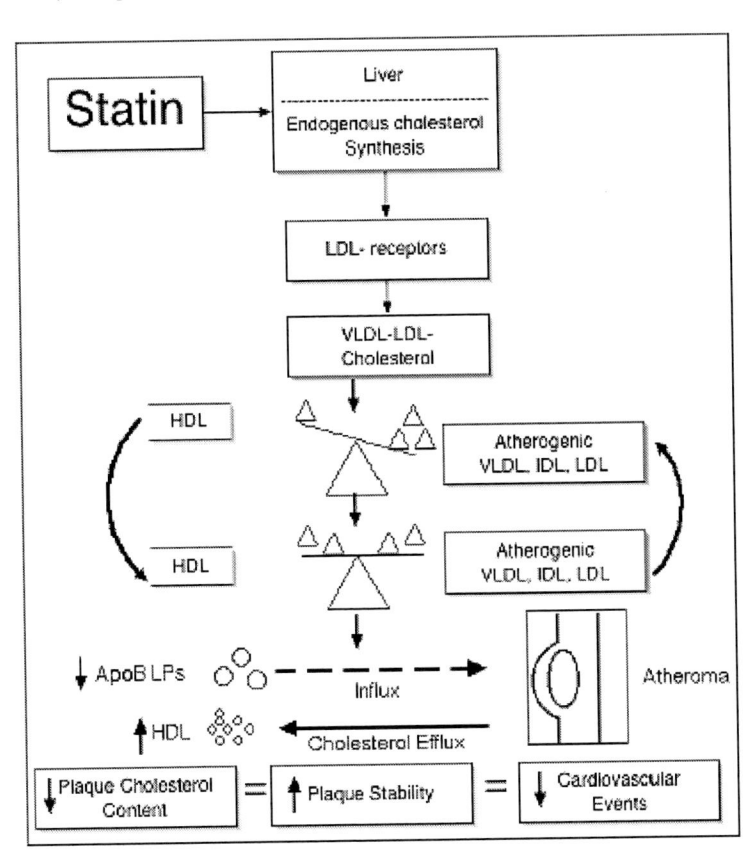

Figure 10. Action mechanism of statines in cholesterol methabolism (From Sposito, A,C.; Chapman, M.J. Arterioscler Thromb Vasc Biol 2002, 22,1524-1534).

10.3. Acetylsaliscilic Acid (Hsal)

Since 50 years ago, HSal has produced favorable effects at cardiovascular level; also showing potential anti-inflammatory properties. HSal inhibits irreversibly the cyclooxigenase; which is in charge of tromboxane A2 and prostaglandine synthesis. These molecules promote the aggregation of plaquetes as an important part of atherosclerosis physiopathology [127]. HSal also stops atherosclerosis evolution from LDL oxidation defense [128]. In apparently healthy people, HSal has shown to reduce the risk of a first infarction and, as a consequence, it is suggested for patients with middle and high infarction risk [129]. Some studies have shown that HSal reduces the risk of death in patients with coronary disease [130, 131]. Actually, Hsal is medicated for primary and secondary prevention [132].

10.4. New Therapies

A better knowledge of physiopathological atherosclerosis aspects, where inflammatory and immunologic mechanisms are involved and interrelated, has focused the research toward new drugs of prevention and coronary artery disease treatment [133].

10.4.1. Pentoxifiline

This phosphodiesterase inhibitor has been modulated the immunological atherosclerosis response. It is known that pentoxifiline inhibits the Th1 and the T-lymphocytes activity. In animals, pentoxifiline has reduced the size of atherosclerotic lesions [134]

In a clinical study with 64 patients presenting acute coronary syndrome, pentoxifiline against a placebo has reduced CRP and TNF-α; incrementing IL-10 after 6 months of observation [135]. Pentoxifiline also reduces the expression of IL-6 [136]. However, it is not possible to give a clinical prognostic conclusion because of the low number of patients involved in this study.

10.5. Other Drugs

An immune-suppression medication could represent a possible option for an acute coronary syndrome treatment [137]

Immune-suppressive drugs like cyclosporine and sirolimus can block the activation of T-cells and the spreading of lyse muscle cells [138)

Stents covered with drugs (sirulimus and paclitaxel), are actually used for getting down restenosis risk after coronary revascularization [139]. Sirulimus and paclitaxel have anti-inflammatory and anti-spreading immune-modulate properties. They promote the reendotelizacion. Paclitaxel inhibits proliferation and migration of smooth muscle cells and, as a consequence, the neointimal hyperplasia. The latter is one of the main mechanisms of restenosis after angioplasty. Sirolimus is a macrolide antibiotic (rapamicine) with immune-suppressive properties. It is also an inhibitor of smooth muscle cells [140].

IL-10 ability for inhibit pro-inflammatory cytokines, has increased the interest in this molecule as a possible therapeutic option for IC. IL-10 in cellular growths inhibits IL-1, IL-6, IL-8, TNF-a and growing factors synthesis [141]. IL-10 also limits atherosclerotic lesions [142]. In animals, IL-10 lacking mice were more vulnerable to atherosclerosis than normal mice [143].

Precautionary actions like vaccination against diverse antigens related with atherosclerosis have promising aspects [144]. Experiments in animals, have stated benefits of the vaccination against oxidized LDL, Apo-B100 and thermal shock proteins from biosynthesis of antibodies [145]. It should be expected that some infections related with atherosclerosis might be prevented with vaccination (see Table 7). Vaccination has also focused on counteract divers effects from cellular growing factors getting into angiogenesis. The latter one is a process that contributes to formation and progression of the atherosclerotic plaque. In animal models, Hauer et al [145], have induced immunity against cells that present overexpression of the receptor 2 of the vascular endothelial growing factor (VEGFR2) from a vaccine containing living attenuated bacteria of Salmonella typhimurium. This has reduced the atherosclerotic progression.

Nonetheless the previous promising results upwards described, we need to improve the actual knowledge of immunologic implied mechanisms in IC and to test the benefit of their medication.

Table 7. Effects of Immune Deficiendy and Immunomodulation on Atherosclerosis*

Experiment	Immune defect	Immune phenotype	Atherosclerosis model	Effect on disease
Compound KO	RAG-1	SCID	ApoE	↓Athero
Compound KO	RAG-2	SCID	Apo-E+fatty diet	
Compound KO	SCID/SCID	SCID	Apo-E	↓Athero
Compound KO	IFN-γ rec	Defective Th1	Apo-E	↓Athero
Ivlg inj		Immunosuppression	Apo-E	↓Athero
Anti-CD40 inj		Immunosuppression	LDLR	↓Athero
Compound KO	CD40L	Reduced immune activation	Apo-E	↓Athero
IFN-γ inj		Increased Th1	Apo-E	↑Athero
KO on B6 background	TNF-α	Defective inflammation	Fat feeding	↓Fatty streaks
KO on B6 background	IL-10	Increased proinflammatory cytokines, ↑Th1	Fat feeding	↑Fatty streaks

*Taken from Hansson, G.K. *Arterioscler Thromb Vasc Biol* 2001, 21, 1876-1890.

11. Conclusion

Atherosclerosis is a chronicle vascular disease that is produced for several genetic and environmental factors. In clinic and in epidemiological poblational studies, these factors are used for predicting the atherosclerosis evolution. In the last years, it has been found good evidences of immune system involvement in atherosclerosis progress from experimental models and clinical studies. Some oxidized lipoproteins like LDL promote activation of the innate and adaptive immune system. As a consequence, an immune dysregulation is characteristic of immunological disease. This immune dysregulation continues inflammatory process of atherosclerosis. Some cells modulate the immune response activation. These cells are known as regulating T-lymphocytes. It has been found the cooperation of iNKT cells in atherosclerosis and, as a consequence, it is possible to consider another regulating T-lymphocytes in atherosclerosis evolution. Nowadays, any research study is looking for these cells. The knowledge that the immune system is involved in atherosclerosis evolution has been useful, because some molecules have been used for determining atherosclerosis existence and progression. The final stage of atherosclerosis, the ischemic cardiopathy (IC) has been also envisaged from these molecules. This knowledge has been also important for focusing therapeutic possibilities. Recently, the relevance of immune system modulation in atherosclerosis pharmacological medication has been increased because they represent a good advance in diagnostic, prognostic and medication of ischemic cardiopathy.

12. References

[1]   Rosamond, W.; Flegal, K. et al. *Circulation* 2007, 115, 69-171.
[2]   Thomas, T; Nancy H.; *Circulation* 2006, 113, 85-151.
[3]   Badimon, L; Badimon, J.J.; Turitto, V.T.; Vallabhajosula, S.; Fuster, V. *Circulation* 1988, 78, 1432-1442.
[4]   Davies, M.J.; *Thrombosis and Coronary Atherosclerosis in Thrombolysis in Cardiovascular Disease*; Marcel Dekker Inc: New York, NY, 1989; 25-43.
[5]   Libby, P. *J Intern Med* 1999, 247, 349-358.
[6]   Ramírez-Velázquez, C.; et al. *Revista de Alergia* 2007, 54, 7-13.
[7]   Quain, R.; *Med Chr Trans* 1850, 33, 1217.
[8]   Herrick, J.B. *JAMA* 1912, 59, 2015-2020.
[9]   Branwood, A.W.; Montgomery, G.L. *Scott Med J* 1956, 1, 367.
[10]   Erhardt, L.R.; Lundman, T.; Mellstedt, H. *Lancet* 1973, 1, 387-390.
[11]   Roberts, W.; Buja, L.M. *Am J Med* 1972, 52, 425-443.
[12]   Dewood, M.A.; Spores, J.; Notske, R.; et al. *New Engl J Med* 1980, 303, 897-902.
[13]   Bresnahan, D.R.; Davis, D.R.; Holmes, Jr. D.R.; Smith, H.C. *J Am Coll Cardiol* 1985, 6, 285-289.
[14]   Ambrose, J.A. *J Am Coll Cardiol* 1992, 19, 1653-1658.
[15]   Gillum, R.F.; Fortmann, S.P.; Prineas, R.J.; Kottke, T.E. *Am Heart J* 1984, 108, 150-158.
[16]   McKeon, T.; Lowe, C.R. *Introducción a la medicina social*; Siglo XXI: México, DF, 1986.
[17]   Dodu, S.R.A. *Cardiology* 1988, 75, 56-64.
[18]   Murria, C.L.; Lopez, A. *Lancet* 1997, 349, 1498-1504.
[19]   Ramírez-Velázquez, C.; Lozano-Nuevo, J.J.; Rubio-Guerra, A.F. *Med Int Mex* 2004, 20, 437-450.
[20]   Health Panamerican Organization; *La salud en las Américas*; Organización Panamericana de la Salud: Washington, DC, 2002; Vol. I.
[21]   Yach, D.; Hawkes, C.; Gould, C.L.; Hofman, K.J.; *JAMA* 2004, 291, 2616-2622.
[22]   Rosamond, W.; Flegal, K. et al. *Circulation* 2008, 117, 1-123.
[23]   Medrano, M.J. *Bol Epidemiol Semanal* 1998, 6, 149-153.

[24] Tunstall, H.; Kuulasmaa, K.; Mahonen, M.; Tolonen, H.; Ruokokoski, E.; Amouyel, P. *Lancet* 1999, 353, 1547-1557.

[25] Keys, A.*J Mt Sinai Hosp* 1953, 20, 118-139.

[26] Keys, A.; *Seven Countries: A Multivariate Analysis of Death and Coronary Heart Disease*; Harvard University Press: Cambridge, MA, 1980.

[27] Marmot, M.; Syme, S.L.; Kagan, A.; Kato, H.; et al. *Am J Epidemiol* 1975, 102, 514-525.

[28] Dawber, T.R.; *The Framingahm Study. The epidemiology of atherosclerotic disease. Cambridge*; Harvard University Press: Cambridge, MA, 1980.

[29] Dawber, T.R.; Meadors, G.F.; Moore, F.E. Jr. *Am J Public Health* 1951, 41, 279-286.

[30] Kannel, W.B.; Dawber, T.R.; Kagan, A.; Revotskie, L.; Stokes, J. *Ann Intern Med* 1961, 55, 33-50.

[31] Goldbourt, U.; Neufeld, H. N. *Arteriosclerosis* 1998, 6, 357-377.

[32] Wilson, P.W.; Schaefer, E.J.; Larson, M.G. *Arterioscler Thromb Vasc Biol* 1996, 16, 1250–1255.

[33] Boer, J.M.; Fesken, E.J.; Verschuren, W.M.; Seidell, J.C.; Kromhout, D. *Epidemiology* 1999, 10, 767–770.

[34] Hawe, E.; Talmud, P.J.; Miller, G.J.; Humphries, S.E. *Ann Hum Genet* 2002, 6, 188-196.

[35] Marenberg, M.E.; Risch, N.; Berkman, L.F.; Floderus, B.; de Flaire, U. *N Engl J Med* 1994, 330, 1041–1046.

[36] Heath, K.E.; Humphries, S.E. *Eur J Hum Genet* 2001, 9, 244–252.

[37] Lusis, A.J. *Nature* 2000, 407, 233-241.

[38] Hansson, G. K. NEJM 2005, 352, 1685-1695.

[39] Hansson, G. K.; Libby, P.; Schonbeck, U.; Yan, Z-Q. *American Heart Association* 2002, 91, 281-291.

[40] Rajavashisth, T.B.; Andalibi, A.; Territo, M.C.; Berliner, J.A.; Navab, M.; Fogelman, A.M.; Lusis, A.J. *Nature* 1990, 344, 254-257.

[41] Heinecke, J.W. *J Lab Clin Med* 1999, 133, 321-325.

[42] Sugiyama, S.; Okada, Y.; Sukhova, G.K.; Virmani, R.; Heinecke, J.W.; Libby, P. *Am J Pathol* 2001, 158, 879-891.

[43] Cybulsky, M.I.; Iiyama, K.; Li, H.; Zhu, S.; Chen, M.; Iiyama, M.; Davis, V.; Gutierrez-Ramos J.C.; Connelly, P.W.; Milstone, D.S. *J Clin Invest* 2001, 107, 1255-1262.

[44] Smith, J.D.; Trogan, E.; Ginsberg, M.; Grigaux, C.; Tian, J.; Miyata, M. *Proc Natl Acad Sci USA* 1995, 92, 8264-8268.

[45] Peiser, L.; Mukhopadhyay, S.; Gordon, S. *Curr Opin Immunol* 2002, 14, 123-128.

[46] Janeway, C.A. Jr.; Medzhitov, R. *Annu Rev Immunol* 2002, 20, 197-216.

[47] Xu, Q. *Arterioscler Thromb Vasc Biol* 2002, 22, 1547-1559.

[48] Miller, Y.I.; Chang, M.K.; Binder, C.J.; Shaw, P.X.; Witztum, J.L. *Curr Opin Lipidol* 2003, 14, 437-445.

[49] Edfeldt, K.; Swedenborg, J.; Hansson, G.K.; Yan, Z.Q. *Circulation* 2002, 105, 1158-1161.

[50] Bjorkbacka, H.; Kunjathoor, V.V.; Moore, K.J.; et al. *Nat Med* 2004, 10, 416-421.

[51]   Tupin, E.; Nicoletti, A.; Elhage, R.; et al. *J Exp Med* 2004, 199, 417-422.
[52]   Hansson, G.K. *Arterioscler Thromb Vasc Biol* 2001, 21, 1876-1890.
[53]   Ludewig, B.; Freigang, S.; Jaggi, M.; et al. *Proc Natl Acad Sci USA* 2000, 97, 12752-12757.
[54]   Szabo, S.J.; Sullivan, B.M.; Peng, S.L.; Glimcher, L.H. *Annu Rev Immunol* 2003, 21, 713-758.
[55]   Topper, J. N. and Gimbrone, M. A. Jr. *Mol. Med. Today* 1999, 5, 40-46.
[56]   de Caterina, R.; et al. *J. Clin. Invest* 1995, 96, 60-68.
[57]   Mulvihill, N T.; Foley, J. B. *Heart* 2002, 87, 201-204.
[58]   Thygesen, K.; Alpert, J.S.; Harvey, W.H.D. *Circulation* 2007, 116, 2634-2653.
[59]   Panteghine, M.; *Chest* 2002, 122, 1428-1435.
[60]   Ohman, E.; Armstrong, P.; Christenson, R.; et al. *N Engl J Med* 1996, 335, 1333-1341.
[61]   Ohman, E.M.; Armstrong, P.W.; White, H.D.; et al. *Am J Cardiol* 1999, 84, 1281-1286.
[62]   Lindahl, B.; Diderholm, E.; Lagerqvist, B.; Venge, P.; Wallentin, L. *J Am Coll Cardiol* 2001, 38, 979-986.
[63]   Giannitsis. E.; Müller-Bardorff, M. *Circulation* 2001, 104, 630-635.
[64]   Macintyre, S.S. *Methods Enzymol* 1988, 163, 383-399.
[65]   Tillett, W.S.; Francis, T. *J Exp Med* 1930, 52, 561-571.
[66]   Ridker, P.M. *Circulation* 2003, 107, 363-369.
[67]   Zouki, C.; Beauchamp, M.; Baron, C.; Filep, J.G. *J Clin Invest* 1997, 100, 522-529.
[68]   Torzewski, M. ; Rist, C. ; Mortensen, R.F. ; et al. *Arterioscler Thromb Vasc Biol* 2000, 20, 2094-2099.
[69]   Cermak, J.; Key, N.S.; Bach, R.R.; et al. *Blood* 1993, 82, 513-520.
[70]   Verma, S.; Wang, C.H.; Li, S.H.; et al. *Circulation* 2002, 106, 913-919.
[71]   Kuller, L.H.; Tracy, R.P.; Shaten, J.; et al. *Am J Epidemiol* 1996, 144, 537-547.
[72]   Jager, A.; van Hinsbergh, V.W.M.; Kostense, P.J.; et al. *Arterioscler Thromb Vasc Biol* 1999, 19, 3071-3078.
[73]   Cushman, M.; Arnold, A.M.; Psaty, B.M.; et al. *Circulation* 2005, 112, 25-31.
[74]   Ridker, P.M.; Cannon, C.P.; Morrow, D.; et al. *N Engl J Med* 2005, 352, 20-28.
[75]   Smith, S.C. Jr.; Anderson, J.L. *Circulation* 2004, 110, 550-553.
[76]   Ridker, P.M.; Cook, N. *Circulation* 2004, 109, 1955-1959.
[77]   Gaubatz, J.W.; Heideman, C.; Gotto, A.M.; et al. *J Biol Chem* 1983, 258, 4582-4589.
[78]   Loscalzo, J.; Weinfeld, M.; Fless, G.M.; et al. Arteriosclerosis 1990, 10, 240-245.
[79]   Hervio, L.; Durlach, V.; Girard-Globa, A.; et al. *Biochemistry* 1995, 34, 13353-13358.
[80]   Kang, C.; Dominguez, M.; Loyau, S.; et al. *Arterioscler Thromb Vasc Biol* 2002, 22, 1232-1238.
[81]   Anglés-Cano, E.; de la Peña, A.; Loyau, S. Ann NY Acad of Sci 2001, 936, 261-275.
[82]   Hobbs, H.H.; White, A.L. *Curr Opin Lipidol* 1999, 10, 225-236.
[83]   Carmena, R.; Duriez, P.; Fruchart, J.C. *Circulation* 2004, 109, III-2 - III-7.
[84]   Berglund, L.; Ramakrishnan, R. *Arterioscler Thromb Vasc Biol* 2004, 24, 2219-2226.
[85]   Danesh, J.; Collins, R.; Peto, R. *Circulation* 2000, 102, 1082-1085.
[86]   Mangoni, A.A.; Jackson, S.H. *Am J Med* 2002, 112, 556-565.
[87]   Boushey, C.J.; Beresford, S.A.; Omenn, G.S.; et al. *JAMA* 1995, 274, 1049-1057.
[88]   Clarke, R.; Collins, R.; et al. *JAMA* 2002, 288, 2015-2022.

[89]   Al-Obaidi, M.K.; Stubbs, P.J.; Collinson, P.; et al. J Am Coll Cardiol 2000, 36, 1217-1222.

[90]   Danesh, J.; Collins, R.; Appleby, P.; et al. *JAMA* 1998, 279, 1477-1482.

[91]   Maresca, G.; Di Blasio, A.; Marchioli, R.; et al. *Arterioscler Thromb Vasc Biol* 1999, 19, 1368-1377.

[92]   Goldstein, J.L.; Hazzard, W.R.; Schrott, H.G.; Bierman, E.L.; Motulsky, A.G. *J Clin Invest* 1973, 52, 1533–1543.

[93]   Castelli, W.P.; Garrison, R.J.; Wilson, P.W.F.; Abbott, R.D.; Kalousdian, S.; Kannel, W.B. *JAMA* 1986, 256, 2835–2838.

[94]   Sacks, F.M.; Pfeffer, M.A.; Moye, L.A.; et al. *N Engl J Med* 1996, 335, 1001-1009.

[95]   Jessup, W.; Kritharides, L.; Stocker, R. *Biochem Soc Trans* 2004, 32, 134 -138.

[96]   Holvoet, P.; Vanhaecke, J.; Janssens, S.; van de Werf, F.; Collen, D. *Circulation* 1998, 98, 1487–1494.

[97]   Toshima, S.; Hasegawa, A.; Kurabayashi, M.; et al. *Arterioscler Thromb Vasc Biol* 2000, 20, 2243–2247.

[98]   Holvoet, P.; Mertens, A.; et al. *Thromb. Vasc. Biol* 2001, 21, 844-848.

[99]   Huang, Y.; Mironova, M.; Lopes-Virella, M.F. *Arterioscler Thromb Vasc Biol* 1999, 19, 2640 –2647.

[100] Xu, X.P.; Meisel, S.R.; et al. *Circulation* 1999, 99, 993–998.

[101] Koenig, W.; Khuseyinova, N. *Arterioscler Thromb Vasc Biol* 2007, 27, 15-26.

[102] Rattazzi, M.; Puato, M.; et al. *J Hypertens* 2003, 21, 1787–1803.

[103] Schieffer, B.; Schieffer, E.; et al. *Circulation* 2000, 101, 1372–1378.

[104] Maier, W.; Altwegg, L.A.; et al. *Circulation* 2005, 111, 1355–1361.

[105] Ridker, P.M.; Rifai, N.; Stampfer, M.J.; Hennekens, C.H. *Circulation* 2000, 101, 1767-1772.

[106] Volpato, S.; Guralnik, J.M.; et al. *Circulation* 2001, 103, 947–953.

[107] Harris, T.B.; Ferrucci, L.; et al. *Am J Med* 1999, 106, 506 –512.

[108] Biasucci, L.M.; Liuzzo, G.; et al. *Circulation* 1999, 99, 2079 –2084.

[109] Lindmark, E.; Diderholm, E.; Wallentin, L.; Siegbahn, A. *J Am Med Assoc* 2001, 286, 2107–2113.

[110] Blake, G.J.; Ostfeld, R.J.; et al. *Arterioscler Thromb Vasc Biol* 2003, 23, e11 - e14.

[111] Hulley, S.; Grady, D.; Bush, T.; et al. *JAMA* 1998, 280, 605-613.

[112] Davignon, J.; Laaksonen, R. *Curr Opin Lipidol* 1999, 10, 543–559.

[113] Cannon, C.P.; Braunwald, E.; McCabe, C.H.; et al. *N Engl J Med* 2004, 350, 1495-1504.

[114] Topol, E.J. *N. Engl J Med* 2004, 350, 1562-1564.

[115] Sacks, F.M. *JAMA* 2004, 291, 1132-1134.

[116] Nissen, S.E.; Tuzcu, E.M.; Schoenhagen, P.; et al. *JAMA* 2004, 291, 1071-1080.

[117] McCarey, D.W.; McInnes, I.B.; Madhok, R.; et al. *Lancet* 2004, 363, 2015-2021.

[118] Ehrenstein, M.R.; Jury, E.C.; Mauri, C. *N Engl J Med* 2005, 352, 73-75.

[119] Kwak, B.; Mulhaupt, F.; Myit, S.; Mach, F. *Nat Med* 2000, 6, 1399-1402.

[120] Youssef, S.; Stuve, O.; Patarroyo, J.C.; et al. *Nature* 2002, 420, 78-84.

[121] Nissen, S.E.; Tuzcu, E.M.; Schoenhagen, P.; Crowe, T.; et al. *N Engl J Med* 2005, 352, 29-38.

[122] Waters, D. *Am J Cardiol* 2003, 92, 692-695.

[123] Yilmaz, A.; Reiss, C.; et al. *Atherosclerosis* 2004, 172, 85–93.

[124] Lee, C.H.; Evans, R.M. *Trends in Endoc and Metab* 2002, 13, 331-335.

[125] Chinetti-Gbaguidi, G.; Fruchart, J.C.; Staels, B. *Curr Opin Pharmacol* 2005, 5, 177-183.

[126] Adamieca, R.; Gacka, M.; et al. *Atherosclerosis* 2007, 194, e108 - e115.

[127] Jneid, H.; Bhatt, D.L.; et al. *Arch Intern Med* 2003, 163, 1145-1153.

[128] Steer, K.A.; Wallace, T,M.; Bolton, C.H.; Hartog, M. *Heart* 1997, 77, 333–337.

[129] Eidelman, R.S.; Hebert, P.R.; Weisman, S.M.; Hennekens, C.H. *Arch Intern Med* 2003, 163, 206-201.

[130] Lewis, H.D.; Davis, J.; Archibald, D.; et al. *N Engl J Med* 1983, 309, 396–403.

[131] Theroux, P.; Ouimet, H.; McCans, J.; et al. *N Engl J Med* 1988, 319, 1105-1111.

[132] Awtry, E.H.; Loscalzo, J. *Circulation* 2000, 101, 1206-1218.

[133] Hansson, G.K. *N Engl J Med* 2005, 352, 1685-1695.

[134] Laurat, E.; Poirier, B.; Tupin, E.; et al. *Circulation* 2001, 104, 197–202.

[135] 136.   Fernandes,   J.L.;   et   al.   *Atherosclerosis*   2006,   doi: 10.1016/j.atherosclerosis.2006.11.032

[136] 137. Ramani, M.; Khechai, F.; Ollivier, V.; et al. *FEBS Lett* 1994, 356, 86–88.

[137] Libby, P.; Aikawa, M. *Nat Med* 2002, 8, 1257-1262. [Erratum, *Nat Med* 2003, 9, 146]

[138] 139. Jonasson, L.; Holm, J.; Hansson, G.K. *Proc Natl Acad Sci USA* 1988, 85, 2303-2306.

[139] Marx, S.O.; Marks, A.R. *Circulation* 2001, 104, 852-855.

[140] Leon, M.B.; Bakhai, A. *Am Heart J* 2003, 146, S13–S17.

[141] de Waal, M.R.; Abrams, R.J.; et al. *J Exp Med* 1991, 174, 1209-1220.

[142] Suttles, J.; Milhorn, D.M.; et al. *J Biol Chem* 1999, 274, 5835-5842.

[143] Mallat, Z.; Besnard, S.; Duriez, M.; et al. *Arterioscler Thromb Vasc Biol* 2005, 25, 18-28.

[144] Zhou, X.; Caligiuri, G.; Hamsten, A.; Lefvert, A.K.; Hansson, G.K. *Arterioscler Thromb Vasc Biol* 2001, 21, 108-114.

[145] Hauer, A.D.; van Puijvelde, G.H.; et al. *Arterioscler Thromb Vasc Biol* 2007, 27, 2050-2057.

In: Angina Pectoris: Etiology, Pathogenesis and Treatment
Editors: A. P. Gallo, M. L. Jones

ISBN: 978-1-60456-674-1
© 2008 Nova Science Publishers, Inc.

Chapter X

Atherosclerosis, Inflammation and Chlamydia Pneumoniae

Giovanni Fazio, Maria Giovino, Loredana Sutera, Giuseppina Novo, and Salvatore Novo

Division of cardiology - University of Palermo, Italy

Coronary heart disease is the single most common cause of illness and death in the developed world.

Coronary atherosclerosis is by far the most frequent cause of ischemic heart disease, and plaque disruption with superimposed thrombosis is the main cause of the acute coronary syndromes of unstable angina, myocardial infarction, and sudden death. Atherosclerosis is the result of a complex interaction between blood elements, disturbed flow, and vessel wall abnormality, involving several pathological processes: inflammation, with increased endothelial permeability, endothelial activation, and monocyte recruitment; growth, with smooth muscle cell proliferation, migration, and matrix synthesis; degeneration, with lipid accumulation; necrosis, possibly related to the cytotoxic effect of oxidized lipid; calcification/ossification, which may represent an active rather than a dystrophic process; and thrombosis, with platelet recruitment and fibrin formation.

Approximately one third of patients with CAD do not have traditional risk factors. New evidence shows that systemic markers of inflammation are a strong predictor of cardiovascular events, adding independently to traditional risk factors. Inflammation systemically or locally within atherosclerotic plaque is believed to play a major role in the initiation and progression of CAD and the precipitation of acute coronary events. Cardiovascular events may most commonly arise from sites of "nonsignificant" stenosis, suggesting that plaque instability rather than the degree of stenosis is the key risk factor. This plaque instability is believed related to inflammation within the plaque, with activated macrophages releasing inflammatory mediators, activating matrix metalloproteinases, and breaking down the protective fibrous cap. The source of this inflammation may include noninfectious triggers (e.g., oxidized low-density lipoprotein [LDL], oxidation products of smoking, endothelial injury, genetics, etc.) or from a number of proposed infectious triggers.

Now it is known that local and systemic inflammatory processes play an important role in the genesis and development of atheroclerotic lesions and in the pathophysiology of acute coronary syndromes. This hypothesis is supported by findings of elevated parameters of the inflammatory reaction in the blood of atherosclerotic patients and of histopathological characteristic of unstable plaque (thin fibrous cap, large necrotic core, less smooth muscle cells and abundant foamy cells and lymphocytes). Besides several studies have demonstrated that inflammation has an determining role in the rupture of the coronaric plaque, and have been carried out to identify the etiopatogenetic moment of the inflammation itself, trying to correlate coronaric atherosclerosis and its development with some infectious agents.

Potentially, acute or chronic infections could initiate and promote CAD in the absence of traditional risk factors. More likely, infections act to augment CAD risk in the presence of other risk factors. A number of mechanisms have been proposed which could link infection to atherosclerosis.

Understanding the pathogenesis of atherosclerosis and the role of inflammation, first requires knowledge of mentions of the structure and biology of the normal artery and its indigenous cell types.

Anatomy

Normal arteries have a well-developed trilaminar structure.The innermost layer, the tunica intima is a monolayer of endothelial cells abutting directly on a basal lamina and constitutes the crucial contact surface with blood. Arterial endothelial cells possess many highly regulated

mechanisms of capital importance in vascular homeostasis that often go awry during the pathogenesis of arterial diseases.The internal elastic membrane serves as the border between the intimal layer and the underlying tunica media. The media of elastic arteries such as the aorta have well-developed concentric layers of smooth muscle cells, interleaved with layers of elastin-rich extracellular matrix. This structure appears well adapted to the storage of the kinetic energy of left ventricular systole by the walls of great arteries. The lamellar structure also doubtless contributes to the structural integrity of the arterial trunks. In the media of smaller muscular arteries usually have smooth muscle cells reside within the surrounding matrix in a more continuous than lamellar array. In the normal artery the smooth muscle cells are generally quiescent from the standpoint of growth control and there is a state of homeostasis of extracellular matrix.The external elastic lamina forming the border with the adventitial layer.The adventitia contains collagen fibrils and cellular population such as fibroblasts and mast cells. Vasa vasorum and nerve endings localize in this outermost layer of the arterial wall.

Pathophysiology

The pathogenesis of atherogenesis and of its development remain largely conjectural. One of the first ultrastructural alterations is an accumulation of small lipoprotein particles

(LDL) in the intima, where bindings lipoproteins to proteoglycan and tend to coalesce into aggregates. This process is supported by permeability of the endothelial monolayer. Lipoprotein particles bound to proteoglycan appear to exhibit increased susceptibility to oxidative or other chemical modifications such as enzymatic processing and glycation which can modify LDL in the intima. The second morphologically definable event in the initiation of atheroma is leukocyte recruitment and accumulation; they adhere to the endothelium, by means of Adhesion molecules, and diapedese between endothelial cell junctions to enter the intima, where they begin to accumulate lipids and transform into foam cells. In addition to the monocyte, T lymphocytes also tend to accumulate in early atherosclerotic lesions. The current concept of directed migration of leukocytes involves the action of protein molecules known as chemoattractant cytokines, or chemokines, produced by the endothelium and smooth muscle in response to oxidized lipoprotein and other stimuli.

Until now the natural history of the atherosclerotic process is not totally cleared. Some have invoked a multicentric origin hypothesis of atherogenesis, positing that atheromas arise as benign leiomyomas of the artery wall. However, the location of sites of lesion predilection at proximal portions of arteries after branch points or bifurcations at flow dividers suggests a hydrodynamic basis for early lesion development. Locally disturbed flow could induce alterations that promote the steps of early atherogenesis; alternatively, the laminar flow may elicit antiatherogenic homeostatic mechanisms (atheroprotective functions). This hypothesis is supported by vitro data suggest that laminar shear stress can augment the expression of genes that may protect against atherosclerosis, including forms of the enzymes superoxide dismutase (reduce oxidative stress by catabolizing the reactive and injurious superoxide anion) or nitric oxide synthase (produces nitric oxide, a endogenous vasodilator and anti-inflammatory agent).

Whereas the early events in atheroma initiation involve primarily altered endothelial function and recruitment and accumulation of leukocytes, the subsequent evolution of atheroma into more complex plaques involves smooth muscle cells as well. Some smooth muscle cells likely migrates from the underlying media into the intima, actracted by molecules such as platelet-derived growth factor, secreted by activated macrophages and overexpressed in atherosclerosis. These smooth muscle cell begin to replication herself; besides, death of these cells may also participate in complication of the atherosclerotic plaque. The vascular smooth muscle cell produces extracellular matrix molecules which makes up much of the volume of an advanced atherosclerotic plaque. These matrix is catalyzed in part by enzymes known as MMP. This dissolution also likely plays a role in arterial remodeling that accompanies lesion growth. During the first part of the life history of an atheromatous lesion, growth of the plaque is outward, in an abluminal direction, rather than inward. The smooth muscle cell is not alone in its proliferation and migration within the evolving atherosclerotic plaque. Endothelial migration and replication also occur as plaques develop in microcirculation, characterized by plexuses of newly formed vessels. The microvascularization of plaques may also allow growth of the plaque overcoming diffusion limitations on oxygen and nutrient supply, Finally, the plaque microvessels may be friable and prone to rupture. Hemorrhage and thrombosis in situ could promote a local round of smooth muscle cell proliferation and matrix accumulation in the area immediately adjacent to the microvascular disruption. Plaques often develop areas of calcification as they evolve.

The process of initiation and evolution of the atherosclerotic plaque generally takes place over many years, during which the affected person often has no symptoms. After the plaque burden exceeds the capacity of the artery to remodel outward, encroachment on the arterial lumen begins. Eventually the stenoses may progress to a degree that impedes blood flow through the artery. The development of chronic stable angina pectoris or intermittent claudication on increased demand is a common presentation of this type of atherosclerotic disease. However, several kinds of clinical observation suggest that most myocardial infarctions result not from critical blockages but from lesions that produce stenoses that do not limit flow. Instead of progressive growth of the intimal lesion to a critical stenosis, we now recognize that thrombosis, complicating a not necessarily occlusive plaque, most oftencauses episodes of unstable angina or acute myocardial infarction. Thrombosis is the consequence of a fracture of the plaque's fibrous cap, or of a superficial erosion of the intima.

Risk Factors

The "risk factor" is a characteristic or feature of an individual or population that is present early in life and is associated with an increased risk of developing future cardiovascular disease. The risk factor of interest may be a behavior (e.g., smoking), an inherited trait (e.g., family history), or a laboratory measurement (e.g., cholesterol). It can discern of the conventional atherosclerotic risk factors such as hyperlipidemia, smoking, hypertension, insulin resistance and diabetes, physical activity, obesity, and hormone status, and novel atherosclerotic risk factors, including homocysteine, fibrinogen, lipoprotein(a) (Lp[a]),as well as infective agent, markers of inflammation (e.g. high-sensitivity C-reactive protein), indices of fibrinolytic function (e.g., tissue-type plasminogen activator [t-PA] and plasminogen activator inhibitor 1 [PAI-1]).

Dyslipidemia

Dyslipidemia encompasses disorders that include average total plasma cholesterol levels, particularly LDL, but low HDL. Several studies point out relationship between low-density lipoproteins (LDL) and possibly very low-density lipoproteins (VLDL) and coronary artery disease. The role of high-density lipoproteins (HDL) as a protective fraction also emerged. Cholesterol play as an important role in atherosclerosis process, actually it is a main constituent of the plaque. Besides the presence of small, dense LDL particles may be related to features of the "metabolic syndrome," characterized by the presence of abdominal obesity, peripheral insulin resistance, high blood pressure, and a dyslipoproteinemia with elevated plasma triglycerides and reduced HDL-C levels.

Smoking

Cigarette consumption constitutes the single most important modifiable risk factor for coronary artery disease. Smoking affects atherothrombosis by several mechanisms. In addition to accelerating atherosclerotic progression, long-term smoking may enhance oxidation of LDL-C and reduce levels of HDL-C. Smoking also impairs endothelium-dependent coronary artery vasodilation; has multiple adverse hemostatic effects; actually increases inflammatory markers such as CRP, soluble intercellular adhesion molecule (ICAM-1), and fibrinogen, causes spontaneous platelet aggregation and increases monocyte adhesion to endothelial cells.

Hypertension

Hypertension is often a silent cardiovascular risk factor. The risk increases in the presence of other cardiovascular risk factors such as insulin resistance and obesity. This cluster of metabolic and cardiovascular risk factor is named "Metabolic Syndrome" and includes as well dyslipidemia, protrombotic state and inflammatory state.

Insulin Resistance and Diabetes

Diabetic patients have a greater atherosclerotic burden both in the major arteries and in the microvascular circulation. Insulin resistance also produces a prothrombotic state due to increased levels of PAI-1 and fibrinogen. In addition to these systemic metabolic abnormalities, hyperglycemia causes accumulation of advanced glycation end products inculpated in vascular damage. Furthermore, diabetic patients have markedly impaired endothelial and smooth muscle function and appear to have increased leukocyte adhesion to vascular endothelium, a critical early step in atherogenesis.

Exercise and Obesity

Regular physical exercise reduces myocardial oxygen demand and increases exercise capacity, both of which are associated with lower levels of coronary risk. The mechanisms by which exercise lowers cardiovascular risk remain uncertain but likely include favorable effects on blood pressure weight control, lipid profiles, and improved glucose tolerance. Exercise also improves endothelial function, enhances fibrinolysis, reduces platelet reactivity, and reduces propensity for in situ thrombosis.

Controversy remains as to whether obesity itself is a true risk factor for cardiovascular disease or whether its impact on vascular risk is mediated solely through interrelations with glucose intolerance, insulin resistance, hypertension, physical inactivity, and dyslipidemia.

Mental Stress

The adrenergic stimulation of mental stress can clearly augment myocardial oxygen requirements, can cause coronary vasoconstiction, particularly in atherosclerotic coronary arteries, and hence can influence myocardial oxygen supply as well. Catecholamines can also promote alterations in thrombosis

Estrogen Status

Before menopause, women have lower age-adjusted incidence and mortality rates for coronary heart disease than men. This effect results from beneficial actions of estrogen on lipid fractions, but also is due to direct vascular mechanisms such as improved endothelial-dependent vasomotion, reduced LDL oxidation, altered adhesion molecule levels, increased fibrinolytic capacity, and enhanced glucose metabolism.

Despite these data, exogenous estrogen use among young women as a form of oral contraception is associated with increased rates of intravascular thrombosis; these effects are particularly prominent among smokers.

Several novel markers of atherothrombotic risk have emerged from epidemiological studies and might prove useful clincially.

Homocysteine

Hyperhomocystinemia is linked to atherosclerosis. The mechanisms that account for these effects remain uncertain but may include endothelial toxicity, accelerated oxidation of LDL-C, impairment of endothelial-derived relaxing factor, and reduced flow-mediated arterial vasodilation. Until now there is not agreement on possible role of Homocysteine such as cardiovascular risk factor.

Fibrinogen

Plasma fibrinogen critically influences platelet aggregation and blood viscosity, interacts with plasminogen binding, and in combination with thrombin mediates the final step in clot formation. In addition, fibrinogen associates positively with age, obesity, smoking, diabetes, and LDL-C and inversely with HDL-C, alcohol use, physical activity, and exercise level. Several studies consider fibrinogen an independent marker of risk for coronary heart disease.

Lipoprotein(A)

The normal function of Lp(a) is unknown, the close homology between Lp(a) and plasminogen has raised the possibility that this unusual lipoprotein may inhibit endogenous fibrinolysis by competing with plasminogen for binding on the endothelial surface. More recent data demonstrate accumulation of Lp(a) and co-localization with fibrin within atherosclerotic lesions, both in stable patients and among those with unstable angina pectoris. Apo(a) may also induce monocyte chemotactic activity in the vascular endothelium, whereas Lp(a) may increase release of PAI. Thus, several mechanisms may contribute to a role for Lp(a) in atherothrombosis. Yet, many studies do not establish the importance of Lp (a) as a marker for all future cardiovascular events or whether any increased risk is restricted to those with the highest levels or an absence of other traditional risk factors.

Markers of Fibrinolytic Function

A role for either t-PA or PAI-1 in the development of venous thrombosis remains controversial, by contrast, a highly consistent series of studies have linked abnormalities of fibrinolysis to increased risk of arterial thrombosis. Finally, several studies indicate that levels of D-dimer also predict myocardial infraction, peripheral atherothrombosis, and recurrent coronary events. Despite these data, the clinical use of fibrinolytic markers to determine coronary risk may offer little marginal value.

Markers of Inflammation and Infection

Recently, interest has increased in the possibility that infections, and perhaps chronic infection, may cause atherosclerosis. Inflammation characterizes all phases of atherosclerosis from foam cell formation to plaque progression and rupture.

Actually, there are a lot of data about it; atherosclerotic lesion are heavily infiltred by cellular components associated whit inflammation, expecially lymphocytes (T cells of both the helper (CD4+) and cytotoxic/suppressor(CD8+) immunologically activated), macrophages, and foam cells. it is evident that plaque complexities, especially intraplaque hemorrhages, were connected with the intensity of inflammation; several studies showed a link between baseline elevations of CRP, or other acute phase protein, and the risk of future cardiac events and the evaluation of this marker of infection and inflammation may be of importance for an effective prevention of cardiovascular events.

However, the potential mechanisms of infection-induced atherosclerosis remain speculative.

Inflammation may promote process by acting both directly and indirectly. Infection could indirectly influence this process without infiltrating the artery wall. Host defenses to extravascular infections usually elicit proinflammatory cytokines and stimulate increased expression of cellular adhesion molecules, enhancing leukocyte adhesion. These cytokines could elicit a second wave or "echo" from inflammatory cells already at sites of atherogenesis, such as arterial wall cells or macrophages. Circulating microbial products such as endotoxin can also produce an echo. Similarly, cytokines induced by extravascular infection (specifically interleukin-6) characteristically elicit hepatic synthesis of acute-phase reactants, some of which might promote atheromata complicated by thrombosis. Accordingly, levels of the acute-phase reactant fibrinogen correlate prospectively with risk for coronary events, and plasminogen activator inhibitor can promote clot stability by interfering with fibrinolysis. Still, direct infection of the arterial wall could promote evolution of atherosclerotic lesions or precipitate acute cardiovascular events as suggested by histological findings in unstable coronary plaques evidence of systemic release of thromboxanes and leukotrienes, and the presence of activated circulating leucocytes.

The earliest lesions of atherogenesis consist of altered endothelial permeability (endothelial dysfunction) - can be induced by haemodynamic forces, by a variety of vasoactive substances, by mediators from blood cells, and directly from risk factors for atherosclerosis - with arterial intimal accumulations of leukocytes, foam cells (primarily lipid-laden macrophages) and T lymphocytes intermixed with smooth muscle cells. After crossing the surface of the endothelium, the leukocytes accumulate within the intima. As the process continues, monocytes are converted to activated macrophages and take up oxidized low-density lipoprotein particles, thus becoming foam cells. The formation and accumulation of foam cells within the intima create the fatty streaks of atherosclerotic lesions. If the precipitating risk factors or offending agents are not removed, this process continues and leads to complex lesions. These complex lesions contain layers of smooth muscle, connective tissues, macrophages, and T lymphocytes. The presence of activated T lymphocytes in the atherosclerotic plaque suggests a local immune response, and it has been postulated that such a response may be directed against local antigens in the plaque. Activated T lymphocytes secrete growth factors and cytokines that may affect other cell types and the process of atherosclerosis. Interleukins, complement factor fragments, and tumour necrosis factors (TNF) can enhance monocyte adhesiveness and chemotaxis and so form an amplification mechanism for recruitment of further monocytes into the lesion. Following endothelial adhesion and transmigration into the arterial intima, these cells express markers of activation. Furthermore, released mitogens, such as macrophage derived growth factor, may play a key role in smooth muscle cell migration and subsequent proliferation and hence the progression of plaques. Activation of circulating leucocytes may be facilitated at the endothelium covering an atherosclerotic plaque, with upregulation of adhesion molecules and tethering of circulating cells. These inflammatory responses may further promote the infiltration of activated leucocytes into the atherosclerotic lesion, which in turn may directly activate smooth muscle cells, macrophages, and T cells inside the vessel wall. Lesional macrophages produce proteolytic enzymes which include members of the metalloproteinase family that contributes to weakness of the protective fibrous cap of the plaque and hence promotes the propensity of those plaques to rupture and trigger thrombosis. Over time, fibrous caps, consisting of smooth muscle, collagen, and elastic fibers, form to cover the complex lesions and intrude into the arterial wall. Along with impeding blood flow in the lumen, these fibrous plaques may rupture, causing thrombus formation, plaque progression, or death.

Raised concentrations of low density lipoprotein (LDL) and possibly lipoprotein(a) (Lp(a)) may attract monocytes to adhere to endothelium and induce their transformation into macrophages. The proinflammatory effects of oxidised LDL involve peroxides and other reactive oxygen intermediates generated by the oxidation of LDL. These molecules activate nuclear transcription factor κB (NF-κB), which plays a key role in the orchestration of inflammatory and immune responses by controlling the transcription of the genes encoding several of the adhesion molecules, interleukins, TNFα, class II antigen, and antibodies. NF-κB recognises various activators, among which are the proinflammatory cytokines and CRP.

Most important is the role of cytochines such as tumour necrosis factor α (TNFα) or IL-1 isoforms can stimulate the expression of IL-6, IL-8, and leucocyte-platelet adhesion molecules such as intercellular adhesion molecule (ICAM-1). These cytokines are produced by neutrophils and macrophages which are located in atheromatous plaques. They may be derived from non-vascular sources and reflect generalised inflammatory states, such as chronic infection, which have been linked to atherogenesis and its clinical manifestations. The contribution of vascular and extravascular sources of inflammatory cytokines may vary between individuals. Primary cytokines (TNFα, IL-1) stimulate the production by endothelial and other cells of adhesion molecules, procoagulants, and other mediators that may be released in soluble form into circulating blood. Primary cytokines also stimulate the production of messenger cytokine, IL-6, which induces expression of hepatic genes encoding acute phase reactants found in the blood, including CRP and serum amyloid A. Nonetheless, CRP may activate complement and thus participate in sustaining inflammation. Serum amyloid A can bind to HDL particles, perhaps rendering them less protective against vascular inflammation.

Inflammatory cytokines modulate the homeostatic properties of the endothelium. The local effects of inflammatory cells on digestion of the fibrous cap lead to plaque disruption and thrombus formation. Tissue factor is normally expressed in exposed intima and activates factor VII which in turn activates factors IX and X. Collagen in exposed intima binds von Willebrand factor, which mediates platelet adherence by binding to the glycoprotein Ib/V/IX platelet surface receptor complex under high shear stress conditions. von Willebrand factor itself is the carrier protein for factor VIII, an essential component of the amplifying mechanism of the factor X–Xa conversion. Furthermore, platelets activated by adhesion adhere to the other platelets through the glycoprotein IIb/IIIa receptor and its ligand, von Willebrand factor and fibrinogen. Such activated platelets release PAI-1, which locally inhibits the fibrinolytic mechanism.

Inflammation may promote thrombosis by acting both locally and systemically. Local mechanisms include the cytokine stimulated expression of tissue factor by endothelial cells and macrophages. Indirectly, inflammation may act locally to induce thrombosis by weakening the fibrous cap of the atheromatous plaque, leading to plaque rupture. However, this role of inflammation, and specifically the role of macrophages, remains controversial. Inflammation can affect systemic haemostatic activity by IL-6 mediated stimulation of hepatocytes to produce acute phase reactants. These include certain coagulation factors, such as increased levels of fibrinogen and PAI-1, which induce a prothrombotic state. An enhanced CD40L–CD40 interaction also promotes thrombotic activity by enhancing tissue factor expression in macrophages and through the direct regulation of endothelium procoagulant activity. Intravascular fibrinolysis induced by tissue type plasminogen activator may contribute to atherosclerosis by inducing P-selectin and platelet activating factor, as well as to plaque rupture by activating metalloproteinases. Oxidised LDL also induces tissue factor expression in macrophages and decreases the anticoagulant activity of endothelium by interfering with thrombomodulin expression and inactivating tissue factor pathway inhibitor. Its expression is upregulated in circulating and endothelium adherent monocytes, and tissue factor has been found to be increased in coronary tissue of the culprit lesion from patients with unstable angina.

It is also now accepted that platelets may promote inflammatory responses. Studies have shown that activated platelets may mediate the homing of leucocytes by interaction with the subendothelial matrix under shear stresses that do not allow neutrophil adhesion. They may also contribute to the oxidative modification of LDL, provide a source of lipids for foam cell generation, and contribute to smooth muscle cell proliferation.

Now it is know that the acute cardiovascular events are linked with a non stenotic plaque, but a vulnerable plaque. The difference between the mature and the unstable plaque regard core and fibrous cap. The first consist of two main components, a soft lipid-rich atheromatous gruel and hard collagen-rich sclerotic tissue. The second containing a core of soft atheromatous gruel that is separated from the vascular lumen by a thin cap of fibrous tissue. The fibrous cap is infiltrated by foam indicating ongoing disease activity. Such a thin and macrophage-infiltrated cap is probably very weak and vulnerable, and it was indeed disrupted nearby, explaining why erythrocytes can be seen in the gruel just beneath the macrophage-infiltrated cap. Sclerosis is relatively innocuous because fibrous tissue appears to stabilize plaques, protecting them against disruption. In contrast, the usually less voluminous atheromatous component is the more dangerous component, because the soft atheromatous gruel destabilizes plaques, making them vulnerable to rupture, whereby the highly thrombogenic gruel is exposed to the flowing blood, leading to thrombosis—a potentially life-threatening event.

The risk of plaque disruption is related to intrinsic properties of individual plaques (their vulnerability) and extrinsic forces acting on plaques (rupture triggers). Plaque disruption occurs most frequently where the fibrous cap is thinnest, most heavily infiltrated by foam cells, and therefore weakest. The vulnerability to rupture depends on size and consistency of the atheromatous core, thickness and collagen content of the fibrous cap covering the core, inflammation within the cap and the cap "fatigue" caused by cyclic stretching, compression, bending, flexion, shear, and pressure fluctuations. About the cap's inflammation, an important role had Macrophages that are capable of degrading extracellular matrix by phagocytosis or by secreting proteolytic enzymes such as plasminogen activators and a family of matrix metalloproteinases such as collagenases, gelatinases, and stromelysins that may weaken the fibrous cap, predisposing it to rupture, and also promoting thrombin generation and luminal thrombosis through the tissue factor pathway. Neutrophils are also capable of destroying tissue by secreting proteolytic enzymes, but neutrophils are rare in intact plaques. They may occasionally be found in disrupted plaques beneath coronary thrombi, probably entering these plaques shortly after disruption, and neutrophils may also migrate into the arterial wall shortly after reperfusion of occluded arteries in response to ischemia/reperfusion. The rupture of cap is linked, presumably, with digestion by macrophages but also with senescense or apoptosis of smooth muscle cells caused by inflammatory cytochines.

Coronary plaques are constantly stressed by a variety of biomechanical and hemodynamic forces that may precipitate or "trigger" disruption of vulnerable plaques. The circumferential wall tension (tensile stress) caused by the blood pressure establish a stress which is redistributed to adjacent structures and may be concentrated at critical points; The consistency of the gruel may be important for this stress redistribution, as also the characteristic of cap; actually the thinner the fibrous cap, the higher the stress that develops in it. Furthermore, mechanical shear stresses may develop in plaques at the interface between tissues of different stiffnesses, resulting in shear failure, calcified plates and adjacent noncalcified tissue, for example.

Plaque disruption may occur when increase the intraplaque pressure, caused by vasospam, bleeding from vasa vasorum, plaque edema, and/or collapse of compliant stenoses. Vasospasm reduces the circumferential tension in fibrous caps by narrowing the lumen (Laplace's law). Nevertheless, spasm could theoretically rupture plaques by compressing the atheromatous core, "blowing" the fibrous cap out into the lumen. Bleeding and/or transudation (edema) into plaques from the thin-walled new vessels originating from vasa vasorum and frequently found at the plaque base could theoretically increase the intraplaque pressure, with resultant cap rupture from the inside. The high-grade stenosis may be subjected to strong compressive forces due to the accelerated velocities in the throat. Collapse of severe but compliant stenoses due to negative transmural pressures may produce highly concentrated compressive stresses from buckling of the wall with bending deformation, preferentially involving plaque edges, and theoretically, this could contribute to plaque disruption.

An other factor important for the rupture is the propagating pulse wave during the cardiac cycle that causes changes in lumen size and shape whit deformation and bending of plaques, and particularly of eccentric plaques.

Onset of acute coronary syndromes does not occur at random; actually, a large fraction appear to be triggered by external factors or conditions such as emotional stress, vigorous exercise or cold. The pathophysiological mechanisms responsible for the nonrandom and apparently often triggered onset of infarction are unknown but probably related to (1) plaque disruption, most likely caused by surges in sympathetic activity with a sudden increase in blood pressure, pulse rate, heart contraction, and coronary blood flow; (2) thrombosis, occurring on previously disrupted or intact plaques when the systemic thrombotic tendency is high because of platelet hyperaggregability, hypercoagulability, and/or impaired fibrinolysis ; and (3) vasoconstriction, occurring locally around a coronary plaque or generalized.

The possibility that various microbial agents may trigger a cascade of reactions leading to inflammation, atherogenesis, and thrombotic events in vascular system has been raised in last two decades. Chronic infection with various agents both bacteria and viruses like Chlamydia pneumoniae, CMV, HSV, Helicobacter pylori, Mycoplasma pneumoniae, anaerobic periodontal organisms, etc., have been implicated in the pathogenesis of coronary artery disease. Specific agents have been proposed as direct initiators or accelerators of atherosclerosis, through nonspecific stimulation of the inflammatory cascade. However the role of these infection agents must be proved; actually there is often confounding factors should be carefully considered. Although it is quite plausible that infections may potentiate the action of traditional risk factors.

Chlamydia Pneumoniae

Chlamydia Pneumoniae is an important respiratory pathogen associated with 5% to 10% of community-acquired cases of pneumoniae, pharyngitis, bronchitis, and sinusitis. It is an obligatory intracellular bacterium that has the tendency to cause persistent infection, may drive a chronic inflammatory reaction in coronary vasculature or other tissues. C. pneumoniae has been proposed as an etiologic factor for atherosclerosis, contributing either directly or indirectly, by modifying traditional risk factors.

In particular, cytokines produced by Cp-infected macrophages, located in coronary atherosclerotic plaques, may trigger an ongoing inflammatory response, and thus an increased prothrombotic state and smooth muscle cell proliferation, all of which favor atherothrombotic complications and restenosis after stent. Lines of evidence associating C. pneumoniae with atherosclerosis include seroepidemiologic studies, direct detection of bacterial components in atherosclerotic lesions by Polymerase Chain Reaction or Electron Microscopic studies, occasional isolation of viable organisms from coronary and carotid atheromatous tissue, and in vitro and animal experiments. The strongest evidence associating C. pneumoniae with atherosclerotic CVD has been detection of bacterial components in atherosclerotic lesions. C. pneumoniae appears to have a tropism for atheromata. Besides it is rarely found in normal arteries.

C. pneumoniae may infect circulatory components, which may attach to the endothelium and smooth muscle cells and kill them by apoptosis. The probably molecular mechanism of atherosclerosis pathogenesis can be explained by up-regulation of expression of heat shock protein 60 (HSP-60) by C. pneumoniae infection, which induces production of cytochines such as TNF-a, IL-1β and IL-6, and matrix-degrading metalloproteinases (MMPs) by macrophages. Besides C. pneumoniae could lead to elevation of CRP and contribute to instability or progression of atherosclerotic plaques. The bacterium replicates in endothelial and smooth muscle cells and macrophages, and it can activate CD4+ and CD8+ T lymphocytes. C. pneumoniae initiates inflammatory activation via the nuclear factor-κB pathway, resulting in increased expression of vascular cell adhesion molecule-1,enhancing recruitment of inflammatory leukocytes to the vessel wall, impaired activity of endothelial nitric oxide, increased platelet adhesion to and procoagulant activity in endothelial cells TNF and also caused oxidation of LDL-C. Therefore chronic infection may contribute to the risk of CHD by a high level of immunologic activity by raising triglyceride levels and decreasing HDL levels and by increasing the concentrations of acute-phase reactants such as fibrinogen, C-reactive protein, and sialic acid.

Specific microbial products such as lipopolysaccharides, heat-shock proteins, or other virulence factors might act locally at the level of the artery wall to potentiate atherosclerosis in infected lesions. Extravascular infection might also influence the development of atheromatous lesions and provoke their complication. For example, circulating endotoxin or cytokines produced in response to a remote infection can act locally at the level of the artery wall to promote the activation of vascular cells and of leukocytes in pre-existing lesions, producing an "echo" at the level of the artery wall of a remote infection. Also, the acute phase response to an infection in a nonvascular site might affect the incidence of thrombotic complications of atherosclerosis by increasing fibrinogen or plasminogen activator inhibitor-

1 (PAI-1) or otherwise altering the balance between coagulation and fibrinolysis. Such disturbance in the prevailing prothrombotic, fibrinolytic balance may critically influence whether a given plaque disruption will produce a clinically inapparent transient or nonocclusive thrombus or sustained and occlusive thrombi that could cause an acute coronary event. Acute infections might also produce hemodynamic alterations that could trigger coronary events such as the tachycardia, that increased metabolic demands of fever could augment the oxygen requirements of the heart, precipitating ischemia in an otherwise compensated individual. Infectious processes, either local in the atheroma or extravascular, might aggravate atherogenesis, particularly in preexisting lesions or in concert with traditional risk factors.

The presence of C. pneumoniae in atherosclerotic lesions raises the possibility that antibiotic treatment might have a favourable effect on the course of CAD. However, few of the large randomized antibiotic trials did not show any beneficial effect of long term antibiotic therapy (azithromycin and rifampin) suggesting the large randomized antibiotic trials may not show clinical benefit in patients with established acute or chronic CAD. After failure of antibiotic trials, it was postulated that C. pneumoniae has a pathogenetic role in early development of atherosclerosis. It is possible, therefore, that infection with C pneumoniae is part of the initiation of atherosclerosis early on in life; however, once plaque and inflammation are established, antichlamydial antibiotics can not alter the progression of coronary disease.

Other infectious agents

Specific infectious agents further C. pneumoniae have the potential to play a role in atherosclerosis as demonstrated by experimental models, the presence of organisms within plaque and inflammatory cells, and by seroepidemiologic associations.

Several investigators suggested a role for other bacteria and viruses in cardiovascular disease such as oral infections caused by Porphyromonas gingivalis, Bacteroides forsythus, Campylobacter rectus, Fusobacterium nucleatum, Treponema spp., and Prevotella species. Like C. pneumoniae, oral bacteria might affect atherosclerosis through direct invasion of vascular endothelial cells or indirectly through products that stimulate proinflammatory and prothrombotic functions of vascular cells.

The literature linking H. pylori, HIV, HSV-1, and HSV-2 to atherogenesis is less extensive than for C. pneumoniae or CMV.

CMV, a herpes-family DNA virus, is a common human pathogen and a candidate atherogenic organism. CMV also can accelerate atherosclerosis in animal models. Infection may have induced a systemic inflammatory response that promotes atherosclerosis.

CMV may contribute to CAD by several mechanisms, including impaired fibrinolysis, increased lipoprotein(a), enhanced procoagulant activity, and upregulation of the macrophage oxidized LDL scavenger receptor.CMV can inactivate p53, an apoptosis-related protein, facilitating excessive proliferation of vascular smooth muscle cells.

The presence of any chronic bacterial infection (e.g., respiratory, urinary, dental, or other) increased considerably the risk of developing atherosclerosis.

H. pylori the etiologic organism of peptic ulcer disease, also has received attention as a potential pathogen in atherosclerosis, although the early positive serologic associations have not been confirmed. H. pylori have not been demonstrated in atherosclerotic plaques, nor have animal models demonstrated a pathologic role. However, H. pylori infection can increase CRP and fibrinogen and promote platelet aggregation. Thus, a role for H. pylori in atherogenesis also remains to be established.

Sign and Symptoms

Atherosclerosis is usually asymptomatic until onset of plaque's complication such as growth and critical stenosis, rupture, thrombosis and embolism. The consequence is ischemic heart disease.

Prevention and Therapy

The best way to prevent cardiovascular disease is the prevention of atherosclerosis and its development through removal of risk factor. Statins are the best therapeutic option to modulate inflammation, actually several studies showed their anti-inflammatory, antioxidant and plaque-stabilizing effects than to their cholesterol-lowering effects. In addition treatments to hypertension, diabetes, weight loss, exercise and smoking cessation are most important measures.

References

Antibodies against Chlamydia pneumoniae and their relation to lymphocyte population levels. González-Castañeda C, Pérez-Castrillón JL, Romero-Gómez M, Herreros-Fernández V. *Int. J. Cardiol.* 2002 Mar.

Association between carotid atherosclerosis, inflammatory markers and Chlamydia pneumoniae infection. Kaźmierski R, Podsiadły E, Tylewska-Wierzbanowska S, Kozubski W. *Neurol. Neurochir. Pol.* 2005 Jul-Aug.

Association of infection with coronary artery disease. Rajesh Vijayvergiya. *Indian J. Med. Res.* February 2007

Background and current knowledge of Chlamydia pneumoniae and atherosclerosis. Grayston JT. *J. Infect. Dis.* 2000 Jun.

Braunwald's Heart Disease - A Textbook Of Cardiovascular Medicine. Douglas P. Zipes MD, MACC; Peter Libby MD; Robert O. Bonow MD; Eugene Braunwald MD, MD (Hon), ScD (Hon), FRCP. Elsevier.

Carotid artery atherosclerotic plaque: clinical and morphological-immunohistochemical correlation. Aurunas Lastas; Vida Graziene; Egidijus Barkauskas; Giedrius Salkus; Arvydas Rimkevicius. *Med. Sci. Monit.*, October 2004.

Chlamydia pneumoniae accompanied by inflammation is associated with the progression of atherosclerosis in CAPD patients: a prospective study for 3 years. Kim DK, Kim HJ, Han SH, Lee JE, Moon SJ, Kim BS, Kang SW, Choi KH, Lee HY, Han DS. *Nephrol. Dial. Transplant.* 2007 Oct.

Chlamydia pneumoniae and cytomegalovirus seropositivity, inflammatory markers, and the risk of myocardial infarction at a young age. Gattone M, Iacoviello L, Colombo M, Castelnuovo AD, Soffiantino F, Gramoni A, Picco D, Benedetta M, Giannuzzi P. *Am. Heart J.* 2001 Oct.

Chlamydia pneumoniae antibody response in patients with acute myocardial infarction and their follow-up. Mazzoli S, Tofani N, Fantini A, Semplici F, Bandini F, Salvi A, Vergassola R. *Am. Heart J.* 1998 Jan.

Chlamydia pneumoniae immunoreactivity in coronary artery plaques of patients with acute coronary syndromes and its relation with serology. Liu R, Yamamoto M, Moroi M, Kubota T, Ono T, Funatsu A, Komatsu H, Tsuji T, Hara H, Hara H, Nakamura M, Hirai H, Yamaguchi T. *Am. Heart J.* 2005 Oct.

Chlamydia pneumoniae in the atherosclerotic plaques of patients with unstable angina undergoing coronary artery bypass grafting: does it have prognostic implications? Zamorano J, García-Tejada J, Suárez A, Culebras E, Castañón J, Moreno R, Reguillo F, Gil M, Picazo J, Sánchez-Harguindey L. *Int. J. Cardiol.* 2003 Aug.

Chlamydia pneumoniae Infection and Atherosclerotic Coronary Disease. Rosa Sessa, PhD; Marisa Di Pietro, PhD; Iolanda Santino, MD; Massimo del Piano, MD; Maria Penco, MD; Antonio Varveri, MD; Armando Dagianti, *MD. Am. Heart J,* June 1999.

Chlamydial and human heat shock protein 60 homologues in acute coronary syndromes. (Auto-)immune reactions as a link between infection and atherosclerosis. Andrié R, Braun P, Welsch U, Straube E, Höpp HW, Erdmann E, Lüderitz B, Bauriedel G. Z Kardiol. 2003 Jun.

Chronic Chlamydia pneumoniae infection in patients with coronary disease. Relation with increased fibrinogen values. Fernández-Miranda C, Paz M, Aranda JL, Fuertes A, Gómez De La Cámara A. *Med. Clin.* (Barc). 2002 Nov.

Coinfection with Mycoplasma pneumoniae and Chlamydia pneumoniae in ruptured plaques associated with acute myocardial infarction. Higuchi Mde L, Reis MM, Sambiase NV, Palomino SA, Castelli JB, Gutierrez PS, Aiello VD, Ramires JA. *Arq. Bras. Cardiol.* 2003 Jul.

Comparison of coronary plaque rupture between stable angina and acute myocardial infarction: a three-vessel intravascular ultrasound study in 235 patients. Hong MK, Mintz GS, Lee CW, Kim YH, Lee SW, Song JM, Han KH, Kang DH, Song JK, Kim JJ, Park SW, Park SJ. *Circulation.* 2004 Aug.

Comparison of levels of serum matrix metalloproteinase-9 in patients with acute myocardial infarction versus unstable angina pectoris versus stable angina pectoris. Fukuda D, Shimada K, Tanaka A, Kusuyama T, Yamashita H, Ehara S, Nakamura Y, Kawarabayashi T, Iida H, Yoshiyama M, Yoshikawa J. *Am. J. Cardiol.* 2006 Jan.

Confirmed previous infection with Chlamydia pneumoniae (TWAR) and its presence in early coronary atherosclerosis. Davidson M, Kuo CC, Middaugh JP, Campbell LA, Wang SP, Newman WP 3rd, Finley JC, Grayston JT. *Circulation.* 1998 Aug.

Coronary Plaque Disruption. Erling Falk, MD, PhD; Prediman K. Shah, MD; Valentin Fuster, MD, PhD. Circulation. 1995 American Heart Association, Inc.

Does Chronic Chlamydia pneumoniae Infection Increase the Risk of Myocardial Injury? Insights From Patients With Non-ST-Elevation Acute Coronary Syndromes. Brian Y. L. Wong, MD; Judy Gnarpe, PhD; Koon K. Teo, MB; E. Magnus Ohman, MD; Connie Prosser, PhD; W. Brian Gibler, MD; Anatoly Langer, MD; Wei-Ching Chang, PhD; Paul W. Armstrong, *MD. Am. Heart J.*, June 2002.

High Prevalence of Chlamydia Pneumoniae Antibodies and Increased High-Sensitive C-Reactive Protein in Patients with Vascular Dementia. Hideki Yamamoto; Takuya Watanabe; Akira Miyazaki; Takashi Katagiri; Tsunenori Idei; Takashi Iguchi; Masaru Mimura; Kunitoshi Kamijima. *J. American Geriatric Society* April 2005.

Infection and coronary atherosclerosis: the role Chlamydia pneumonia. Paz M, de Otero J, Codinach P, Ferrer-Ruscalleda F, Gayà M, Ibernón M.. *Rev. Esp. Cardiol.* 1998 Nov.

Infectious Agents In Coronary Atheromas: A Possible Role In The Pathogenesis Of Plaque Rupture And Acute Myocardial Infarction. Maria de Lourdes Higuchi; Jose A. F. Ramires. Rev. Inst. Med. trop. S. Paulo vol.44 no.4 São Paulo July/Aug. 2002

Infectious features of atherosclerosis. Wyplosz B, Capron L. Med Sci (Paris). 2004 Feb.

Inflammatory and thrombotic mechanisms in coronary atherosclerosis. D. Tousoulis; G. Davies; C. Stefanadis; P. Toutouzas; J.A. Ambrose. *Heart*. 2003 September.

Intima-media thickening and asymptomatic carotid plaque as markers of future cerebro- and cardiovascular events. Prof. S. Novo , Prof. F. Gennaro. *E-Journal of Cardiology Practice.*

Involvement of Chlamydia pneumoniae in Atherosclerosis: More Evidence for Lack of Evidence. Margareta M. Ieven; Vicky Y. Hoymans. *Journal of Clinical Microbiology*, January 2005.

Joint Effects of Chlamydia Pneumoniae Infection and Classic Coronary Risk Factors on Risk of Acute Myocardial Infarction. Kunihiro Kinjo, MD; Hiroshi Sato, MD; Hideyuki Sato, MD; Yozo Ohnishi, MD; Eiji Hishida, MD; Daisaku Nakatani, MD; Hiroya Mizuno, MD; Nobuhisa Ohgitani, MD; Mitsuaki Kubo, MD; Takashi Shimazu, MD; Noriyuki Akehi, MD; Hiroshi Takeda, MD; Masatsugu Hori, MD; Osaka Acute Coronary Insufficiency Study (OACIS) *Group. Am. Heart J.*, August 2003

Markers of Inflammation and Infection Influence the Outcome of Patients With Baseline Asymptomatic Carotid Lesions. Egle Corrado, MD; Manfredi Rizzo, MD; Rosalba Tantillo, MD; Ida Muratori, MD; Francesca Bonura, MD; Giustina Vitale, MD Salvatore Novo, MD. *Stroke.* 2006 American Heart Association, Inc.

Metabolic Syndrome, C-Reactive Protein, and Prognosis in Patients With Established Coronary Artery Disease. David Aguilar, MD; Marian R. Fisher, PhD; Christopher M. O'Connor, MD; Michael W. Dunne, MD; Joseph B. Muhlestein, MD; Louis Yao, MD; Sandeep Gupta, MD; Rebecca J. Benner, PhD; Thomas D. Cook, PhD; Dearborn Edwards, MD; Marc A. Pfeffer, MD, *PhD. Am. Heart J.*, September 2006.

Mycoplasma pneumoniae and Chlamydia pneumoniae are associated to inflammation and rupture of the atherosclerotic coronary plaques. Ramires JA, Higuchi Mde L. *Rev. Esp. Cardiol.* 2002.

Novel Risk Factors for Atherosclerotic Disease. Lauren S. Schlesselman, PhD. Conference Coverage, January 2001.

Potential Infectious Etiologies of Atherosclerosis: A Multifactorial Perspective. Siobhán O'Connor; Christopher Taylor; Lee Ann Campbell; Stephen Epstein; Peter Libby. *Emerg. Infect .Dis.*, September 2001.

Presence and severity of Chlamydia pneumoniae and Cytomegalovirus infection in coronary plaques are associated with acute coronary syndromes. Liu R, Moroi M, Yamamoto M, Kubota T, Ono T, Funatsu A, Komatsu H, Tsuji T, Hara H, Hara H, Nakamura M, Hirai H, Yamaguchi T. *Int. Heart J.* 2006 Jul.

Prevalence of Chlamydia pneumoniae in the atherosclerotic plaque of patients with unstable angina and its relation with serology. Zamorano J, Suarez A, Garcia Tejada J, Culebras E, Castañón J, Picazo J, Moreno R, Sanchez-Harguindey L. *Int. J. Cardiol.* 2003 Jun.

Relation of secretory phospholipase A(2) and high-sensitivity C-reactive protein to Chlamydia pneumoniae infection in acute coronary syndromes. Miya N, Oguchi S, Watanabe I, Kanmatsuse K. *Circ J.* 2004 Jul.

Rupture of the atherosclerotic plaque: is chlamydia an possible agent? Fazio G, Sutera L, Zito R, Cascio C, Briguglia D, Taormina S, Giammanco A, Assennato P, Novo S. G Ital. Cardiol. (Rome). 2006 Dec

Serologic Markers of Persistent Chlamydia Pneumonia Infection and Long-Term Prognosis After Successful Coronary Stenting. Michael N. Zairis, MD; Olga A. Papadaki, MD; Paraskevi K. Psarogianni, MD; Maria A. Thoma, MD; George K. Andrikopoulos, MD; Pelagia C. Batika, RN; Christina G. Poulopoulou, MD; Kyriaki G. Trifinopoulou, MD; Christopher D. Olympios, MD; Stefanos G. Foussas, MD, FESC, FACC. *Am. Heart J.*, December 2003.

The Role of Infection in the Pathogenesis of Cardiovascular Disease. James S. Zebrack, MD, Jeffrey L. Anderson, *MD. Prog. Cardiovasc. Nurs.*, January 2003.

Using statins to treat inflammation in acute coronary syndromes: are we there yet?. Mehdi H. Shishehbor, DO, MPH; Taral Patel, MD; Deepak l. Bhatt, MD. *Cleveland Clinic Journal Of Medicine* August 2006.

Viewpoint: Chlamydia pneumonia and Heart Disease: Are Antibiotics Protective? Jacqueline A. Hart, MD. Medscape Family Medicine September 2005.

Vulnerable Atherosclerotic Plaque. A Multifocal Disease. Ward Casscells, MD; Morteza Naghavi, MD; James T. Willerson, MD. Circulation. 2003 American Heart Association, Inc.

In: Angina Pectoris: Etiology, Pathogenesis and Treatment   ISBN: 978-1-60456-674-1
Editors: A. P. Gallo, M. L. Jones   © 2008 Nova Science Publishers, Inc.

Chapter XI

Nitrate Tolerance and Cross-Tolerance in Long-Term Treatment of Patients with Stable Angina Pectoris

Marek A. Kosmicki [*]

Second Department of Coronary Artery Disease, Institute of Cardiology;
ul.Spartanska 1; PL.02-637 Warszawa, Poland

Descriptive Abstract

Nitrates, apart from beta-blockers and calcium antagonists, are the mainstays of antianginal drug therapy in patients with stable angina pectoris. All patients with angina should receive a prescription for sublingual nitroglycerin (NTG) and instructions on its use. The pharmacological and physiological benefits of nitrates in coronary artery disease, and also some potentially harmful mechanisms are discussed in the paper. Organic nitrates are considered as valuable symptomatic agents, improving the quality of life of patients with angina pectoris. Although, these nitrates are effective anti-anginal drugs during initial treatment, their therapeutic value is compromised by the rapid development of tolerance during sustained therapy. Thus, their major disadvantage is connected with the occurrence of tolerance, which means that their clinical efficacy is decreased during long-term use. A widely accepted method of preventing tolerance is intermittent administration. Sublingual tablets or sprays are suitable for the immediate relief of effort or rest angina and can be used prophylactically before exercise. In patients with stable angina treated with high doses of oral nitrates in long-term therapy, sublingual NTG maintains its full anti-ischemic effect both after initial oral ingestion and after intermittent long-term oral administration (eg once daily). However, sublingual NTG attenuates this effect during continuous treatment (eg administration every 6h), when tolerance to oral nitrates occurs, and this is called cross-tolerance between sublingual and long-lasting nitrates. The relationship between nitrate tolerance and cross-tolerance is a positive phenomenon. Thus, when high doses of nitrates in sustained-release medications are chosen, they should be given once daily. This method of

[*] Tel. (+4822) 3434016; Tel./Fax (+4822) 8449510; E-mail: Marek.7372069@pharmanet.com.pl.

treatment should be used not only to maintain antianginal efficacy of nitrate in the prophylaxis of angina pectoris, but also to effectively relieve angina after sublingual NTG ingestion during chest pain. Long-acting nitrates are considered third-line therapy because a nitrate-free interval is required to avoid the development of tolerance. Therefore, nitrates should be considered for patients who cannot tolerate or fail to respond adequately to beta-blockers and calcium antagonists. All long-acting nitrates seem to be equally effective, but the duration of antianginal effects of pentaerythritol tetranitrate (PETN) in lower doses are not known. A relatively recent development is the suggestion that organic nitrates vary considerably in their potential to induce the development of tolerance. In particular, it has been suggested that PETN may induce minimal release of a superoxide anion, and hence may result in minimal tolerance. During long-lasting nitrate therapy (except PETN), one can observe the development of reactive oxygen species (ROS) inside the muscular cell of a vessel wall, and these bind with nitric oxide (NO). This leads to decreased NO activity, thus, nitrate tolerance. PETN has no tendency to form ROS, and therefore nitrate tolerance is absent. One would expect that prolonged exposure to PETN does not lead to diminution of responses to other organic nitrates such as sublingual NTG. Thus, during long-term PETN therapy, there is probably no tolerance or cross-tolerance, as during treatment with other organic nitrates.

Abbreviations and Acronyms

ALDH2 or mtALDH	= mitochondrial aldehyde dehydrogenase-2
cGMP	= cyclic guanosine monophosphate
ECG	= electrocardiogram
ISDN	= isosorbide dinitrate
IS-2-MN	= isosorbide-2-mononitrate
IS-5-MN	= isosorbide-5-mononitrate
MASS-II study	= The medicine, angioplasty, or surgery study
NO	= nitric oxide
NOS	= endothelial nitric oxide synthase
NTG	= nitroglycerin
$\cdot O_2^-$	= vascular superoxide anion
PCI	= percutaneous coronary intervention
PETN	= pentaerythritol tetranitrate
ROS	= reactive oxygen species

Introduction

Myocardial ischemia, which produces angina pectoris, the principal symptom of coronary heart disease, results from a relative lack of coronary blood flow, generally due to partial obstruction of a large coronary artery. Atherosclerotic fixed obstruction is often worsened in a given patient by superimposed spasm, whereas collateral coronary blood flow into the ischemic area is variable from time to time as well as from patient to patient. Both the typical and variant (vasospastic or Prinzmetal's) forms of angina may be manifested by sudden, severe, pressing substernal pain that radiates to the left shoulder and along the flexor surface of the left arm. However, the location and character of chest pain may vary.

Typical angina pectoris (stable angina) is commonly induced by exercise, emotion, or eating and is often associated with depression of the ST segment of the electrocardiogram (ECG). Typical angina is usually due to advanced atherosclerosis of the coronary vasculature. In contrast, variant angina is caused by vasospasm of the coronary vessels and may not be associated with severe atherosclerosis. Patients with Prinzmetal's angina may develop chest pain while at rest and exhibit elevation of the ST segment of the ECG.

Anginal attacks may recur for years or may rapidly increase in their frequency (unstable angina). They result from temporary ischemia of the myocardium, such that blood flow is insufficient to maintain adequate oxygenation. This can be due to a decrease in myocardial blood flow, an increase in the requirement of the myocardium for oxygen, or both. Thus, myocardial ischemia results from an imbalance between myocardial oxygen supply and demand. Factors that influence energy supply and energy demand in the myocardium were showed in figure 1.

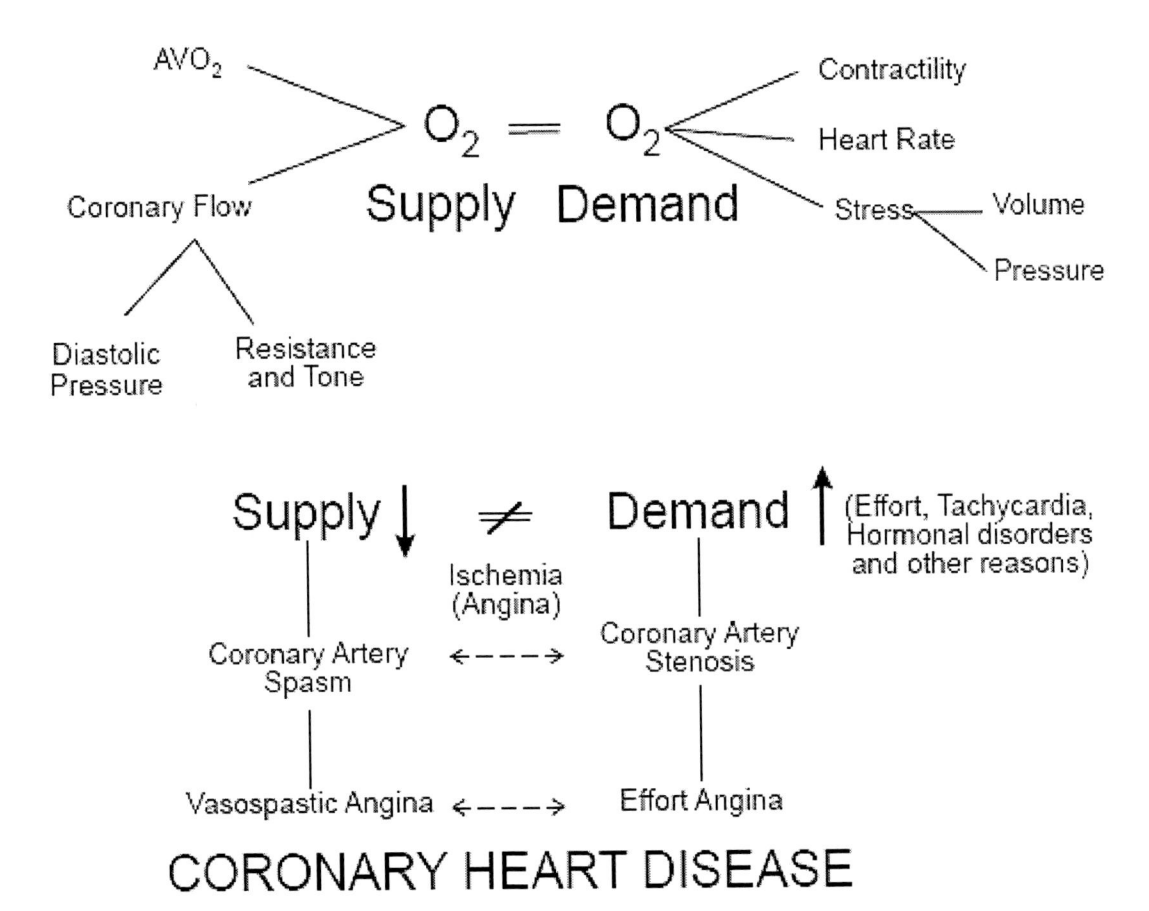

Figure 1. Physiology and pathophysiology of coronary circulation. (AVO_2 = arteriovenous oxygen content difference).

Figure 1. illustrates that an imbalance between oxygen supply and demand can result from a diminished supply in the face of normal demands or increased demands that outstrip the blood supply. Primary, or variant, angina represents 'primary' decrease in the energy supply usually the result of a vasospastic problem. Secondary, or typical, angina represents a 'secondary' increase in myocardial oxygen demands exceeding the blood supply, thus resulting in myocardial ischemia.

The goals of pharmacological treatment of stable angina pectoris are to improve quality of life by reducing the severity and/or frequency of symptoms and to improve the prognosis of the patient. Pharmacotherapy is a viable alternative to invasive strategies for the treatment of most patients with stable angina pectoris and was actually associated with fewer complications than surgery or percutaneous coronary intervention (PCI) during a 1-year follow-up of MASS-II study [1]. An invasive treatment strategy may be reserved for patients at high risk or patients with symptoms that are poorly controlled by medical treatment.

The strategy for pharmacological relief of angina is based on improvement of the balance between myocardial oxygen supply and demand. For typical exertional angina (stable angina), this necessitates increasing the blood flow to heart or decreasing its work load. Treatment of variant angina is directed at reduction of vasospasm of the coronary vessels. Thus, symptoms of angina pectoris and signs of ischemia (also silent ischemia) may be reduced by drugs that reduce myocardial oxygen demand and/or increase blood flow to the ischemic area. Commonly used antianginal drugs are beta-blockers, calcium antagonists, and organic nitrates [2,3].

This chapter deals with some problems of organic nitrates. They have been for many years the cornerstone of antianginal therapy. However, nitrates have been also a source of numerous controversies related to their real efficacy and the mode of administration. The major controversies are connected with the occurrence of tolerance, and cross-tolerance which means that their clinical efficacy is decreased during long-term use.

History of Organic Nitrates

Organic nitrates have been used in the treatment of angina pectoris for over one hundred years. Nitroglycerin (NTG) was first synthesized in 1846 by Ascanio Sobrero, who observed that a small quantity of the oily substance placed on the tongue elicited a severe headache. Constantin Hering, in 1847, developed the sublingual dosage form for NTG, which he advocated for a number of diseases. The eminent English physician T. Lauder Brunton was unable to relieve severe recurrent anginal pain except when he bled his patient, and he believed that phlebotomy provided relief by lowering arterial blood pressure. The concept that reduced cardiac afterload and work are beneficial continues to present day. In 1857, Brunton administered amyl nitrite, a known vasodepressor, by inhalation, and he noted that anginal pain was relieved within 30 to 60 seconds. The action of amyl nitrite was transitory, however, and the dosage was difficult to adjust.

NTG was used by Alfred Nobel to manufacture dynamite. It was in Nobel's dynamite factories in the late 1860s that the antianginal effect of NTG was discovered. Two interesting observations were made. First, factory workers on Monday mornings often complained of headaches that disappeared over the weekends. Second, factory workers suffering from angina pectoris or heart failure often experienced relief from chest pain during the work week, but which recurred on weekends. Both effects were attributed to the vasodilator action of NTG, which quickly became apparent to the physicians and physiologists in local communities.

In 1879, William Murrell decided that the action of NTG mimicked that of amyl nitrite, he established the use of sublingual NTG for relief of the acute anginal attack and as a prophylactic agent to be taken prior to exertion [4]. Recently its antianginal efficacy following sublingual administration has been well established [5].

The other organic nitrates such as isosorbide dinitrate (ISDN), erythrityl tetranitrate, pentaerythritol tetranitrate (PETN) and manitol hexanitrate were developed and introduced into clinical practice when it was realized that the effect of sublingual NTG is short-lasting and that the effect of oral NTG is limited and unpredictable. ISDN, developed by Krantz in the first part of 20th century [6], has been used, like NTG, to relieve anginal symptoms. This agent can be administered by various routes, and in oral administration it has been confirmed as an effective antianginal drug [7]. Later, when the pharmacokinetic profile of the various nitrates was better understood and the therapeutic requirements in different cardiovascular diseases were better defined, new agents, such mononitrates, were developed and studied.

The use of organic nitrates in prophylactic clinical practice has largely been delayed by a conclusion made by group of investigators and reported first in 1972 and repeated thereafter. Needleman and co-workers [8] reported that orally administered organic nitrates were ineffective because of complete first-pass hepatic metabolism. Based on this thesis the use of long-acting organic nitrates declined markedly. It took almost a decade until the pharmacokinetic and pharmacodynamic profiles of ISDN and its metabolites (mononitrates) were fully understood. Only then was it possible for Needleman's thesis to be rejected on a strong scientific basis [9].

Isosorbide-5-mononitrate (IS-5-MN) is one of two major metabolites of ISDN, the other being isosorbide-2-mononitrate (IS-2-MN). It was initially pursued as a clinically useful agent as a result of suggestions that vascular effects of the parent drug were comparatively minor compared to those of these two metabolites. Subsequent work demonstrated that all three compounds are pharmacologically active and that elimination half-life of IS-5-MN is considerably longer than either the parent drug or the alternative metabolite. It has a number of advantages over ISDN including better absorption after oral administration and lack of first-pass hepatic metabolism. IS-5-MN was released in Germany in 1981 and has been widely used in clinical practice in Europe and in the other continents since than [10,11].

Nicorandil is an agent with a double cellular mechanism of action, acting both as a potassium channel activator and as a nitrate [3]. Therefore, it can be expected to cause less tolerance than nitrates do, and also cross-tolerance with classical nitrates does not seem to be a problem. In Japan, nicorandil is a standard antianginal drug, but it is not available in all countries.

The empirical observation that organic nitrates could be used safely for the rapid, dramatic alleviation of the symptoms of angina pectoris led to their widespread acceptance by the medical profession. However, in 1999 Nakamura et al. [12] have suggested that nitrate therapy may worsen the prognosis and survival in ischemic heart disease, although further studies are required to confirm these findings.

Recently nitrates, apart from beta-blockers and calcium antagonists, are still the mainstays of antianginal drug therapy. According to present European and American guidelines, all patients with angina should receive a prescription for sublingual NTG and instructions on its use. Long-acting nitrates should be considered for patients who cannot tolerate or fail to respond adequately to beta-blockers and calcium antagonists [2,3,13].

Chemistry of Organic Nitrates

Organic nitrates are polyol esters of nitric acid, whereas organic nitrites are esters of nitrous acid. Nitrate esters (-C-O-NO$_2$) and nitrite esters (-C-O-NO) are characterized by a sequence of carbon-oxygen-nitrogen, whereas nitro compounds possess carbon-nitrogen bonds (C-NO$_2$). Thus, glyceryl trinitrate is not a 'nitro' compound, and it is erroneously called nitroglycerin (NTG). However, this nomenclature is both widespread and official. Chemical structures of some organic nitrates of pharmacological interest were showed in figure 2.

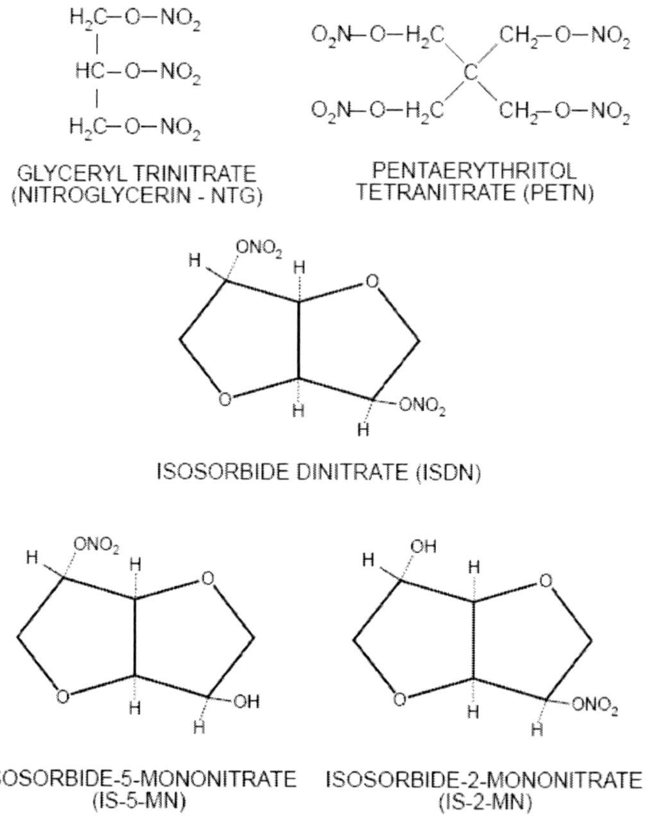

Figure 2. Chemical structures of some organic nitrates of pharmacological interest.

Amyl nitrite is a highly volatile liquid that is administered by inhalation. Organic nitrates of low molecular weight (such as NTG) are moderately volatile, oily liquids, whereas the high-molecular-weight nitrate esters (e.g., erythrityl tetranitrate, PETN, ISDN) are solids. The fully nitrated polyols are lipid soluble, whereas their incompletely nitrated metabolites are soluble in water. In the pure form (without an inert carrier such as lactose), NTG is explosive. The organic nitrates and nitrites and several other compounds that are capable of conversion to nitric oxide (NO) have been collectively termed 'nitrovasodilators'. NO is thought to be the active intermediate in the action of this broad class of agents [14].

Cardiovascular Effects

The action of organic nitrates is to relax vascular smooth muscle. Their vasodilator effects are evident in both systemic arteries (including coronary) and veins in normal subjects and in patients with ischemic heart disease, but they appear to be predominant in the venous circulation.

The venodilator effect reduces ventricular preload, which in turn reduces myocardial wall tension and O_2 requirements. The action of nitrates in reducing both preload and afterload makes them useful in the treatment of heart failure, as well as angina pectoris [15]. By reducing the heart's mechanical activity, volume, and O_2 consumption, in patients with exertional angina, nitrates improve exercise tolerance and extend the time to onset of angina and ischemia during exertion. When used in combination with calcium antagonists and/or beta-blockers, the antianginal effects appear greater.

Nitrates can reduce or reverse coronary vasospasm [16]. Thus, patients with primarily vasospastic angina or a large vasoconstrictor component to their angina can benefit from the direct coronary action of nitrate therapy.

Nitrates also indirectly improve subendocardial blood flow as the reduction in left ventricular end-diastolic pressure induced by systemic venous dilatation decreases the resistance to coronary blood flow from epicardium to endocardium [17]. In addition, nitrates may lower the resistance to collateral vessel blood flow [18].

Nitrates have also an antithrombotic and antiplatelet effect. However, the clinical importance of these potentially beneficial effects is unclear [19]. Stimulation of platelet guanylate cyclase by nitrates prevents fibrinogen binding to platelet IIb/IIIa receptors, which is essential for platelet aggregation [20]. Transdermal nitroglycerin has been shown to inhibit platelet aggregation and thrombus formation in patients with angina [21].

Mechanism of Action of Nitrates

In the late 1970s and early 1980s, the vasodilator effect of NTG was discovered to be caused by NO, which was apparently generated from NTG in vascular smooth muscle [22-24]. These early observations on NO culminated less than 10 years later, in 1986, with the discovery that mammalian cells synthesize NO [25]. NO has been shown to be an extremely important signaling molecule in the cardiovascular system. In 1998, about 130 years after

Alfred Nobel's invention of dynamite and the first observed clinical benefit of NTG, Furchgott, Ignarro and Murad were awarded the Nobel Prize in Medicine and Physiology "for their discoveries concerning nitric oxide as a signaling molecule in the cardiovascular system". Despite these achievements, the precise molecular mechanism by which NO is generated from nitroglycerin remained elusive until the work of Chen et al. [26].

Previous studies showed that the bioactivation of NTG somehow involved thiols or sulfhydryl-containing compounds, and that NO or NO-containing compounds constituted the biologically active species [22-25,27]. The earliest studies suggested that an interaction between nitroglycerin and sulfhydryl (-SH)-containing cellular receptors was necessary for vascular smooth muscle relaxation to occur and that repeated administration of nitroglycerin caused sulfhydryl depletion (via oxidation) and consequent tolerance to further vasodilation [27-29]. Subsequent studies addressing the activation of cytosolic guanylate cyclase by organic nitrate esters (nitroglycerin), organic nitrite esters (isoamyl nitrite), and nitroso compounds revealed that a chemical reaction occurred between the nitro compound and a thiol to generate an intermediate *S*-nitrosothiol, which then decomposed with the liberation of NO [24]. Tolerance to NTG was explained simply by thiol utilization and depletion in the presence of excess nitroglycerin, thereby resulting in deficient production of *S*-nitrosothiol and NO. This working hypothesis was supported by animal and clinical studies showing that the administration of relatively large doses of cysteine or *N*-acetylcysteine could prevent or reverse the tolerance to the vasodilator action of repeated administration of NTG. There were many unanswered questions associated with these earlier studies, however. The molecular mechanism of the interaction between nitroglycerin and thiol to generate *S*-nitrosothiol and NO remained an enigma. Moreover, the basis of the earlier hypotheses was activation of cytosolic guanylate cyclase in enzyme reaction mixtures and not vascular smooth muscle relaxation [24]. Isolated enzyme reaction mixtures or broken cell preparations are very different from intact cells or tissues. The early work with cellular extracts did not address the likely possibility that the reaction between nitroglycerin and thiol might be enzymatic in nature. In fact, the evidence was in favor of a nonenzymatic chemical reaction [24]. Subsequent studies suggested that one or more enzymatic mechanisms might be responsible for the bioactivation of NTG [30-36]. However, none of these enzyme systems could catalyze the selective formation of 1,2-glyceryl dinitrate from NTG and no correlation could be found between tolerance to NTG action and tolerance to enzyme activities. Chen et al. [26] uncovered the role of mitochondrial aldehyde dehydrogenase-2 (ALDH2 or mtALDH), which specifically generates 1,2-glyceryl dinitrate from NTG, in the bioactivation of NTG to elicit vasorelaxation and in the development of tolerance to NTG.

Chen et al. [26] used several ingenious approaches to elucidate the enzymatic mechanism of bioactivation of nitroglycerin: a source of large numbers of cells so that the lack of starting material would not be a limiting factor. By using mouse macrophages grown in cell culture, physiologically relevant, relatively low concentrations of nitroglycerin (0.1 μM) were shown to generate 1,2-glyceryl dinitrate through the catalytic action of an enzyme that was virtually identical to mouse mtALDH. ALDH2 purified from bovine liver showed identical catalytic properties to the mouse enzyme. Inhibitors of mtALDH, such as cyanamide and chloral hydrate, blocked the formation of 1,2-glyceryl dinitrate from nitroglycerin. ALDH2 possesses esterase activity [37] in addition to the classical NAD^+-dependent dehydrogenation activity, and the catalytic action on NTG was analogous to its esterase activity, with the important exception that nitrite (NO_2^-) rather than nitrate (NO_3^-) was a product of the enzymatic reaction. Thus, these observations were in agreement with the earliest biological findings that NTG is metabolized by tissues to inorganic nitrite or NO_2^- [24-25,27-29]. The classical sulfhydryl requirement for vascular smooth muscle relaxation by NTG [27] was explained as a chemical reaction between nitroglycerin and thiol sulfhydryl group to generate an intermediate *S*-nitrosothiol species, which then decomposed with the liberation of NO [24]. Other explanations and hypotheses were offered, but none of them could be replicated or confirmed across different tissues [38,39]. Therefore, the selective conversion of 1,2,3-glyceryl trinitrate (nitroglycerin) to 1,2-glyceryl dinitrate plus nitrite, together with the dependence on a reducing thiol cofactor, made mtALDH a compelling choice for the elusive enzyme pathway responsible for NTG bioactivation in vascular smooth muscle [40].

Nitrate Tolerance

The organic nitrates are effective antianginal drugs during initial treatment, but their therapeutic value is compromised by the rapid development of tolerance during sustained therapy. This means that repeated and prolonged administration of NTG and other organic nitrate esters causes the development of desensitization of vascular smooth muscle to further vasorelaxation by nitrates. This phenomenon has become a serious limitation to the chronic use of organic nitrate esters to treat angina pectoris. Thus, the potential for gradual attenuation of the pharmacological and therapeutic effects of organic nitrates during prolonged, and particularly continuous therapy, commonly designated 'nitrate tolerance' induction, represents the Achilles heel of this group of drugs [41]. Numerous studies have shown that acute administration of various organic nitrates leads to impressive amelioration of myocardial ischaemia, and there is increasing evidence that they may play a pivotal role in the initial management of acute pulmonary oedema [42,43]. On the other hand, after prolonged administration of many, if not all, organic nitrates, beneficial effect is minimal [44].

Mechanisms of Nitrate Tolerance

How nitrate tolerance occurs is incompletely understood. It is due to attenuation of the vascular effect of nitrates, not to altered pharmacokinetics [15]. Understanding the molecular mechanisms associated with the development of 'nitroglycerin tolerance' would undoubtedly lead to the discovery either of ways to avoid tolerance or of new NO-generating drugs that do not cause tolerance. At least several, not mutually exclusive, mechanisms have been proposed to explain the development of nitrate tolerance – see table 1.

Accumulating data support the hypothesis that increased generation of vascular superoxide anion ($\cdot O_2^-$) is central to the process of nitrate tolerance [45,46]. There are multiple possible contributors to generation of oxygen free radicals, including effects of NTG on endothelial nitric oxide synthase (NOS) and counterregulatory neurohormonal activation.

Table 1. Proposed mechanisms of nitrate tolerance [26,45-53]

1. Increased generation of vascular superoxide anion ($\cdot O_2^-$) [45,46]
2. Plasma volume expansion [46]
3. Impaired biotransformation of nitrates to NO [26,47]
4. Decreased end-oxygen responsiveness to NO [48-50]
5. Neurohormonal activation [46,51-53]

The consequences of increased superoxide anion formation are also multiple and include plausible links to many of the proposed mechanisms of nitrate tolerance.

Several studies reported that nitrate therapy causes plasma volume expansion. This observation led to the hypothesis that increased circulating volume and, subsequently, filing pressures, would counteract the NTG-induced decrease in preload, thus causing nitrate tolerance [46].

Impaired biotransformation of nitrates to NO is nitrate-specific and is not seen with non-nitrate sources of NO such as nitroprusside [47]. Consistent with this theory are the experimental observations that there is no tolerance to the effect of S-nitrosothiols and that the activity of mtALDH, the enzyme required for metabolism of nitrates to 1,2-glyceryl dinitrate in markedly reduced [26]. The same findings can be induced by inhibitors of mtALDH [26]. Chen *et al.* [26] demonstrated that in vascular tissue made tolerant to the vasorelaxant effect of NTG, a comparable decrease occurs in both mtALDH activity and tissue cyclic guanosine monophosphate (cGMP) accumulation [26]. Consistent with this observation is the report that mtALDH activity is markedly inhibited in patients undergoing chronic administration of NTG and other organic nitrate esters [39]. These findings also are consistent with previous reports that NTG tolerance in patients can sometimes be overcome by administration of *N*-acetylcysteine [25,47]. Chen *et al.* [26] showed that mtALDH is at least partially responsible for the bioactivation of NTG and is likely to be the target of nitroglycerin tolerance. Moreover, by understanding the molecular mechanism of nitroglycerin bioactivation and tolerance, it may now be possible to design and develop novel nitrovasodilator drugs that do not cause tolerance. One approach might be to develop drugs that do not engage mtALDH for the generation of NO. Ideally, the most appropriate kind of NO-donor drug might be one that is targeted to an enzyme that is selectively distributed to the vascular smooth muscle and acts as a substrate with only limited capacity to inhibit catalytic activity. Such a drug would be an effective vasodilator that could be used in combination with other drugs for the symptomatic treatment of hypertension. To be useful for the symptomatic treatment of angina pectoris, however, the drug would need to be targeted more to venous than arterial smooth muscle. Despite the desire to avoid tolerance, it may be a difficult task, indeed, to come up with an overall better antianginal drug than the 130-year-old NTG [40]. A relatively recent development is the suggestion that organic nitrates vary considerably in their potential to induce the development of tolerance. In particular, it has been suggested that PETN and possibly nicorandil may induce minimal release of superoxide anion, and hence minimal tolerance [41].

Consistent with a theory of decreased end-oxygen responsiveness to NO [48] is the finding in an animal study that vascular and hemodynamic tolerance to nitrates occurred despite high levels of NO and rates of NO formation that were similar in those animals that were not tolerant [49]. Also in support of this hypothesis is that transgenic animals that overexpress NOS have chronically elevated NO release, which is associated with reduced vascular reactivity to NO-mediated vasodilators [50].

Neurohormonal activation means an activation of the vasoconstrictor renin-angiotensin-aldosterone and sympathetic nervous systems in response to nitrate-induced vasodilation [51,52]. There is also increased peripheral sensitivity to these vasoconstrictors, an effect that can be reversed by angiotensin converting enzyme inhibition [51]. Abnormal coronary vasoconstrictor responses have also been described with continuous nitrate exposure [53].

A secondary implication of these emerging findings is that extended treatment with organic nitrates may have unfavorable consequences (free radical generation, endothelial dysfunction, and sympathetic activation) that could adversely affect long-term clinical outcomes. Such data raise a cautionary note that warrants additional investigation.

Prevention of Nitrate Toleance

The major drawback of long-term nitrate therapy is the development of tolerance. However, nitrate sensitivity in patients can be restored daily after a nitrate-free period of 8-12 hours [54-55]. Therefore, the only widely accepted method of preventing tolerance is the use of intermittent administration, independently of the type of preparation or route of administration [56-61].

Authors most frequently state that nitrate administration should be at 8 to 12 hour intervals, without specifying to what extent the length of interval is dependent on the type of nitrate and its pharmaceutical form and its dose [56-61]. However, in one study [62] it was showed that an almost linear dependence can be found between the duration of nitrate-free interval and the level of dose in oral administration of ISDN in sustained-release form. It should be 12 hr. nitrate-free interval for ISDN 40 mg; 18 hr. for ISDN 80 mg and 24 hr. for ISDN 120 mg.

There are, however, two concerns regarding intermittent therapy:

1. A time-zero effect, which refers to a deterioration in exercise performance relative to placebo prior to the morning dose of nitrates.
2. Rebound angina, which refers to an increase in angina during the nitrate-free interval. There may result from a supersensitivity of the vessel wall to vasoconstrictors [63] or an increased vasomotor response to acetylcholine, suggesting the development of endothelial dysfunction [64].

Whether these effects occur to a clinically significant degree remains unclear [60]. Several other methods have been proposed to reduce nitrate tolerance, although none is as yet used clinically. Among them it could be mentioned, that co administration of nitrates with other vasodilators, such as captopril and hydralazine, may avoid the development of nitrate tolerance in patients with congestive heart failure [61].

Cross-Tolerance

Nitrate tolerance is still an important limiting factor in the treatment of coronary heart disease. An additional clinical problem, which has not been fully resolved, is whether the development of tolerance to one organic nitrate in sustained therapy is connected with significant attenuation of the acute anti-ischemic effects of sublingual NTG. This is particularly relevant, because nitrate tolerance not only causes a decrease in the effectiveness of nitrates in the prevention of chest pain, but it may also restrict the effects of sublingual nitrates during anginal attacks. While nitrate tolerance is a widely known and treatable phenomenon, cross-tolerance, which can develop during concomitant therapy with two nitrate formulas, is less frequently acknowledged [41,55,65].

A recent development is the suggestion that cross-tolerance exists and could be clinically important [65]. Initial exposure to either ISDN or NTG led to marked prolongation of time to development of ischemic ECG changes; furthermore the acute effects of these agents were additive. Chronic continuous exposure to ISDN led to abolition of anti-ischemic effects, with simultaneous loss of effects of sublingual NTG. This demonstration cross-tolerance between ISDN and NTG is clinical evidence for the potentially damaging implications of this problem [65].

If the suggestion that PETN and possibly nicorandil may induce minimal tolerance is true, one would expect that prolonged exposure to PETN or nicorandil

would not lead to diminution of responses to other organic nitrates such as NTG (that is, there would be no 'cross-tolerance'). However, further studies are needed to confirm this suggestion.

Conclusion

A major problem with the use of nitrates is the development of nitrate tolerance, which has been demonstrated with all forms of nitrate administration delivering continuous, relatively stable blood levels of the drug. Several mechanisms of nitrate tolerance have been proposed. One of them is the hypothesis that increased generation of vascular superoxide anion is central to the process. However, there is the suggestion that PETN and possibly nicorandil may induce minimal tolerance. The only practical strategy to manage nitrate tolerance is to prevent it by providing a 'nitrate-free' interval. The optimal interval should be not shorter than 12-hour. A common form of nitrate withdrawal (rebound) is observed in patients whose angina is intensified after discontinuation of large doses of long-acting nitrates. Concomitant administration of other anti-anginal drugs could be resolution of the problem. In patients with stable angina treated with high doses of oral nitrates in long-term therapy, sublingual NTG maintains its full anti-ischemic effect both after initial oral ingestion and after intermittent long-term oral administration. However, sublingual NTG attenuates this effect during continuous treatment, when tolerance to oral nitrates occurs, and this is called cross-tolerance between sublingual and long-lasting nitrates. Long-acting nitrates are considered third-line therapy because a nitrate-free interval is required to avoid the development of tolerance. Therefore, nitrates should be considered for patients who cannot tolerate or fail to respond adequately to beta-blockers and calcium antagonists.

References

[1] Hueb, W., Soares, P.R., Gersh, B.J., Cesar, L.A., Luz, P.L., Puig, L.B. et al. (2004). The medicine, angioplasty, or surgery study (MASS-II): a randomized, controlled clinical trial of three therapeutic strategies for multivessel coronary artery disease: 1 year results. *J Am Coll Cardiol, 43,* 1743-1751.

[2] Fox, K., Garcia, M.A.A., Ardissino, D., Buszman, P., Camici, P.G., Crea, F., Daly, C., De Backer, G., Hjemdahl, P., Lopez-Sendon, J., Marco, J., Morais, J., Pepper, J., Sechtem, U., Simoons, M. & Thygesen, K. (2006). The Task Force on the Management of Stable Angina Pectoris of the European Society of Cardiology. Guidelines on the management of stable angina pectoris: executive summary. *Eur Heart J, 27,* 1341-1381. doi:10.1093/eurheartj/ehl001.

[3] Fox, K., Garcia, M.A.A., Ardissino, D., Buszman, P., Camici, P.G., Crea, F., Daly, C., De Backer, G., Hjemdahl, P., Lopez-Sendon, J., Marco, J., Morais, J., Pepper, J., Sechtem, U., Simoons, M. & Thygesen, K. (2006). The Task Force on the Management of Stable Angina Pectoris of the European Society of Cardiology. Guidelines on the management of stable angina pectoris: full text. *Eur Heart J,* doi:10.1093 /eurheartj /ehl002.

[4] Murrell, W. (1879). Nitro-glycerine as a remedy for angina pectoris. *Lancet, 1,* 80-1, 113-5, 151-2, 225-7, 284, 642-6.

[5] Wight, L.J., VandenBurg, M.J., Potter, C.E. & Freeth, C.J. (1992). A large scale comparative study in general practice with nitroglycerin spray and tablet formulations in elderly patients with angina pectoris. *Eur J Clin Pharmacol, 42,* 341-342.

[6] Krantz, J.C., Carr, C.J., Forman, S.E., et al. (1940). Mechanism and action of organic nitrates. *J Pharmacol Exp Ther, 70,* 323-327.

[7] Thadani, U., Fung, H-L., Drake, A.C., et al. (1982). Oral isosorbide dinitrate in angina pectoris: comparison of duration of action and dose-response relation during acute and sustained therapy. *Am J Cardiol, 49,* 411-419.

[8] Needleman, P., Land, S. & Johnson, E.M. (1972). Organic nitrates: Relationship between biotransformation and rational angina pectoris therapy. *J Pharmacol Exp Ther, 182,* 56-62.

[9] Schneeweiss, A. & Weiss, M. (1988). *Advances in nitrate therapy.* Berlin Heidelberg: Springer-Verlag.

[10] Tauchert, M. & Jansen, W. (1986). Development of mononitrates. *Cardiology, 74(suppl 1),* 3-5.

[11] Rezakovic, Dz.E. & Alpert, J.S. (1993). *Nitrate therapy and nitrate tolerance: Current concepts and controversies.* Basel: S. Karger AG.

[12] Nakamura, Y., Moss, A.J., Brown, M.W., Kinoshita, M. & Kawai, C. (1999). Long-term nitrate use may be deleterious in ischemic heart disease: A study using the

databases from two large-scale postinfarction studies. Multicenter Myocardial Ischemia Research Group. *Am Heart J, 138,* 577-585.

[13] Fihn, S.D., Williams, S.V., Daley, J. & Gibbons, R.J. (2001). Guidelines for the management of patients with chronic stable angina: treatment. *Ann Intern Med,135,* 616-632.

[14] Murad, F. (1986). Cyclic guanosine monophosphate as a mediator of vasodilation. *J Clin Invest, 78,* 1-5.

[15] Parker, J.D. & Parker, J.O. (1998). Nitrate therapy for stable angina pectoris. *N Engl J Med, 338,* 520-531.

[16] Ginsburg, R., Lamb, I., Schroeder, J.S., et al. (1982). Randomized double-blind comparison of nifedipine and isosorbide dinitrate therapy in variant angina pectoris due to coronary arterial spasm. *Am Heart J, 103,* 44-48.

[17] Bache, R.J., Ball, R.M., Cobb, F.R., et al. (1975). Effects of nitroglycerin on transmural myocardial blood flow in the unanesthetized dog. *J Clin Invest, 55,* 1219-1228.

[18] Cohen, M.V., Downey, J.M., Sonnenblick, E.H. & Kirk, E.S. (1973). The effects of nitroglycerin on coronary collaterals and myocardial contractility. *J Clin Invest, 52,* 2836-2847.

[19] Knight, C.J., Pansear, M., Wilson, D.J., et al. (1997). Different effects of calcium antagonists, nitrates, and beta blockers on platelet function. Possible importance for the treatment of unstable angina. *Circulation, 95,* 125-132.

[20] Loscalzo, J. (1992). Antiplatelet and antithrombotic effects of organic nitrates. *Am J Cardiol, 70,* 18B-22B.

[21] Lacoste, L., Theroux, P., Lidon, R., Colucci, R. & Lam, J.Y.T. (1994). Antithrombotic properties of transdermal nitroglycerin in stable angina pectoris. *Am J Cardiol, 73,* 1058-1062.

[22] Arnold, W. P., Mittal, C. K., Katsuki, S. & Murad, F. (1977). Nitric oxide activates guanylate cyclase and increases guanosine 3':5'-cyclic monophosphate levels in various tissue preparations. *Proc Natl Acad Sci USA, 74,* 3203-3207.

[23] Murad, F., Mittal, C. K., Arnold, W. P., Katsuki, S. & Kimura, H. (1978). Guanylate cyclase: activation by azide, nitro compounds, nitric oxide, and hydroxyl radical and inhibition by hemoglobin and myoglobin. *Adv Cyclic Nucleotide Res, 9,* 145-158.

[24] Ignarro, L. J., Lippton, H., Edwards, J. C., Baricos, W. H., Hyman, A. L., Kadowitz, P. J. & Gruetter, C. A. (1981). Endothelium-drived relaxing factor produced and released from artery and vein is nitric oxide. *Pharmacol Exp Ther, 218,* 739-749.

[25] Ignarro, L. J. (1989). Biological actions and properties of endothelium-derived nitric oxide formed and released from artery and vein. *Circ Res, 65,* 1-21.

[26] Chen, Z., Zhang, J. & Stamler, J. S. (2002). Identification of the enzymatic mechanism of nitroglycerin bioactivation. *Proc Natl Acad Sci USA, 99,* 8306-8311.

[27] Needleman, P., Jakschik, B. & Johnson, E. M., Jr. (1973). Sulfhydryl requirement for relaxation of vascular smooth muscle. *J Pharmacol Exp Ther, 187,* 324-331.

[28] Needleman, P. (1976). Organic nitrate metabolism. *Annu Rev Pharmacol, 16,* 81-93.

[29] Tsuchida, S., Maki, T. & Sato, K. (1990). Purification and characterization of glutathione transferases with an activity toward nitroglycerin from human aorta and heart: Multiplicity of the human class Mu forms. *J Biol Chem, 265,* 7150-7157.

[30] Yeates, R. A., Schmid, M. & Leitold, M. (1989). Antagonism of glyceryl trinitrate activity by an inhibitor of glutathione S-transferase. *Biochem Pharmacol, 38*, 1749-1753.

[31] Millar, T. M. , Stevens, C. R. , Benjamin, N. , Eisenthal, R. , Harrison, R. & Blake, D. R. (1998). Xanthine oxidoreductase catalyses the reduction of nitrates and nitrite to nitric oxide under hypoxic conditions. *FEBS Lett, 427*, 225-228.

[32] McDonald, B. J. & Bennett, B. M. (1990). Cytochrome P-450-mediated biotransformation of organic. nitrates. *Can J Physiol Pharmacol, 68*, 1552-1557.

[33] McDonald, B. J. & Bennett, B. M. (1993). Biotransformation of glyceryl trinitrate by rat aortic. cytochrome P450. *Biochem Pharmacol, 45*, 268-270.

[34] Seth, P. & Fung, H. L. (1993). Biochemical characterization of a membrane-bound enzyme responsible for generating nitric oxide from nitroglycerin in vascular smooth muscle cells. *Biochem Pharmacol, 46*, 1481-1486.

[35] McGuire, J. J., Anderson, D. J., McDonald, B. J., Narayanasami, R. & Bennett, B. M. (1998). Inhibition of NADPH-cytochrome P450 reductase and glyceryl trinitrate biotransformation by diphenyleneiodonium sulfate. *Biochem Pharmacol, 56*, 881-893.

[36] Mukerjee, N. & Pietruszko, R. (1994). Inactivation of human aldehyde dehydrogenase by isosorbide dinitrate. *J Biol Chem, 269*, 21664-21669.

[37] Boesgaard, S., Aldershville, J., Poulsen, H. E., Loft, S., Anderson, M. E. & Meister, A. (1994). Nitrate tolerance in vivo is not associated with depletion of arterial or venous thiol levels. *Circ Res, 74*, 115-120.

[38] Munzel, T., Sayegh, H., Freeman, B. A., Tarpey, M. M. & Harrison, D. G. (1995). Evidence for enhanced vascular superoxide anion production in nitrate tolerance: a novel mechanism underlying tolerance and cross-tolerance. *J Clin Invest, 95*, 187-194.

[39] Towell, J., Garthwaite, T. & Wang, R. (1985). Erythrocyte aldehyde dehydrogenase and disulfiram-like side effects of hypoglycemics and antianginals. *Alcohol Clin Exp Re, 9*, 438-442.

[40] Ignarro, L. J. (2002). After 130 years, the molecular mechanism of action of nitroglycerin is revealed. *Proc Natl Acad Sci USA, 99*, 7816-7817.

[41] Horowitz, J.D. (2004). Tolerance induction during therapy with long-acting nitrates: how extensive is the "collateral damage"? *Cardiovasc Drugs Ther, 18*, 11-12.

[42] Cotter, G., Metzkor, E., Kaluski, E., et al. (1998). Randomised trial of high-dose isosorbide dinitrate plus low-dose furosemide versus high-dose furosemide plus low-dose isosorbide dinitrate in severe pulmonary oedema. *Lancet, 351*, 389–393.

[43] Beltrame, J.F., Zeitz, C.J., Unger, S.A., et al. (1998). Nitrate therapy is an alternative to morphine-furosemide therapy in the management of acute cardiogenic pulmonary edema. *J Card Fail, 4*, 271–279.

[44] ISIS 4. (1995). A randomised factorial trial assessing early oral captopril, oral mononitrate, and intravenous magnesium sulphate in 58,050 patients with suspected acute myocardial infarction. *Lancet, 345*, 669–685.

[45] Gori T. & Parker J.D. (2002). The puzzle of nitrate tolerance: pieces smaller than we though? *Circulation, 106*, 2404-2408.

[46] Gori T. & Parker J.D. (2002). Nitrate tolerance: a unifying hypothesis. *Circulation, 106,* 2510-2513.

[47] Sage, P. R., de la Lande, I. S., Stafford, I., Bennett, C. L., Phillipov, G., Stubberfield, J. & Horowitz, J. D. (2000). Nitroglycerin tolerance in human vessels: evidence for impaired nitroglycerin bioconversion. *Circulation, 102,* 2810-2815.

[48] Mangione, N.J., Glasser, S.P. (1994). Phenomenon of nitrate tolerance. *Am Heart J, 128,* 137-146.

[49] Laursen, J.B., Mulsch, A., Boesgaard, S., et al. (1996). In vivo nitrate tolerance is not associated with reduced bioconversion of nitroglycerin to nitric oxide. *Circulation, 94,* 2241-2247.

[50] Ohashi, Y., Kawashima, S., Hirata, Ki., et al. (1998). Hypotension and reduced nitric oxide-elicited vasorelaxation in transgenic mice overexpressing endothelial nitric oxide synthetase. *J Clin Invest, 102,* 2061-2071.

[51] Heitzer, T., Just, H., Brockhoff, C., et al. (1998). Long-term nitroglycerin treatment is associated with supersensitivity to vasoconstrictors in men with stable coronary artery disease: Prevention by concomitant treatment with captopril. *J Am Coll Cardiol, 31,* 83-88.

[52] Parker, J.O. & Parker, J.D. (1992). Neurohormonal activation during nitrate therapy: A possible mechanism for tolerance. *Am J Cardiol, 70,* 93B-97B.

[53] Caramori, P.R.A., Adelman, A.G., Azevedo, E., et al. (1998). Therapy with nitroglycerine increases coronary vasoconstriction in response to acetylcholine. *J Am Coll Cardiol, 32,* 1969-1974.

[54] Parker, J. Farrell, B. Lahey, K. et al. (1987). Effect of intervals between doses on the development of tolerance to isosorbide dinitrate. *N Engl J Med, 316,* 1440-1444.

[55] Elkayam, U. (1991). Tolerance to organic nitrates: evidence, mechanisms, clinical relevance, and strategies for prevention. *Ann Intern Med, 114,* 667-677.

[56] Fung, H.L., McNiff, E.F., Ruggirello, D. et al. (1981). Kinetics of isosorbide dinitrate and relationship to pharmacological effects. *Br J Clin Pharmacol, 11,* 579-90.

[57] Glasser, S.P. (1999). Prospects for therapy of nitrate tolerance. *Lancet, 353,* 1545-6.

[58] Amsterdam, E.A. (1992). Rationale for intermittent nitrate therapy. *Am J Cardiol, 70,* 55G-59G; Discussion 59G-60 G.

[59] Parker, J.O., Amies, M.H., Hawkinson, R.W. et al., and the Minitran Efficacy Study Group. (1995). Intermittent transdermal nitroglycerin therapy in angina pectoris clinically effective without tolerance or rebound. *Circulation, 91,* 1368-74.

[60] Glasser, S.P. (1998). Clinical mechanisms of nitrate action. *Am J Cardiol, 81(1A),* 49A-53A.

[61] Fung, H.L. (1993). Clinical pharmacology of organic nitrates. *Am J Cardiol, 72,* 9C-13C; discussion 14C-15C.

[62] Kosmicki, M., Sadowski, Z., Szwed, H. & Kowalik, I. (2000). What intervals in oral therapy of isosorbide dinitrate in various doses are sufficient to prevent nitrate tolerance? *Med Sci Monit, 6,* 763-768.

[63] Hebert, D. & Lam, J.Y. (2000). Nitroglycerin rebound associated with vascular, rather than platelet, hypersensitivity. *J Am Coll Cardiol, 36,* 2311-2316.

[64] Azevedo, E.R., Schofield, A.M., Kelly, S. & Parker, J.D. (2001). Nitroglycerin withdrawal increases endothelium-dependent vasomotor response to acetylcholine. *J Am Coll Cardiol, 37*, 505-509.

[65] Kosmicki, M.A., Szwed, H. & Sadowski, Z. (2004). Anti-ischemic response to sublingual nitroglycerin during oral administration of isosorbide dinitrate in patients with stable angina pectoris: when does cross–tolerance occur? *Cardiovasc Drugs Ther, 18*, 47-55.

In: Angina Pectoris: Etiology, Pathogenesis and Treatment
Editors: A. P. Gallo, M. L. Jones

ISBN: 978-1-60456-674-1
© 2008 Nova Science Publishers, Inc.

Chapter XII

Tako-Tsubo-Like Left Ventricular Dysfunction: Transient Left Ventricular Apical Ballooning Syndrome

E. Vizzardi, * *G. Zanini, E. Antonioli, I. Bonadei, C. Fiorina, E. Chiari,
A. D'Aloia, S. Nodari, and L. Dei Cas*
Section of Cardiovascular Disease. Department of Applied Experimental Medicine.
Department of Cardiology. Brescia, University Study of Brescia, Italy

Introduction

Tako-tsubo cardiomyopathy (TC) is a recently described acute cardiac syndrome that mimics acute myocardial infarction and is characterized by ischemic chest symptoms, an elevated ST segment on electrocardiogram, increase levels of cardiac disease markers and transient left apical and middle ventricular walls disfunction (apical "ballooning"). In contrast to the acute coronary arterial syndromes (ACS), patients with TC have no angiographically detectable or nonobstructive coronary arterial disease [1]

This syndrome can be triggered by profound psychological stress and is also known as "stress cardiomyopathy" or "broken-heart syndrome" [2]

The TC was initially recognized in the Japanese population (first described in 1991) but has recently been reported in the USA and Europe.[3] The term "tako-tsubo" was proposed by Dote et al and means "fishing pot for trapping octopus," and the left ventricle disfunction, in this syndrome, resembles that shape [4] (Figure 1). The true prevalence of the apical ballooning syndrome remains uncertain. In the last few years, the number of published reports of patients presenting with this syndrome is constantly increasing. Only six series

* Corrispondine author: Dott Vizzardi Enrico, Department of Cardiology, University of Brescia Italy, Pzzle Spedali Civili 1 25124 Brescia, Tel 049303995659, Email: enrico.vizzardi@tin.it.

assessed the prevalence of this syndrome among consecutive patients presenting with suspected ACS.

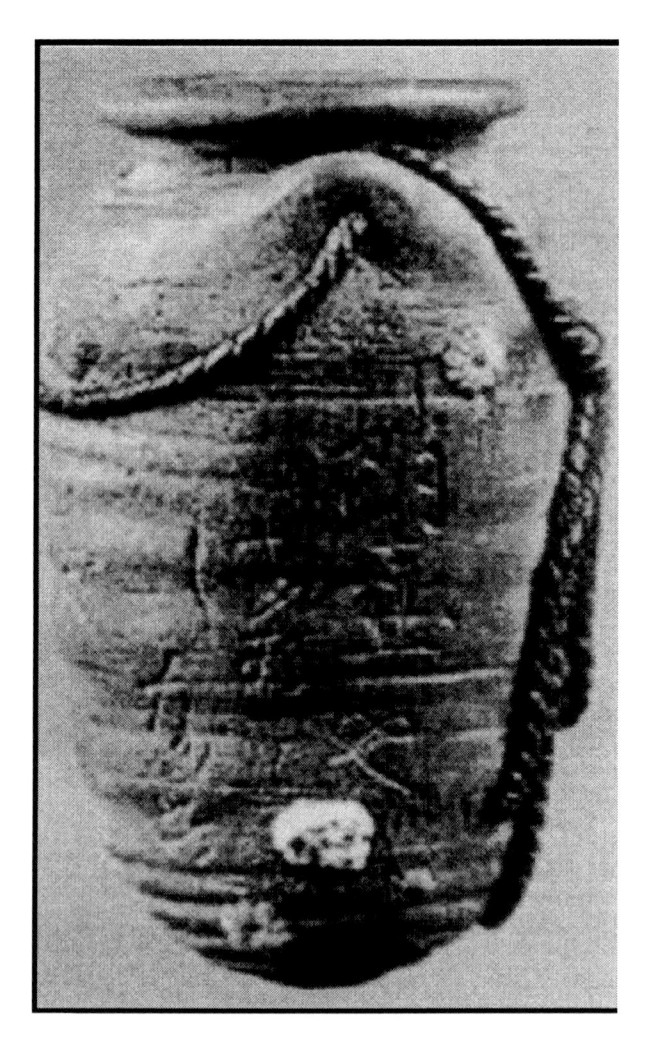

Figure 1. an antique TakoTsubo.

Klinceva M et al. evaluated the prevalence of stress-induced myocardial stunning during a four-year period (2002-2005), and it was estimated as 0.07% and the annual population incidence of this disorder was as 0.00006%;[5] also Pillière et al. assess same results [6]. In a study from the USA, Bybee et al. [7] reported that the apical ballooning syndrome accounted for 2.2% of the ST-segment elevation ACS presenting to the investigators' institution. Three series evaluated the prevalence of this syndrome in Japan. Among patients presenting with suspected ACS, Ito et al. [8] reported that the apical ballooning syndrome accounted for 1.7% of cases and Matsuoka et al. [9] for 2.2%. Akashi et al. [10] diagnosed apical ballooning syndrome in 2.0% of patients with sudden onset of heart failure and abnormal Q waves or ST-T changes suggestive of acute MI on admission.

This cardiomyopathy has been documented prevalently postmenopausal women of an advanced age and the explanation for this gender and age incidence is still unresolved.[11]

Table 1.

Physical stress (60%)
External injury
Heavy labor
Travel
Electrophysiologic study
Emotional stress (35%)
Human relations
Death of spouse
Public performance
Medical examination (5%)

In a recent review, Gianni et al.[1] reported a history of hypertension in 43% of patients, diabetes in 11.0%, dyslipidaemia in 25.45% and current or past smoking in 23%. The most common presenting clinical symptoms were chest pain and dyspnoea. Chest pain was reported to be a cardinal presenting symptom in 67.8%, and dyspnoea in 17.8%. However, more serious clinical presentations such as cardiogenic shock and ventricular fibrillation are frequent, 4.2% and 1.5% respectively. In one case there was a fatal left ventricular rupture.[12] Isolated cases of syncope as the presenting symptom have been reported[7].

The onset of the transient LV apical ballooning syndrome is often preceded by emotional or physical stress. An emotional stressor, such as unexpected death of a relative or friend, domestic abuse, a catastrophic medical diagnosis, devastating business, or gambling losses, was identified and a physical stressor, such as exhausting work, asthma attack, gastric endoscopy, and exacerbated systemic disorders in about 70% (Table 1). However in 30% there was no preceding emotional or physical stressful event identified.

Electrocardiographic Features and Cardiac Biomarkers

Electrocardiographic changes in the acute phase comprise ST-elevations. These elevations may be present only for several hours. Then, normalization of the ST- segment occurs, followed by negative T-waves in V1-V6, I and aVL, which persist for weeks to months. The QT interval is initially often prolonged and may shorten over weeks.[13,14] ST-elevation was detected in 81.6%,, usually involving the precordial leads (83.9%); T wave abnormalities were seen in 64.3% patients and Q waves were present in 31.8% patients. Only rarely ST – depression and the development of Q waves have been observed [15] (Figure 2A e 2B). Six studies measured serum levels of troponin I and three CK-MB fraction levels. Troponin I was positive in 86.2% and CK-MB levels were elevated in 73.9% However, in this particular syndrome cardiac biomarker levels were usually only slightly elevated compared to the extension of segment involved with a rapid decrease to normal enzymatic plasmatic level suggesting a reversible myocardial dysfunction, compared to the ordinary kinetic of a "normal" acute myocardial infarction.

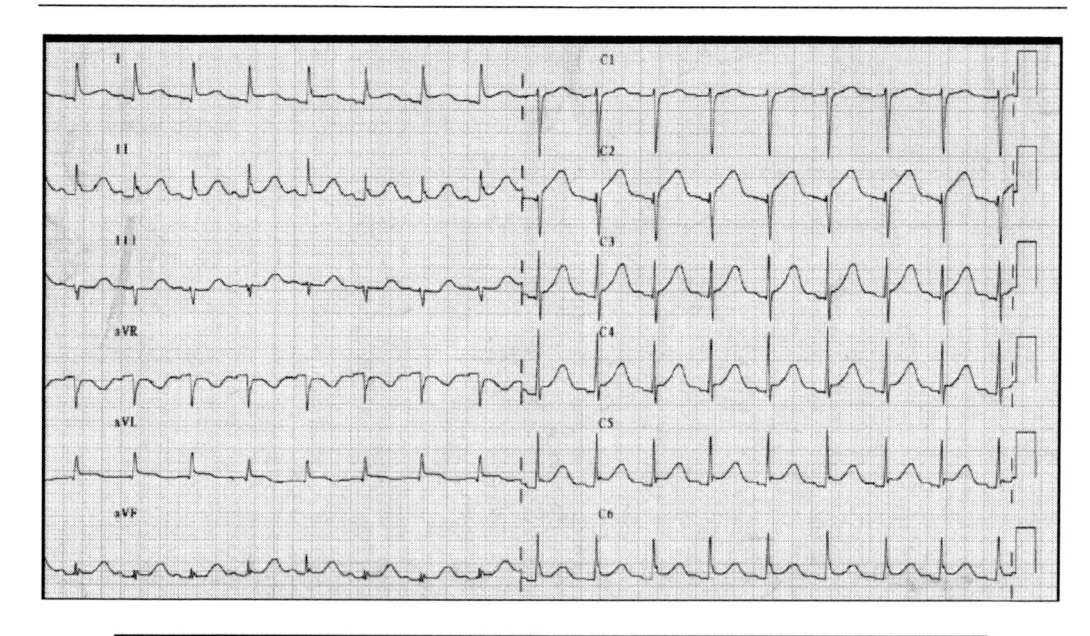

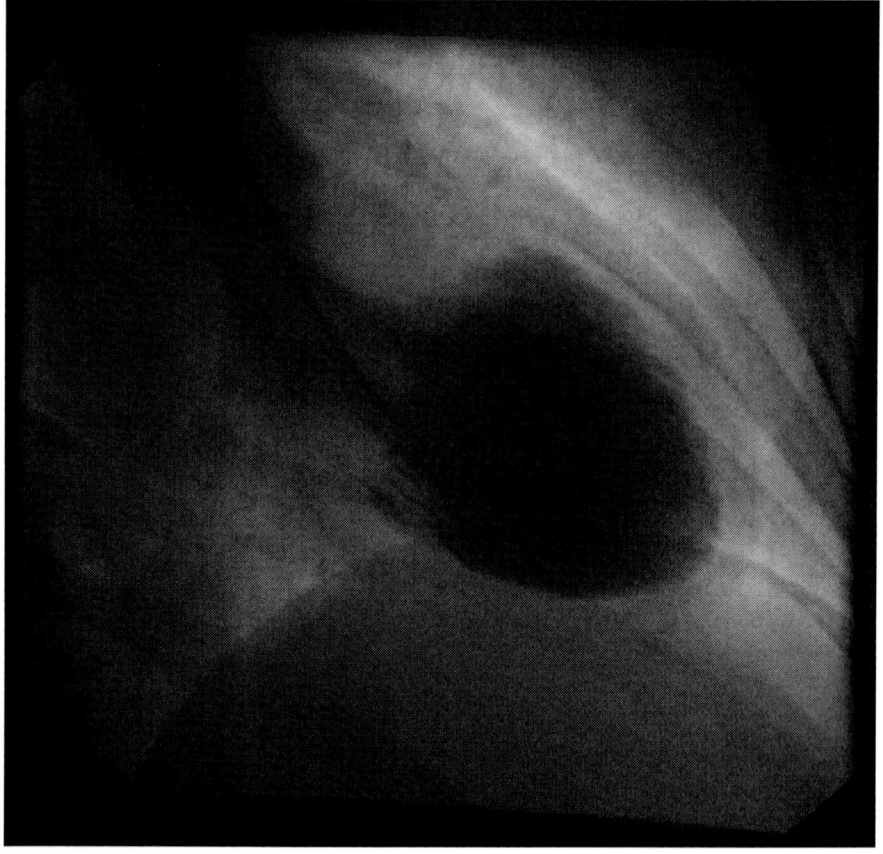

Figure 2A-2B. example of tako-tsubo syndrome electrocardiogram of one patient at admission and demission.

Frequently, an increase of plasma brain natriuretic peptide can be observed in the acute phase[10] but is not associated with a poor prognosis in this condition.[16]

Cardiac Catheterization and Echocardiography

The coronary angiographic pattern usually shows the absence of coronary disease or only mild coronary atherosclerosis (<50%); coronary spasm may be visible or may be provoked by acetylcholine or ergonovine administration in up to 80% of patients.[17] Left ventriculography documents akinesis in the apical, diaphragmatic and/or anterolateral segments, and hyperkinesis in the basal segments (Figure 3A/3B). According to the proposed diagnostic criteria, demonstration of ruptured atherosclerotic plaques in the major coronary arteries by angiography or intracoronary ultrasound examination (IVUS) formally excludes tako-tsubo.

During the acute phase, all patients had an abnormal left ventricular ejection fraction (mean, 0.39 to 0.49) that improve rapidly over a period of days to weeks (mean follow- up left ventricular ejection fraction, 0.60 to 0.76).[18]

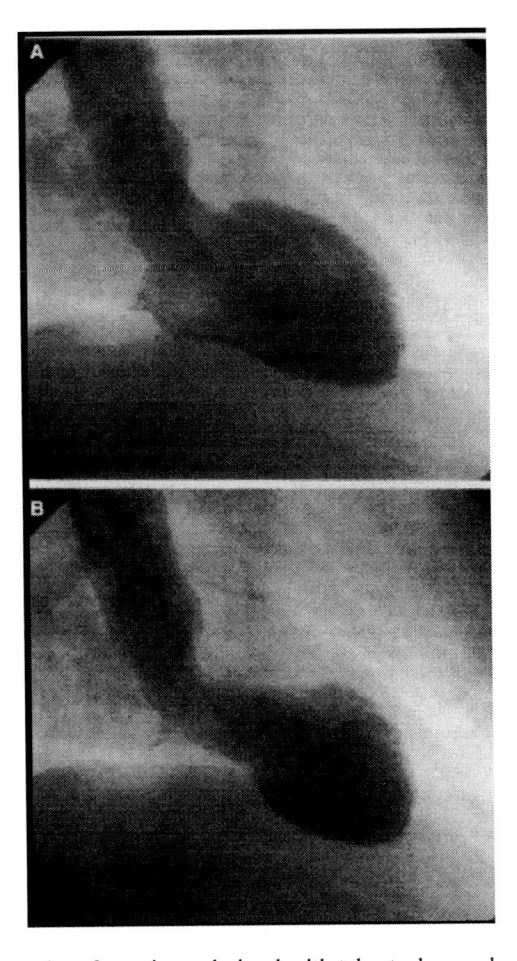

Figure 3A-3B. Ventriculography of a patient admitted with tako-tsubo syndrome.

Echocardiogram shows also the apical ballooning of the left ventricle akinesis or diskinesis with the basal function preserved or hyperkinetic (Figure 4). The akinesia is more extensive than the area supplied by any one coronary vessel.[19] Occasionally, a left intraventricular gradient with high velocity in the basal segment may be detected.[20] Mid-ventricle and apical wall-motion abnormalities completely resolved in all surviving patients.

Some studies evidenced that reversible right ventricular dysfunction is common in this syndrome and involves about one-quarter of patients. Its presence seems to be associated with a more severe impairment in LV function. Pleural effusion, especially when significant or bilateral, is a reliable clinical indicator of RV involvement.[21]

Clinical experience with cardiovascular magnetic resonance (CMR) in this entity is still limited. CMR may be a valuable tool in the diagnosis work up of patients with classical as well as variant tako-tsubo cardiomyopathy and seems to be superior to echocardiography in this regard, not only providing information on extent and reversibility of left ventricular wall motion abnormality but may be useful in differentiating this entity from entities with similar clinical presentation such as myocardial infarction and myocarditis which commonly exhibit typical patterns of delayed hyperenhancement. Furthermore, absence of delayed hyperenhancement indicates good functional recovery.[22] There was some criteria for the clinical diagnosis of tako-tsubo syndrome (see Table 2).

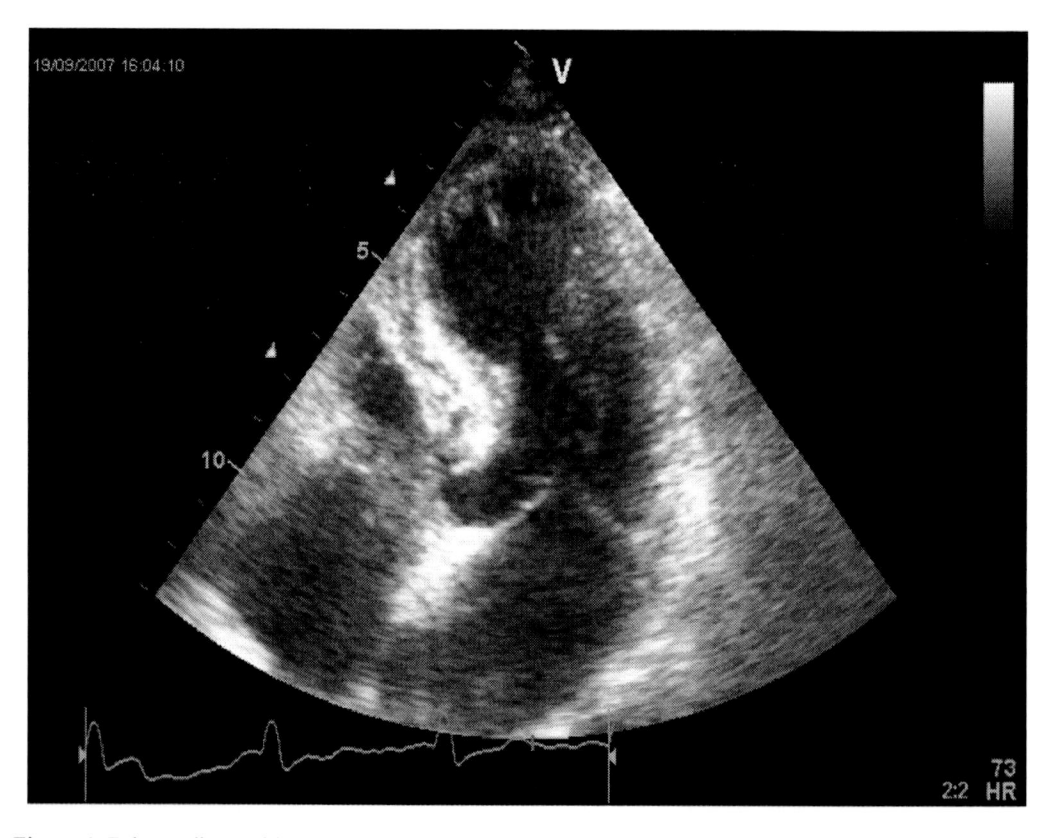

Figure 4. Echocardiographic aspect of tako-tsubo with hypercontractility of the basal segments and akinesia and apical expansion.

Table 2. Proposed Mayo Clinic Criteria for the Clinical Diagnosis of tako-tsubo syndrome

1) Transient hypokinesis, akinesis, or dyskinesis of the left ventricular mid segments with or without apical involvement. The regional wall-motion abnormalities extend beyond a single epicardial vascular distribution.*

2) Absence of obstructive coronary disease or angiographic evidence of acute plaque rupture.†

3) New ECG abnormalities (either ST-segment elevation and/or T-wave inversion) or elevated cardiac troponin.

4) Absence of: recent significant head trauma intracranial bleeding pheochromocytoma myocarditis hypertrophic cardiomyopathy

*There are rare exceptions to these criteria, such as those patients in whom the regional wall-motion abnormality is limited to a single coronary territory.

†It is possible that a patient with obstructive coronary atherosclerosis may also develop tako-tsubo syndrome. However, this is very rare in our experience and in the published literature, perhaps because such cases are misdiagnosed as an acute coronary syndrome.

In both of the above circumstances, the diagnosis of tako-tsubo syndrome should be made with caution, and a clear stressful precipitating trigger must be sought.

Pathophysiological Mechanisms

The cause of the transient left ventricular apical ballooning syndrome is unknown. However, speculatively, it may represent a catecholamine-mediated myocardial stunning that results from a combination of myocardial ischemia related to diffuse microvascular dysfunction and, in some cases, multivessel epicardial spasm and metabolic injury. The explanation for a female predominance of the syndrome is also unclear. However, the reason may be related to postmenopausal alterations of endothelial function in response to reduced estrogen levels [23]and microcirculatory vasomotor reactivity in response to catecholamine-mediated stimuli.[24]

Many studies have evaluated the presence of either spontaneous or provocable multivessel epicardial spasm during angiography. Only few patients experienced spontaneous multivessel epicardial spasm during coronarography (1.4%). Coronary flow reserve, which assesses coronary microvascular function, has been reported in a few patients, and results were conflicting[20,].[25] Frame counts from the Thrombolysis in Myocardial Infarction (TIMI) study, a quantization method of the time required for injected intracoronary contrast to reach predefined distal landmarks, were reported in 2 series. In these reports abnormal TIMI frame counts in all 3 major epicardial coronary arteries during the acute phase of the syndrome; this finding suggests widespread coronary microvascular dysfunction [26][19].

Abe et al. evaluated the coronary microcirculation using Doppler guidewire or contrast echocardiography. Although based only on few patients, their findings suggest that abnormalities in the coronary microcirculation do not contribute significantly to the syndrome[24]. In contrast, Kurisu et al. found that the TIMI frame count, a validated index of coronary blood flow, was significantly higher in patients with transient LV apical ballooning syndrome when compared with controls both during acute phase and follow-up[26]. Bybee et al. confirmed these findings, evaluating coronary angiograms on admission. They also evaluated the TIMI frame counts in 16 patients with this syndrome, who were compared with 16 age- and gender matched controls, without coronary atherosclerosis but who underwent coronary angiography before valve surgery. They found that all patients with transient LV apical ballooning syndrome had significantly abnormal TIMI frame counts in one or more epicardial coronary vessels[27]. These investigators interpreted their findings as indicative of diffuse coronary microvascular dysfunction and suggested that this abnormality may play a significant role in the pathogenesis of this syndrome. However, it remains unclear whether microvascular dysfunction is the primary cause of the syndrome or a secondary phenomenon.

Some investigators used provocative tests, such as infusion of ergonovine or acetylcholine, to evaluate inducible coronary spasm, with conflicting results. Overall 28.6% experienced multivessel spasm after infusion of a provocative agent. Considering only the reports from Japan, where vasospastic ischaemia may be more common, the presence of spontaneous coronary spasm was ranging from 1.8 to 27.7%.

Catecholamines probably play a role in the syndrome. Some researchers have suggested that the syndrome could be a result of catecholamine-associated stunning of the myocardium, which is provoked by emotional or physiologic stress [27] Patients presenting with the syndrome appear to have abnormalities of cardiac sympathetic innervation with evidence of sympathetic hyperactivity at the cardiac apex. Local release of catecholamines from cardiac sympathetic efferent neurons seems to be an unlikely explanation because of the higher norepinephrine content and greater density of sympathetic nerves at the base of the heart when compared with the apex[10,][28] The distribution of apical wall-motion abnormalities in the syndrome is similar to the distribution reported with catecholamine-induced cardiomyopathy.[29] Of note, the wall-motion abnormalities in the syndrome are not typical of those found with subarachnoid or intracranial hemorrhage in which the apex is generally spared and the basal left ventricular segments are affected.[30,31] However, isolated reports describe transient apical systolic dysfunction associated with subarachnoid hemorrhage[30,].[32, 33, 34] Measurements of circulating catecholamine levels in patients presenting with the syndrome have shown inconsistent results[15,28]. In some studies plasma levels of catecholamines and their metabolites were measured and it has been found that catecholamines levels were two to three times higher in patients with transient LV apical ballooning syndrome.[35]

However, several case reports of patients with pheochromocytoma-related cardiomyopathy described a similar distribution of LV wall-motion abnormalities.[36]

Furthermore, there is some evidence suggesting that the apical myocardium may be more responsive to sympathetic stimulation and may be more vulnerable to sudden catecholamine surges. A longitudinal, base-to-apex decline in LV myocardial perfusion, as described in patients with coronary risk factors, was also proposed as a possible alternative explanation. A longitudinal, base-to-apex decline in LV myocardial perfusion, as described in patients with coronary risk factors, was also proposed as a possible alternative explanation.

An acute coronary syndrome with early reperfusion and extensive left ventricular stunning is a further pathogenic theory, substantiated by IVUS per esteso atherosclerotic plaques findings in a small series of Tako-Tsubo patients.[37] This hypothesis need to be tested by further studies comprising a large number of patients.[38]

Four studies evaluated myocardial perfusion using single photon emission computed tomography (SPECT)[8,14,16,20]. Results of these studies showed moderate or severe myocardial ischaemia. Thus, Abe et al. reported that 11 of 13 patients (85%), in whom resting technetium-99m tetrofosmin tomographic myocardial imaging was performed during the acute phase, had decreased radioisotope uptake at the LV apex[20]. Ito et al. reported that myocardial perfusion assessed by the SPECT imaging was impaired immediately after hospital admission, but improved considerably at 3–5 days. They interpreted the nuclear imaging findings of decreased myocardial perfusion in the absence of obstructive coronary lesions as direct evidence for impaired coronary microcirculation as a causative mechanism of this syndrome[8].

Results of these studies showed moderate or severe myocardial ischaemia decreased myocardial perfusion in the absence of obstructive coronary lesions as direct evidence for impaired coronary microcirculation as a causative mechanism of this syndrome.

Penas-Lado et al. suggest a possible role of a transient dynamic left ventricular outflow tract (LVOT) obstruction in the pathogenesis of this syndrome [39]. In fact, a transient dynamic LVOT gradient was detected at initial evaluation in a substantial proportion of the patients described by Tsuchihashi et al. , and in other cases of this syndrome described elsewhere. In these patients, the clinical and hemodynamic situation improved after gradient disappearing. Moreover, in some of the patients presenting with cardiogenic shock, this situation persisted until the dynamic obstruction was diagnosed and specifically treated.[40] Thus, at least in some patients, a possible mechanism for tako-tsubo syndrome could be a dynamic LVOT obstruction preceding the ischemic event. Once present, the dynamic obstruction elevates left ventricular filling pressures, increasing myocardial oxygen demand at the mid-to-apical cavity. If this situation persists, apical hypoperfusion and ischemia may worsen, with eventual apical infarction. In fact, it is well known that, even in normal hearts, exposure to an exogenous catecholamine, such as dobutamine infusion, can precipitate dynamic LVOT obstruction.[41] Some patients, primarily women, may have geometric predisposition (sigmoid interventricular septum, small LVOT, reduced left ventricular volume) to dynamic LVOT obstruction, which may manifest only in the setting of intense adrenergic stimulation or hypovolemia. In these susceptible patients, increate adrenergic tone might produce primary LVOT obstruction leading to secondary ischemia and focal wall-motion abnormalities. Thus, the intense physical or emotional stress that precedes apical ischemia in most patients with apical ballooning syndrome could be the trigger for the acute development of LVOT obstruction capable of producing severe apical ischemia.

Myocarditis could have characteristics similar to those seen with the transient left ventricular apical ballooning syndrome but results of endomyocardial biopsies and paired serum tests for viral serology have been always resulted negative in the patients studied[15,20].

Patients with the transient left ventricular apical ballooning syndrome seem to often present in the setting of an acute mental stress, a time of enhanced sympathetic outflow. This association could be linked to mental stress– induced transient coronary endothelial dysfunction.[42,43] It is unclear why the apex of the heart is affected and the basal segments are spared. However, this may be partly explained by increased adrenergic receptor density in cardiac apical segments or increased apical myocardial responsiveness to adrenergic stimulation.[44] Transient apical and mid-ventricular wall-motion abnormalities have been induced in rats through physical immobilization, a model of emotional stress.[45] In this model, the wall-motion abnormalities could not be reproduced after pretreatment with the α- and β- adrenoreceptor antagonist. Notably estradiol supplementation has been reported to attenuate emotional stress–induced changes in left ventricular function in ovariectomized female rats[25].

In literature there are a lot of cases describing TC activated by a number of different situations. Adrain Ionescu [46] and Merli et al [47] reported that all their patients had mid-septal thickening contribution to the development of subaortic obstruction. Low-dose dobutamine stress echo showed regional stunning. Intraventricular gradients are not universally present thought suggesting a complex, non homogenous pathophysiology. Widespread subendocardial ischaemia (from excess catecholamines and high intracavitary pressures, potentially exacerbated by relative or absolute hypovolemia) may lead to loss of apical ventricular function, perhaps with a contribution from microvascular dysfunction.

Lentschener et al [48]diagnosed transient left ventricular apical wall motion abnormalities after non cardiac surgery; Satoro Sakuragi et al [49] described TC associated with epileptic seizure while Wadi Mawad et al [50]observed this syndrome following transcatheter radiofrequency ablation of the atrioventricular node.

Therapy

In the absence of studies specifically evaluating different therapies, the treatment of this syndrome remains entirely empirical and should be individualized according to the patient characteristics at the time of presentation. No consensus exists regarding appropriate therapy for Takotsubo cardiomyopathy because the number of reported cases is low and the disorder is possibly underdiagnosed. Patients with tako-tsubo syndrome should be monitored like patients with myocardial infarction. Ventilators support may be necessary in up to 77% of the patients due to respiratory failure.[51]

Most data regarding treatment have been derived by observing patients initially treated for STEMI, and diagnosed later as having TC. Since differentiation between this cardiomyopathy and an acute coronary syndrome is often difficult at initial presentation, we tend to treat patients conservatively to avoid complications that might arise by failing to treat an anterior wall myocardial infarction. Patients receive aspirin, β-blockers, angiotensin-converting-enzyme inhibitors, cardiac catheterization and intravenous diuretics if needed.

Whether anticoagulation should be administered in cases with large apical akinesia is controversial [52,53]but short-term anticoagulation may be considered to prevent left ventricular mural thrombus formation in patients with markedly depressed left ventricular function. Patients with TC must be monitored for symptoms of cardiogenic shock, heart failure and arrhythmias. Heart failure may require aggressive pharmacological treatment with inotropics drugs and mechanical circulatory support such as intra-aortic balloon pumps and left ventricular assist devices. Those with hypotension should be evaluated by echocardiography or cardiac catheterization to exclude intra-cavitary gradient, which in this case was exacerbated by dobutamine and resulted in a dynamic left ventricular mid-cavity obstruction. If a dynamic outflow pressure gradient is identified, nitroglycerine, inotropic drugs, and ACE inhibitors should be immediately discontinued to avoid gradient increasing and intravenous beta-blockers should be administered to suppress contractility in basal segments and increase left ventricular diastolic filling time and end-diastolic volume. The optimal long-term management of the syndrome has not been defined[3,7,15,21].[54] Thickening of the mid ventricular septum is reported to be a predisposing factor for developing an intracavitary gradient.

Although no randomized studies are available, it seems reasonable to give beta-blockers to patients in the acute and chronic phases, and possibly indefinitely, to prevent recurrences[51].[55]

Left ventricular apical ballooning may have the same complications of myocardial infarction, adding the early ventricular fibrillation to the previous findings of left ventricular wall rupture, ventricular arrhythmias during hospitalization and complete atrio-ventricular block. Moreover, left ventricular apical ballooning may have different and unusual clinical onsets, including sudden cardiac death due to ventricular tachyarrhythmias in the absence of associated symptoms. [56]

Most patients, however, experience improvements in left ventricular function within 2–4 weeks of symptom onset.

Prognosis

Prognosis seems to be good and the in-hospital death rate ranged from 0% to 8% in the various studies. The largest group, 88 patients, had a 1% death rate[52]. The presence of acute pulmonary oedema or acute heart failure was represented by a variable patient incidence of 3-46% and some of them were treated with aortic counterpulsation. Systolic dysfunction usually regresses in an average time of a few days or weeks, with complete recovery of normal ventricular contractility and geometry.

Only 3.5% of cases experienced a recurrence. However, evaluation of the true recurrence rate is limited, as follow-up is not reported in all patients, and in patients assessed during follow-up, timing of the follow-up assessment varied widely.

There is no evidence in the literature of therapy and short/long-term follow-up yet. The occurrence of a reversible cardiomyopathy in familial member is a sporadic event signalled and it induce to speculate on the possibility of a familial predisposition to this entity or its variants but the association cannot be ascertained until specific genetic tests have evolved and statistical correlation be established with more such observations.

Recently a new syndrome has been described called "inverted Tako-Tsubo syndrome" ("squid syndrome"). This is less frequent than *tako-tsubo* syndrome even more mind boggling syndrome. This syndrome can also be transient and reversible.

How about the inverted tako-tsubo syndrome that has been recently described in patients with severe intra cranial process or with pheochromocytoma crisis. In those rare cases, instead of the tip of the left ventricle becoming stunned and "paralyzed", the tip of the left ventricle is hyperdynamic ("hypercontracting") while it is the base of the heart that is stunned and "paralyzed".

What has not been delved into much is the possibility of a familial predisposition towards stress-induced cardiomyopathy. A review of literature notes the recent observation by Japanese investigators of CD 36 deficiency in a patient with stress-; induced cardiomiopathy [57]suggesting an association between this entity and certain genetic profiles The mutations found in the present patient were previously found in other Japanese patients with type I CD36 deficiency. C478T was the more common of these two mutations, with a frequency of 50% in such patients. Kashiwagi et al. detected heterozygosity of both C478T and 1159insA in 3 of 28 patients with type I CD36 deficiency.5 Recently, ^{123}I-betamethyl-*p*-iodophenyl pentadecanoic acid (^{123}I-BMIPP) has been used in myocardial scintigraphy to evaluate fatty acid metabolism and myocardial viability. Some investigators have reported a lack of BMIPP accumulation in the hearts of patients with heart diseases including ischemic heart diseases, hypertrophic cardiomyopathy, and dilated cardiomyopathy. Type I CD36 deficiency is characterized by a lack of BMIPP accumulation. These findings suggest that CD36 deficiency contributes to the pathogenesis of heart diseases and arteriosclerosis via abnormal metabolism of fatty acids and oxidized low-density lipoprotein. CD36 deficiency is observed more frequently in Japanese than in Americans of European descent.10,11 This may be related to the fact that many more cases of tako-tsubo-shaped cardiomyopathy have been reported in Japan than in other countries. Further studies of tako-tsubo-shaped cardiomyopathy and CD36 deficiency may reveal an association between this cardiomyopathy and specific genetic profiles.

Cherien et al. recently reported a case of an older patient who had two episodes with features that satisfy proposed current diagnostic criteria for TC.[58]Her daughter had reversible inferior wall akinesia that did not span the distribution of more than one epicardial coronary artery. Hence this would not be classified today as TC although variant forms have been described in literature very recently.[59] These variant forms or 'acute reversible heart injury syndromes', which have spared the apex, have been multi vessels in distribution. However, since coronary microvascular spasm and/ or cardiac autonomic dysfunction have been shown to be probable mechanisms involved in tako-tsubo cardiomyopathy, they would like to cautiously speculate on the possibility that the younger patient described may have experienced a variant form of tako-tsubo cardiomyopathy involving a smaller portion of myocardium. As in the variant forms, anatomic variations in sympathetic innervation in their younger patient would explain the difference in the portion of the myocardium that was 'stunned'. So in that patient if one were to consider the scenario of a takotsubo-like cardiomyopathy in terms of etiopathogenesis, the question arise.[60]

References

[1] Gianni M, Dentali F, Grandi AM et al. Apical ballooning syndrome or takotsubo cardiomyopathy: a systematic review. *European Heart Journal* (2006) 27, 1523–1529

[2] Pavin D, LeBreton H, Daubert C. Human stress cardiomyopathy mimicking acute myocardial syndrome. *Heart.* 1997;78:509 –511

[3] Desmet WJ, Adriaenssens BF, Dens JA. Apical ballooning of the left ventricle: first series in white patients. *Heart* 2003;89:1027–1031.

[4] Dote K, Sato H, Tateishi H, Uhida T, Ishihara M. Myocardial stunning due to simulataneous multivessel coronary spasm: a review of 5 cases. *J. cardiol.* 1991;21:203–214.

[5] Klinceva M, Widimský P, Pesl L, Stásek J, Tousek F, Vambera M, Bílková D. Prevalence of stress-induced myocardial stunning (Tako-Tsubo cardiomyopathy) among patients undergoing emergency coronary angiography for suspected acute myocardial infarction. *Int .J. Cardiol.* 2007 Sep 3;120(3):411-3.

[6] Pillière R, Mansencal N, Digne F, Lacombe P, Joseph T, Dubourg O. Prevalence of tako-tsubo syndrome in a large urban agglomeration. *Am. J. Cardiol.* 2006 Sep 1;98(5):662-5.

[7] Bybee KA, Prasad A, Barsness GW, Lerman A, Jaffe AS, Murphy JG, Wright RS, Rihal CS. Clinical characteristics and thrombolysis in myocardial infarction frame counts in women with transient left ventricular apical ballooning syndrome. *Am. J. Cardiol.* 2004;94:343-3

[8] Ito K, Sugihara H, Katoh S, Azuma A, Nakagawa M. Assessment of Takotsubo (ampulla) cardiomyopathy using 99mTc-tetrofosmin myocardial SPECT-comparison with acute coronary syndrome. *Ann. Nucl. Med.* 2003;17:115–122.

[9] Matsuoka K, Okubo S, Fujii E, Uchida F, Kasai A, Aoki T, Makino K, Omichi C, Fujimoto N, Ohta S, Sawai T, Nakano T. Evaluation of the arrhythmogenicity of stress-induced 'takotsubo cardiomyopathy' from the time course of the 12-lead surface electrocardiogram. *Am. J. Cardiol.* 2003;92:230–233.

[10] Akashi YJ, Nakazawa K, Sakakibara M, Miyake F, Musha H, Sasaka K. 123I-MIBG myocardial scintigraphy in patients with 'takotsubo' cardiomyopathy. *J. Nucl. Med.* 2004;45:1121–1127.

[11] Lindberg, Terrence F. Longe and Barry J. Maron Scott W. Sharkey, John R. Lesser, Andrey G. Zenovich, Martin S. Maron, Jana Acute and Reversible Cardiomyopathy Provoked by Stress in Women From the United States *Circulation* 2005;111;472-479

[12] Akashi Y, Tejma T et al. Left Ventricular Rupture Associated With Takotsubo Cardiomyopathy Mayo Clin. Proc. 2004;79:821-824

[13] Ogura R, Hiasa Y, Takahashi T et al. Specific findings on the standard 12-lead ECG in patients with Takotsubo cardiomyopathy. Comparison with the findings of acute anterior myocardial infarction. *Circ. J.* 2003; 67: 687-90

[14] Kurisu S, Inoue I, Kawagoe T et al. Time course of electrocardiographic changes in patients with tako-tsubo syndrome. Comparison with acute myocardial infarction with minimal enzymatic release. *Circ. J.* 2004; 68: 77-81

[15] Akashi YJ, Nakazawa K, Sakakibara M et al. The clinical features of takotsubo cardiomyopathy. *QJ. Med.* 2003; 96:563-73

[16] Akashi YJ, Musha H, Nakazawa K, Miyake F. Plasma brain natriuretic peptide in takotsubo cardiomyopathy. *QJM.* 2004 Sep;97(9):599-607

[17] Yamasa T, Ikeda S, Ninomiya A et al. Characteristic clinical findings of reversibile left ventricular dysfunction. *Intern .Med .*2002;41: 789-92

[18] Bybee K, Kara T, Prasad A et al. Systematic Review: Transient Left Ventricular Apical Ballooning: A Syndrome That Mimics ST-Segment Elevation Myocardial Infarction. *Ann. Intern. Med.* 2004;141:858-865.

[19] Abe Y, Kondo M, Matsuoka R et al . Assessment of clinical features in transient left ventricular apical ballooning. *J. Am. Coll. Cardiol.* 2003; 41: 737-42

[20] Villareal RP, Achari A, Wilansky S et al. Anteroapical stunning and left ventricular out flow tract obstruction. *Mayo Clinic Proc.* 2001; 76: 79-83

[21] Haghi D, Athanasiadis A, Papavassiliu T et al. Right ventricular involvement in Takotsubo Cardiomyopathy. *Eur. Heart J.* 2006 Oct;27(20):2433-9.

[22] Haghi D , Fluechter S, Suselbeck T et al. Cardiovascular magnetic resonance findings in typical versus atipical forms of the acute apical ballooning syndrome (Takotsubo cardiomyopathy). *International Journal of Cardiology* 120 (2007) 205–211

[23] Celermajer DS, Sorensen KE, Spiegelhalter DJ, Georgakopoulos D, Robinson J, Deanfield JE. Aging is associated with endothelial dysfunction in healthy men years before the age-related decline in women. *J .Am .Coll. Cardiol.* 1994;24: 471-6.

[24] Ueyama T, Hano T, Kasamatsu K, Yamamoto K, Tsuruo Y, Nishio I. Estrogen attenuates the emotional stress-induced cardiac responses in the animal model of Tako-tsubo (Ampulla) cardiomyopathy. *J. Cardiovasc. Pharmacol.* 2003;42 Suppl 1:S117-9

[25] Ako J, Takenaka K, Uno K, Nakamura F, Shoji T, Iijima K, et al. Reversible left ventricular systolic dysfunction—reversibility of coronary microvascular abnormality. *Jpn Heart* J. 2001;42:355-63

[26] Kurisu S, Sato H, Kawagoe T, Ishihara M, Shimatani Y, Nishioka K, et al. Tako-tsubo-like left ventricular dysfunction with ST-segment elevation: a novel cardiac syndrome mimicking acute myocardial infarction. *Am. Heart J.* 2002;143: 448-55.

[27] Kono T, Morita H, Kuroiwa T, Onaka H, Takatsuka H, Fujiwara A. Left ventricular wall motion abnormalities in patients with subarachnoid hemorrhage: neurogenic stunned myocardium. *J. Am. Coll. Cardiol.* 1994;24:636-40

[28] Owa M, Aizawa K, Urasawa N, Ichinose H, Yamamoto K, Karasawa K, et al. Emotional stress-induced "ampulla cardiomyopathy": discrepancy between the metabolic and sympathetic innervation imaging performed during the recovery course. *Jpn Circ. J.* 2001;65:349-52.

[29] Scott IU, Gutterman DD. Pheochromocytoma with reversible focal cardiac dysfunction. *Am. Heart J.* 1995;130:909-1

[30] Dujardin KS, McCully RB, Wijdicks EF, Tazelaar HD, Seward JB, McGregor CG, et al. Myocardial dysfunction associated with brain death: clinical, echocardiographic, and pathologic features. *J. Heart Lung Transplant.* 2001; 20:350-7.

[31] Zaroff JG, Rordorf GA, Ogilvy CS, Picard MH. Regional patterns of left ventricular systolic dysfunction after subarachnoid hemorrhage: evidence for neurally mediated cardiac injury. *J. Am .Soc. Echocardiogr.* 2000;13:774-9.

[32] Yoshikawa D, Hara T, Takahashi K, Morita T, Goto F. An association between QTc prolongation and left ventricular hypokinesis during sequential episodes of subarachnoid hemorrhage. *Anesth. Analg.* 1999;89:962-4

[33] Chang PC, Lee SH, Hung HF, Kaun P, Cheng JJ. Transient ST elevation and left ventricular asynergy associated with normal coronary artery and Tc-99m PYP

Myocardial Infarct Scan in subarachnoid hemorrhage [Letter]. *Int. J. Cardiol.* 1998;63:189-92.

[34] Pollick C, Cujec B, Parker S, Tator C. Left ventricular wall motion abnormalities in subarachnoid hemorrhage: an echocardiographic study. *J. Am. Coll. Cardiol.* 1988;12:600-5.

[35] Wittstein I, Thiemann D, Lima J et al. Neurohumoral Features of Myocardial Stunning Due to Sudden Emotional Stress *N. Engl. J. Med.* 2005;352:539-48.

[36] Sarsedai SH, Mourant AJ, Sivathan Y et al. Pheocromocytoma and catecholamine induced cardiomyopathy presentino as heart failure. *Br. Heart J.* 1990; 63: 234-7

[37] Ibanez B, Navarro F, Cordoba M et al. Tako-tsubo transient left ventricular apical ballooning: is intravascular ultrasound the key to resolve the enigma? *Heart* 2005; 91:102-4

[38] Briguori C, Tobis J, Nishida T et al. Discrepancy between angiography and intravascular ultrasound when analysing small coronary arteries. *Eur .Heart J.* 2002; 23:247-54

[39] Penas-Lado M, Barriales-Villa R, Goicolea J. Transient Left Ventricular Apical Ballooning and Outflow Tract Obstruction JACC Vol. 42, No. 6, 2003 September 17, 2003:1140-6

[40] Haley JH, Sinak LJ, Tajik AJ, Ommen SR, Oh JK. Dynamic left ventricular outflow tract obstruction in acute coronary syndromes: an important cause of new systolic murmur and cardiogenic shock. *Mayo Clin. Proc.* 1999;74:901–6.

[41] Luria D, Klutstein MW, Rosenmann D, Shaheen J, Sergey S, Tzivoni D. Prevalence and significance of left ventricular outflow gradient during dobutamine echocardiography. *Eur. Heart J.* 1999;20:386–92

[42] Spieker LE, Hurlimann D, Ruschitzka F, Corti R, Enseleit F, Shaw S, et al. Mental stress induces prolonged endothelial dysfunction via endothelin-A receptors. *Circulation.* 2002;105:2817-20

[43] Ghiadoni L, Donald AE, Cropley M, Mullen MJ, Oakley G, Taylor M, et al. Mental stress induces transient endothelial dysfunction in humans. *Circulation.* 2000;102:2473-8.

[44] Mori H, Ishikawa S, Kojima S, Hayashi J, Watanabe Y, Hoffman JI, et al. Increased responsiveness of left ventricular apical myocardium to adrenergic stimuli. *Cardiovasc. Res.* 1993;27:192-8.

[45] Ueyama T, Kasamatsu K, Hano T, Yamamoto K, Tsuruo Y, Nishio I. Emotional stress induces transient left ventricular hypocontraction in the rat via activation of cardiac adrenoceptors: a possible animal model of 'tako-tsubo' cardiomyopathy. *Circ. J.* 2002;66:712-3

[46] Ionescu A. Subaortic dynamic obstruction: A contributing factor to hemodynamic instability in tako-tsubo syndrome? *Eur .J .Echocardiogr.* 2007 Jan 3

[47] Merli E, Sutcliffe S, Gori M, Sutherland GG. Tako-Tsubo cardiomyopathy: new insights into the possible underlying pathophysiology. *Eur. J. Echocardiogr.* 2006 Jan;7(1):53-61.

[48] Lentschener C, Vignaux O, Spaulding C, Bonnichon P, Legmann P, Ozier Y. Early postoperative tako-tsubo-like left ventricular dysfunction: transient left ventricular apical ballooning syndrome. *Anesth. Analg.* 2006 Sep;103(3):580-2.

[49] Sakuragi S, Tokunaga N, Okawa K et al. A case of takotsubo cardiomyopathy associated with epileptic seizure: reversible left ventricular wall motion abnormality and ST-segment elevation. *Heart Vessels.* 2007 Jan;22(1):59-63.

[50] Mawad W, Guerra PG, Dubuc M, Khairy P. Tako-tsubo cardiomyopathy following transcatheter radiofrequency ablation of the atrioventricular node. *Europace.* 2007 Nov;9(11):1075-6.

[51] Seth PS, Aurigemma GP, Krasnow JM et al. A syndrome of transient left ventricular apical wall motion abnormality in the absence of coronary disease: a perspective from the United States. *Cardiology* 2003; 100:61.6

[52] Sasaki N, Kinugawa T, Yamawaki M, et al. Transient left ventricular apical ballooning in a patient with bicuspid aortic valve created a left ventricular thrombus leading to acute renal infarction. *Circ. J.* 2004; 68:1081-3

[53] Akashi Yj, Tejima T, Sakurada H, et al. Takotsubo cardiomyopathy with a significant pressure gradient in the left ventricle. *Heart Vessels* 2000; 15:203

[54] Tsuchihashi K, Ueshima K, Uchida T, et al. Angina Pectoris- Miocardial Infarction Investigations in Japan. Transient left ventricular apical ballooning without coronary artery stenosis: aA novel heart syndrome mimicking acute myocardial infarction. *J. Am. Coll. Cardiol.* 2001; 38: 11-8

[55] Kyuma M, Tsuchihashi K, Shinshi Y, et al. Effect of intravenous propanolol on left ventricular apical ballooning without coronary artery stenosis (ampulla cardiomyopathy): Three cases. *Circ. J.* 2002;66:1181-4

[56] Raddino R, Pedrinazzi C, Zanini G et al. Out-of-hospital cardiac arrest caused by transient left ventricular apical ballooning syndrome. *Int .J .Cardiol.* 2007 Aug 9.

[57] Kushiro T, Saito F, Kusama J et al. Takotsubo-shaped cardiomyopathy with type I CD36 deficiency. *Heart Vessels May* 2005;20(3):123–5.

[58] Kevin B, Kara Tomas, Abhiram P, et al. Systematic review: transient left ventricular apical ballooning: a syndrome that mimics ST-segment elevation myocardial infarction. *Ann. Intern. Med.* 2004;141:858–65

[59] Haghi D, Papavassiliu T, Flüchter S, et al. Variant form of the acute apical ballooning syndrome (takotsubo cardiomyopathy): observations on a novel entity. *Heart* 2006;92:392–4.

[60] Cherian J, Angelis D, Filiberti A, Saperia G. Can takotsubo cardiomyopathy be familial? *Int. J. Cardiol.* 2007 Sep 14;121(1):74-5.

Index

C

D

E

F

I

M

N

O

Q

R

S

U

V

ventricle, 21, 284, 290
ventricular arrhythmias, 91, 289
ventricular fibrillation, 281, 289
ventricular septum, 289
ventricular systolic dysfunction, 292
ventricular tachycardia, 107
venules, 95, 119
verapamil, 33
vessels, 13, 25, 27, 29, 31, 40, 63, 81, 105, 185, 186, 225, 245, 253, 263, 264, 276, 290
Victoria, 180
viral hepatitis, 87, 125
viral infection, 87
Virginia, 194
virus(es), 14, 67, 87, 253, 255
virus infection, 67
viscera, 19
viscosity, 192, 248
vitamin B6, 73
vitamin C, 71
vitamin E, 62, 72, 92, 131, 132
vitamin K, 90
vitamins, viii, 49, 58, 62, 72
VLDL, 234, 246
vomiting, 225
vulnerability, 252

W

Wales, 216, 217
walking, 19, 192
warrants, 271
Washington, 44, 238
weakness, 250
weight control, 247
weight loss, 256
weight reduction, 35
white blood cell count, 18
white blood cells, 44
wind, 19
wine, 93
withdrawal, 75, 104, 109, 272, 277
Wolff-Parkinson-White syndrome, 21, 23
women, 16, 17, 27, 59, 74, 101, 163, 214, 248, 287, 291, 292
work absenteeism, 208
workers, 264, 265
workload, 30
World Health Organization, 157
wound healing, 113, 149

Y

yes/no, 169, 170
yield, 51
young adults, 21, 66
young women, 248

Z

zinc, 127
zymogen, ix, 78, 83, 84